# Advanced Materials for Oral Application

# Advanced Materials for Oral Application

Editors

**Laura-Cristina Rusu**
**Lavinia Cosmina Ardelean**

MDPI • Basel • Beijing • Wuhan • Barcelona • Belgrade • Manchester • Tokyo • Cluj • Tianjin

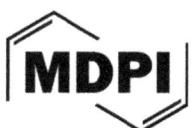

*Editors*
Laura-Cristina Rusu
Oral Pathology
"Victor Babes" University of
Medicine and Pharmacy
Timisoara
Romania

Lavinia Cosmina Ardelean
Technology of Materials and
Devices in Dental Medicine
"Victor Babes" University of
Medicine and Pharmacy
Timisoara
Romania

*Editorial Office*
MDPI
St. Alban-Anlage 66
4052 Basel, Switzerland

This is a reprint of articles from the Special Issue published online in the open access journal *Materials* (ISSN 1996-1944) (available at: www.mdpi.com/journal/materials/special_issues/mater_oral).

For citation purposes, cite each article independently as indicated on the article page online and as indicated below:

LastName, A.A.; LastName, B.B.; LastName, C.C. Article Title. *Journal Name* **Year**, *Volume Number*, Page Range.

**ISBN 978-3-0365-5742-7 (Hbk)**
**ISBN 978-3-0365-5741-0 (PDF)**

© 2022 by the authors. Articles in this book are Open Access and distributed under the Creative Commons Attribution (CC BY) license, which allows users to download, copy and build upon published articles, as long as the author and publisher are properly credited, which ensures maximum dissemination and a wider impact of our publications.

The book as a whole is distributed by MDPI under the terms and conditions of the Creative Commons license CC BY-NC-ND.

# Contents

**About the Editors** . . . . . . . . . . . . . . . . . . . . . . . . . . . . . . . . . . . . . . . . . . . . vii

**Preface to "Advanced Materials for Oral Application"** . . . . . . . . . . . . . . . . . . . . . . . ix

**Laura-Cristina Rusu and Lavinia Cosmina Ardelean**
Advanced Materials for Oral Application
Reprinted from: *Materials* **2022**, *15*, 4749, doi:10.3390/ma15144749 . . . . . . . . . . . . . . . . . . 1

**Anamaria Matichescu, Lavinia Cosmina Ardelean, Laura-Cristina Rusu, Dragos Craciun, Emanuel Adrian Bratu and Marius Babucea et al.**
Advanced Biomaterials and Techniques for Oral Tissue Engineering and Regeneration—A Review
Reprinted from: *Materials* **2020**, *13*, 5303, doi:10.3390/ma13225303 . . . . . . . . . . . . . . . . . . 7

**Barbara Sterczała, Agnieszka Chwiłkowska, Urszula Szwedowicz, Magdalena Kobielarz, Bartłomiej Chwiłkowski and Marzena Dominiak**
Impact of APRF+ in Combination with Autogenous Fibroblasts on Release Growth Factors, Collagen, and Proliferation and Migration of Gingival Fibroblasts: An In Vitro Study
Reprinted from: *Materials* **2022**, *15*, 796, doi:10.3390/ma15030796 . . . . . . . . . . . . . . . . . . 45

**Alessandro Addis, Elena Canciani, Marino Campagnol, Matteo Colombo, Christian Frigerio and Daniele Recupero et al.**
A New Anorganic Equine Bone Substitute for Oral Surgery: Structural Characterization and Regenerative Potential
Reprinted from: *Materials* **2022**, *15*, 1031, doi:10.3390/ma15031031 . . . . . . . . . . . . . . . . . . 57

**Raluca Grigore, Bogdan Popescu, Şerban Vifor Gabriel Berteşteanu, Cornelia Nichita, Irina Doinita Oașă and Gloria Simona Munteanu et al.**
The Role of Biomaterials in Upper Digestive Tract Transoral Reconstruction
Reprinted from: *Materials* **2021**, *14*, 1436, doi:10.3390/ma14061436 . . . . . . . . . . . . . . . . . . 73

**Julian Nold, Christian Wesemann, Laura Rieg, Lara Binder, Siegbert Witkowski and Benedikt Christopher Spies et al.**
Does Printing Orientation Matter? In-Vitro Fracture Strength of Temporary Fixed Dental Prostheses after a 1-Year Simulation in the Artificial Mouth
Reprinted from: *Materials* **2021**, *14*, 259, doi:10.3390/ma14020259 . . . . . . . . . . . . . . . . . . 87

**Yohei Kawajiri, Hiroshi Ikeda, Yuki Nagamatsu, Chihiro Masaki, Ryuji Hosokawa and Hiroshi Shimizu**
PICN Nanocomposite as Dental CAD/CAM Block Comparable to Human Tooth in Terms of Hardness and Flexural Modulus
Reprinted from: *Materials* **2021**, *14*, 1182, doi:10.3390/ma14051182 . . . . . . . . . . . . . . . . . . 99

**João Paulo Mendes Tribst, Alison Flavio Campos dos Santos, Giuliane da Cruz Santos, Larissa Sandy da Silva Leite, Julio Chávez Lozada and Laís Regiane Silva-Concílio et al.**
Effect of Cement Layer Thickness on the Immediate and Long-Term Bond Strength and Residual Stress between Lithium Disilicate Glass-Ceramic and Human Dentin
Reprinted from: *Materials* **2021**, *14*, 5153, doi:10.3390/ma14185153 . . . . . . . . . . . . . . . . . . 113

**Cristina Gasparik, Manuela Maria Manziuc, Alexandru Victor Burde, Javier Ruiz-López, Smaranda Buduru and Diana Dudea**
Masking Ability of Monolithic and Layered Zirconia Crowns on Discolored Substrates
Reprinted from: *Materials* **2022**, *15*, 2233, doi:10.3390/ma15062233 . . . . . . . . . . . . . . . . . . 127

**Isabel Paczkowski, Catalina S. Stingu, Sebastian Hahnel, Angelika Rauch and Oliver Schierz**
Cross-Contamination Risk of Dental Tray Adhesives: An In Vitro Study
Reprinted from: *Materials* **2021**, *14*, 6138, doi:10.3390/ma14206138 . . . . . . . . . . . . . . . . . . 143

**Germain Sfeir, Carla Zogheib, Shanon Patel, Thomas Giraud, Venkateshbabu Nagendrababu and Frédéric Bukiet**
Calcium Silicate-Based Root Canal Sealers: A Narrative Review and Clinical Perspectives
Reprinted from: *Materials* **2021**, *14*, 3965, doi:10.3390/ma14143965 . . . . . . . . . . . . . . . . . . 151

**Diana Eid, Etienne Medioni, Gustavo De-Deus, Issam Khalil, Alfred Naaman and Carla Zogheib**
Impact of Warm Vertical Compaction on the Sealing Ability of Calcium Silicate-Based Sealers: A Confocal Microscopic Evaluation
Reprinted from: *Materials* **2021**, *14*, 372, doi:10.3390/ma14020372 . . . . . . . . . . . . . . . . . . . 173

**Loai Alsofi, Muhannad Al Harbi, Martin Stauber and Khaled Balto**
Analysis of the Morpho-Geometrical Changes of the Root Canal System Produced by TF Adaptive vs. BioRace: A Micro-Computed Tomography Study
Reprinted from: *Materials* **2021**, *14*, 531, doi:10.3390/ma14030531 . . . . . . . . . . . . . . . . . . . 181

**Zsuzsanna Bardocz-Veres, Melinda Székely, Pál Salamon, Előd Bala, Előd Bereczki and Bernadette Kerekes-Máthé**
Quantitative and Qualitative Assessment of Fluorescence in Aesthetic Direct Restorations
Reprinted from: *Materials* **2022**, *15*, 4619, doi:10.3390/ma15134619 . . . . . . . . . . . . . . . . . . 191

**Gabriela Ciavoi, Ruxandra Mărgărit, Liana Todor, Dana Bodnar, Magdalena Natalia Dina and Daniela Ioana Tărlungeanu et al.**
Base Materials' Influence on Fracture Resistance of Molars with MOD Cavities
Reprinted from: *Materials* **2021**, *14*, 5242, doi:10.3390/ma14185242 . . . . . . . . . . . . . . . . . . 201

# About the Editors

**Laura-Cristina Rusu**

Professor Laura Cristina Rusu, DMD, PhD, is a full-time professor and head of the Oral Pathology Department, Faculty of Dental Medicine, "Victor Babes" University of Medicine and Pharmacy, Timisoara, Romania. Her PhD thesis was centered on allergens in dental materials. In 2017, she obtained a Dr Habil and was confirmed as PhD coordinator in the field of dental medicine. She took part in 10 research projects, including FP7 COST Action MP 1005, and authored over 140 peer-reviewed papers. She has published nine books and book chapters as an author and co-author. She has guest-edited five Special Issues in different journals, and edited two books, plus one ongoing book editing project. She currently holds two patents. With a current H-index 12, she is a member in the editorial board of Journal of Science and Art, Medicine in Evolution, topic editor for Materials, and academic editor for Scanning. Her main scientific interests are oral pathology and oral diagnosis in dental medicine, focusing on oral cancer.

**Lavinia Cosmina Ardelean**

Professor Lavinia Cosmina Ardelean, DMD, PhD, is a professor and head of the Department of Technology of Materials and Devices in Dental Medicine, "Victor Babes" University of Medicine and Pharmacy, Timisoara, Romania. She has authored/co-authored sixteen books, twelve book chapters, and over 120 peer-reviewed papers. With a current H-index of 12, she is an editorial board member of numerous journals and a member of reviewer/topic boards of Materials, Coatings, Prosthesis, Metals, Polymers, Journal of Functional Biomaterials, and an academic editor for Scanning. She has guest-edited eight Special Issues in different journals, and two books, plus one ongoing book editing project. Being an active reviewer, with more than 200 reviews to her credit so far, she was awarded with Top reviewers in Cross-Field award 2019, and Top reviewers in Materials Science award 2019. She currently holds one patent. Her research interest includes most areas of dentistry, with a focus on dental materials/biomaterials, dental alloys, resins, ceramics/bioceramics, CAD/CAM milling, 3D printing/bioprinting in dentistry, laser welding, scanning, and oral health care.

# Preface to "Advanced Materials for Oral Application"

The continuous development of dental materials enables dentists and dental technicians to choose from a wide variety. The introduction of new aesthetic materials, digital devices, processing software, and manufacturing and prototyping tools have radically transformed the dental profession. Enhancing the quality of life for dental patients can be achieved by the development and selection of biocompatible, durable, and high aesthetic materials, able to withstand the conditions of the oral environment for a long time. Their physical and chemical properties ensure high-resistant results, as well as the maintenance of the original characteristics of the material. Biocompatibility issues also have to be considered, as dental materials must be well tolerated by the human organism. The main goal of the dental treatment concerns either the regeneration of diseased tissues or their replacement. Recent advances enable tailoring dental materials to specific applications, resulting in progressive materials. Bioactive materials, which play an important role in the regenerative process, and smart materials, capable to react to external stimuli, represent the future of dental materials. "Advanced Materials for Oral Application" aimed a multidisciplinary approach of the subject, focusing on what is new in this attractive field of research.

**Laura-Cristina Rusu and Lavinia Cosmina Ardelean**
*Editors*

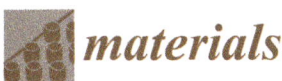

*Editorial*

# Advanced Materials for Oral Application

Laura-Cristina Rusu [1] and Lavinia Cosmina Ardelean [2,*]

1. Department of Oral Pathology, Multidisciplinary Center for Research, Evaluation, Diagnosis and Therapies in Oral Medicine, "Victor Babes" University of Medicine and Pharmacy, 300041 Timisoara, Romania; laura.rusu@umft.ro
2. Department of Technology of Materials and Devices in Dental Medicine, Multidisciplinary Center for Research, Evaluation, Diagnosis and Therapies in Oral Medicine, "Victor Babes" University of Medicine and Pharmacy, 300041 Timisoara, Romania
* Correspondence: lavinia_ardelean@umft.ro

This Special Issue of *Materials* explores the wide variety of dental materials, which enables the dentists and dental technicians to select the most suitable therapeutic solution for each patient. The main goal of dental treatment concerns either the regeneration of diseased tissues or their replacement with prosthesis. Recent advances in this field enable the tailoring of dental materials to specific applications, resulting in progressive materials. The introduction of new aesthetic materials, digital devices, processing software, and manufacturing and prototyping tools has radically transformed the dental profession. Bioactive dental materials, which release specific ions, play an important role in the regenerative process, in preventive and restorative dentistry, and in endodontics or maxillofacial surgery, inducing cell differentiation and stimulation, promoting hard tissue formation, and exerting antimicrobial actions. Smart materials are able to react to pH changes and induce reparative processes in the oral environment [1,2].

This Special Issue aims to focus on the recent advances in this attractive field of research, which encourage a multidisciplinary approach to the subject.

This Special Issue contains a blend of 12 original research articles and 2 review papers from leading scientists across the world, with expertise in materials for dental application.

The reconstruction or repair of oral and maxillofacial functionalities and aesthetics is currently a priority for dental patients, as stated by Matichescu et al. in their review discussing "Advanced Biomaterials and Techniques for Oral Tissue Engineering and Regeneration" [3]. Tissue reconstruction is of utmost importance in oral and maxillofacial surgery, periodontics, orthodontics, endodontics, and even daily clinical practice. It involves a vast array of techniques ranging from the traditional use of tissue grafts to the most innovative regenerative procedures, such as tissue engineering, as well as a wide range of artificial and natural biomaterials and scaffolds, genes, oral stem cells, and growth factors. Due to the high rate of success, the future objective is achieving the regeneration of the entire tooth, which would replace classical dental implants and overcome their disadvantages [3].

Advanced platelet-rich fibrin, due to its concentrations of growth factors, is widely used to stimulate bone and soft tissue regeneration, currently being completely autologous and prepared without any anticoagulants or separators. The study by Sterczala et al. [4] aimed to determine whether combining advanced platelet-rich fibrin with autogenous fibroblasts results in increased release of components involved in the healing processes, such as fibroblast growth factor, vascular endothelial growth factor, transforming growth factor-beta 1 and 2, and collagen. The results have proven that advanced platelet-rich fibrin with autogenous human fibroblasts is a potential connective tissue substitute in the augmentation of keratinized gingiva, and it may considerably enhance the healing of surgical wounds [4].

Anorganic equine bone has been recently introduced as an alternative for bone grafting, used in oral surgery for volume preservation and for augmentation purposes. The aim of

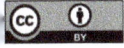

the study performed by Addis et al. [5] was to assess the physicochemical and structural properties of anorganic equine bone and its in vivo performance in mandibular bony defects. The study confirmed that its structural and physicochemical properties match the typical features of heat-treated xenogeneic bone substitutes, and its use as a grafting material yielded bone formation with no presence of inflammatory cell infiltrate [5].

Surgical reconstruction after radical surgery for malignant neoplasia was performed by Grigore et al. in the study "The Role of Biomaterials in Upper Digestive Tract Transoral Reconstruction" [6], aiming to provide novel biomaterials suitable for this purpose. Polydimethylsiloxane with silver nanoparticles was used for surgical reconstruction of the esophagus with templates, aiming to establish its antifungal properties. Following in vitro testing, the conclusion was that the insertion of bacteriostatic agents, such as silver nanoparticles, decreases the fatigue strength, increases flexibility, and offers an optimal local protection solution against fungal development [6].

Among the most recent and performant technologies used in prosthetic dentistry, computer-aided design and computer-aided manufacturing (CAD/CAM) enable subtractive or additive fabrication of various types of dental prostheses and appliances. The in vitro study by Nold et al., titled "Does Printing Orientation Matter? In-Vitro Fracture Strength of Temporary Fixed Dental Prostheses after a 1-Year Simulation in the Artificial Mouth" [7], aimed to compare the fracture resistance of milled and additive manufactured three-unit temporary fixed dental prostheses and bar-shaped specimens. The materials used were polymethylmethacrylate for subtractive manufacturing and a light-curing resin for additive manufacturing. Four different printing orientations were used for additive manufacturing. The subtractive manufactured bars and prostheses showed the highest strength in all experiments. The conclusion of the study was that fracture resistance is significantly affected by the manufacturing technique, the printing orientation, and the applied loading procedure [7].

Recent advances in CAD/CAM technologies have allowed the manufacturing of different types of materials for the CAD/CAM milling process. Contemporary CAD/CAM blocks are categorized into metal-based, ceramic-based, and resin-based. Polymer infiltrated ceramic network (PICN) composites are increasingly popular as CAD/CAM restorative materials because of their mechanical biocompatibility with human enamel. The study by Kawajiri et al. [8], "PICN Nanocomposite as Dental CAD/CAM Block Comparable to Human Tooth in Terms of Hardness and Flexural Modulus", aimed to develop a novel PICN composite CAD/CAM block material comprising a silica skeleton and infiltrated UDMA-based resin. The proposed PICN nanocomposite represents a promising biocompatible material, as it exhibited a similar Vickers hardness to enamel and flexural modulus to dentin, in addition to excellent bond properties with resin cement [8].

Among the ceramic-based CAD/CAM blocks, lithium disilicate glass-ceramic represents a trending topic in prosthodontics due to its multifunctional use and translucency. The clinical performance of a fixed prosthetic restoration is influenced by the cement used to bond it to the dental structures. The aim of the study performed by Tribst et al. [9] was to evaluate the effect of different cement layer thicknesses on immediate and aged microtensile bond strength between lithium disilicate and dentin. The residual stress of polymerization shrinkage was assessed by applying the finite element method. The results showed that the cement layer thickness does not affect the immediate bond strength in lithium disilicate restorations. Thicker cement layers, due to the higher volume of material, induce higher residual stress; in the long term, the bond strength will be dampened. Therefore, to improve bond durability, a thinner cement layer is recommended [9].

Dental zirconia is another frequent choice of ceramic-based CAD/CAM block because of its versatility, combining high strength with acceptable aesthetics. Its lack of translucency has been overcome by the latest generations of 3Y-TZP zirconia, with improved properties and wider indications for both monolithic and veneered restorations. The study by Gasparik et al. [10] aimed to evaluate the masking ability of 1 mm thick monolithic and veneered zirconia crowns on different discolored substrates. Its importance lies in the fact that treating tooth discoloration is challenging, and a successful outcome relies on the material's ability to hide the discolored substrate, as well as matching the color of neighboring teeth. The color measurements were performed using a non-contact dental spectrophotometer in the cervical, middle, and incisal portion of each crown. Despite the fact that the color coordinates of monolithic and veneered crowns were significantly different on all substrates, none of the 1 mm thick 3Y-TZP zirconia crowns showed sufficient masking ability on moderately or severely discolored substrates [10].

Despite the availability of digital impression procedures associated with the CAD/CAM techniques, conventional impressions are still widely used in daily dental practice. The impression material is usually handled by means of a dental tray; in certain cases, an adhesive is needed to provide a chemical adhesion between the material and the tray. The article by Paczkowski et al. [11] aimed to investigate the risk of cross-contamination when using dental tray adhesives with reusable brush systems. The risk of potential transmission for Staphylococcus aureus, Escherichia coli, Pseudomonas aeruginosa, Streptococcus oralis, and Candida albicans was determined for four dental tray adhesives with different disinfectant components. Isopropanol and ethyl acetate proved the most effective disinfectants, while hydrogen chloride and acetone were the least effective; however, all four tested adhesives showed sufficient bactericidal and fungicidal properties [11].

One dental field with great development within the recent time period has been endodontics. The ultimate goal of endodontic treatment is to obtain a three-dimensional, tight canal seal. Characterized by high biocompatibility, low cytotoxicity, and viscosity, tricalcium-silicate-based sealers have been considered to improving canal filling quality.

Nevertheless, as stated by Sfeir et al. in their review article "Calcium Silicate-Based Root Canal Sealers: A Narrative Review and Clinical Perspectives" [12], their dimensional stability is still questionable, with available studies showing contradictory results. Aiming to propose rational indications and help practitioners in selecting the appropriate sealer, the authors have shown that, compared to conventional sealers, calcium-silicate-based root canal sealers show good all-around performance, despite the significant differences between the different formulations. For this reason, their specificities must be considered by the practitioner when selecting the proper material for clinical usage, and slightly modified clinical endodontic protocols should be considered to match their specific behaviors [12].

From this perspective, two new modified calcium-silicate-based sealers, proposed with warm vertical gutta-percha obturation techniques, were evaluated by Eid et al. [13] to determine the impact of the warm vertical compaction on the dentinal tubule penetration. The in vitro study "Impact of Warm Vertical Compaction on the Sealing Ability of Calcium Silicate-Based Sealers: A Confocal Microscopic Evaluation" concluded that warm vertical compaction enhanced the penetration of calcium-silicate-based sealers into the dentinal tubules in comparison with the single cone technique [13].

Three-dimensional cleaning and shaping of the root canal system is the base for a proper obturation. Various nickel–titanium (NiTi) instruments have recently become available on the market. NiTi rotary files may undergo fatigue; novel manufacturing technologies such as reciprocating files or active cutting regions are aimed to overcome this deficiency. Alsofi et al. [14], in the article "Analysis of the Morpho-Geometrical Changes of the Root Canal System Produced by TF Adaptive vs. BioRace: A Micro-Computed Tomography Study", aimed to evaluate and compare, using an ex vivo model, the shaping ability of adaptive reciprocation kinematics and continuous rotation instrumentation movement using TF Adaptive files and BioRace files, respectively. The conclusion was that both rotary systems produced canal preparations with adequate geometrical changes, but none of them could touch all the canal walls [14].

The materials used in restorative dentistry are also subject to continuous improvement, in terms of both physical properties and aesthetic appearance. Direct composite materials are the first choice when aesthetics is the primary goal. A wide choice of such materials is currently available, the match between the appearance of the restoration and the tooth structures depending not only on color but also on fundamental optical properties, such as translucency, opalescence, and fluorescence, indispensable for clinical shade-matching [15]. The article by Bardocz-Veres et al. aimed to investigate the fluorescence of nine different composite resins. They concluded that the fluorescence intensity of the assessed restorative materials shows significant differences compared to dental enamel, presenting lower or higher values. Further, all the tested composite resins showed decreased fluorescence values after six months [15].

Base materials are commonly used in dental practice to replace lost dentin and enable a uniform distribution of the load and tension, thus preventing tooth fracture. The in vitro study by Ciavoi et al. [16] aimed to compare the fracture resistance of teeth presenting medium-sized mesial–occlusal–distal cavities, restored with a light-cured composite resin, using different base materials: zinc polycarboxylate cement, glass ionomer cement, resin-modified glass ionomer cement, and flow composite. The study concluded that, in case of medium-sized mesial–occlusal–distal cavities, the base material with the highest fracture resistance is flow composite, followed by resin-modified glass ionomer cement, glass ionomer cement, and zinc polycarboxylate cement. In the authors' opinion, one possible reason for this might be better compatibility with the final, light-cured restoration material [16].

In summary, this Special Issue of *Materials*, titled "Advanced Materials for Oral Application", compiles a total of 14 cutting-edge research and extensive review articles demonstrating the great potential of novel, durable, and highly aesthetic dental materials in enhancing the quality of life for dental patients. The Special Issue also informs the readers of the current challenges and future directions in this domain. The Guest Editors would like to thank all contributing authors for the success of the Special Issue. This Special Issue would not have been of such quality without the constructive criticism of the Reviewers.

**Funding:** This research received no external funding.

**Acknowledgments:** The Guest Editors would like to thank all contributing authors for the success of the Special Issue, as well as the Reviewers, for their constructive criticism and valuable contribution to the quality of the Special Issue.

**Conflicts of Interest:** The authors declare no conflict of interest.

## References

1. Grecu, A.F.; Reclaru, L.; Ardelean, L.C.; Nica, O.; Ciucă, E.M.; Ciurea, M.E. Platelet-Rich Fibrin and Its Emerging Therapeutic Benefits for Musculoskeletal Injury Treatment. *Medicina* 2019, 55, 141. [CrossRef] [PubMed]
2. Rusu, L.-C.; Ardelean, L.; Negrutiu, M.-L.; Dragomirescu, A.-O.; Albu, M.G.; Ghica, M.V.; Topala, F.I.; Podoleanu, A.; Sinescu, C. SEM for the General Structural Features Assesing of the Synthetic Polymer Scaffolds. *Rev. Chim.* 2011, 62, 841–845.
3. Matichescu, A.; Ardelean, L.C.; Rusu, L.-C.; Craciun, D.; Bratu, E.A.; Babucea, M.; Leretter, M. Advanced Biomaterials and Techniques for Oral Tissue Engineering and Regeneration—A Review. *Materials* 2020, 13, 5303. [CrossRef] [PubMed]
4. Sterczała, B.; Chwiłkowska, A.; Szwedowicz, U.; Kobielarz, M.; Chwiłkowski, B.; Dominiak, M. Impact of APRF+ in Combination with Autogenous Fibroblasts on Release Growth Factors, Collagen, and Proliferation and Migration of Gingival Fibroblasts: An In Vitro Study. *Materials* 2022, 15, 796. [CrossRef] [PubMed]
5. Addis, A.; Canciani, E.; Campagnol, M.; Colombo, M.; Frigerio, C.; Recupero, D.; Dellavia, C.; Morroni, M. A New Anorganic Equine Bone Substitute for Oral Surgery: Structural Characterization and Regenerative Potential. *Materials* 2022, 15, 1031. [CrossRef] [PubMed]
6. Grigore, R.; Popescu, B.; Berteşteanu, Ş.V.G.; Nichita, C.; Oașă, I.D.; Munteanu, G.S.; Nicolaescu, A.; Bejenaru, P.L.; Simion-Antonie, C.B.; Ene, D.; et al. The Role of Biomaterials in Upper Digestive Tract Transoral Reconstruction. *Materials* 2021, 14, 1436. [CrossRef] [PubMed]
7. Nold, J.; Wesemann, C.; Rieg, L.; Binder, L.; Witkowski, S.; Spies, B.C.; Kohal, R.J. Does Printing Orientation Matter? In-Vitro Fracture Strength of Temporary Fixed Dental Prostheses after a 1-Year Simulation in the Artificial Mouth. *Materials* 2021, 14, 259. [CrossRef] [PubMed]
8. Kawajiri, Y.; Ikeda, H.; Nagamatsu, Y.; Masaki, C.; Hosokawa, R.; Shimizu, H. PICN Nanocomposite as Dental CAD/CAM Block Comparable to Human Tooth in Terms of Hardness and Flexural Modulus. *Materials* 2021, 14, 1182. [CrossRef] [PubMed]
9. Tribst, J.P.M.; dos Santos, A.F.C.; da Cruz Santos, G.; da Silva Leite, L.S.; Lozada, J.C.; Silva-Concílio, L.R.; Baroudi, K.; Amaral, M. Effect of Cement Layer Thickness on the Immediate and Long-Term Bond Strength and Residual Stress between Lithium Disilicate Glass-Ceramic and Human Dentin. *Materials* 2021, 14, 5153. [CrossRef] [PubMed]
10. Gasparik, C.; Manziuc, M.M.; Burde, A.V.; Ruiz-López, J.; Buduru, S.; Dudea, D. Masking Ability of Monolithic and Layered Zirconia Crowns on Discolored Substrates. *Materials* 2022, 15, 2233. [CrossRef] [PubMed]

11. Paczkowski, I.; Stingu, C.S.; Hahnel, S.; Rauch, A.; Schierz, O. Cross-Contamination Risk of Dental Tray Adhesives: An In Vitro Study. *Materials* **2021**, *14*, 6138. [CrossRef] [PubMed]
12. Sfeir, G.; Zogheib, C.; Patel, S.; Giraud, T.; Nagendrababu, V.; Bukiet, F. Calcium Silicate-Based Root Canal Sealers: A Narrative Review and Clinical Perspectives. *Materials* **2021**, *14*, 3965. [CrossRef] [PubMed]
13. Eid, D.; Medioni, E.; De-Deus, G.; Khalil, I.; Naaman, A.; Zogheib, C. Impact of Warm Vertical Compaction on the Sealing Ability of Calcium Silicate-Based Sealers: A Confocal Microscopic Evaluation. *Materials* **2021**, *14*, 372. [CrossRef] [PubMed]
14. Alsofi, L.; Al Harbi, M.; Stauber, M.; Balto, K. Analysis of the Morpho-Geometrical Changes of the Root Canal System Produced by TF Adaptive vs. BioRace: A Micro-Computed Tomography Study. *Materials* **2021**, *14*, 531. [CrossRef] [PubMed]
15. Bardocz-Veres, Z.; Székely, M.; Salamon, P.; Bala, E.; Bereczki, E.; Kerekes-Máthé, B. Quantitative and Qualitative Assessment of Fluorescence in Aesthetic Direct Restorations. *Materials* **2022**, *15*, 4619. [CrossRef]
16. Ciavoi, G.; Mărgărit, R.; Todor, L.; Bodnar, D.; Dina, M.N.; Tărlungeanu, D.I.; Cojocaru, D.; Farcaşiu, C.; Andrei, O.C. Base Materials' Influence on Fracture Resistance of Molars with MOD Cavities. *Materials* **2021**, *14*, 5242. [CrossRef] [PubMed]

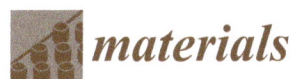 

*Review*

# Advanced Biomaterials and Techniques for Oral Tissue Engineering and Regeneration—A Review

Anamaria Matichescu [1], Lavinia Cosmina Ardelean [2,*], Laura-Cristina Rusu [3], Dragos Craciun [3], Emanuel Adrian Bratu [4,*], Marius Babucea [3] and Marius Leretter [5]

[1] Department of Preventive Dentistry, Community and Oral Health, "Victor Babeș" University of Medicine and Pharmacy Timisoara, 2 Eftimie Murgu Sq., 300041 Timisoara, Romania; matichescu.anamaria@umft.ro
[2] Department of Technology of Materials and Devices in Dental Medicine, "Victor Babeș" University of Medicine and Pharmacy Timisoara, 2 Eftimie Murgu Sq., 300041 Timisoara, Romania
[3] Department of Oral Pathology, "Victor Babeș" University of Medicine and Pharmacy Timisoara, 2 Eftimie Murgu Sq., 300041 Timisoara, Romania; laura.rusu@umft.ro (L.-C.R.); craciun.dragosi@gmail.com (D.C.); babucea.marius@gmail.com (M.B.)
[4] Department of Implant Supported Restorations, "Victor Babeș" University of Medicine and Pharmacy Timisoara, 2 Eftimie Murgu Sq., 300041 Timisoara, Romania
[5] Department of Prosthodontics, "Victor Babeș" University of Medicine and Pharmacy Timisoara, 2 Eftimie Murgu Sq., 300041 Timisoara, Romania; mariusleretter@yahoo.com
* Correspondence: lavinia_ardelean@umft.ro (L.C.A.); ebratu@umft.ro (E.A.B.)

Received: 24 October 2020; Accepted: 19 November 2020; Published: 23 November 2020

**Abstract:** The reconstruction or repair of oral and maxillofacial functionalities and aesthetics is a priority for patients affected by tooth loss, congenital defects, trauma deformities, or various dental diseases. Therefore, in dental medicine, tissue reconstruction represents a major interest in oral and maxillofacial surgery, periodontics, orthodontics, endodontics, and even daily clinical practice. The current clinical approaches involve a vast array of techniques ranging from the traditional use of tissue grafts to the most innovative regenerative procedures, such as tissue engineering. In recent decades, a wide range of both artificial and natural biomaterials and scaffolds, genes, stem cells isolated from the mouth area (dental follicle, deciduous teeth, periodontal ligament, dental pulp, salivary glands, and adipose tissue), and various growth factors have been tested in tissue engineering approaches in dentistry, with many being proven successful. However, to fully eliminate the problems of traditional bone and tissue reconstruction in dentistry, continuous research is needed. Based on a recent literature review, this paper creates a picture of current innovative strategies applying dental stem cells for tissue regeneration in different dental fields and maxillofacial surgery, and offers detailed information regarding the available scientific data and practical applications.

**Keywords:** regenerative medicine; regenerative dentistry; tissue engineering; stem cells; biomaterials; scaffolds; growth factors; additive manufacturing; 3D printing

## 1. Introduction

The traditional standard techniques based on replacing missing or deteriorated tissue with autologous grafts from living donors or even cadavers are still used in dentistry as well as in other medical fields, despite their disadvantages, such as risk of infections and rejection following the transplantation procedure. An innovative alternative is provided by regenerative medicine, which aims to regenerate, repair, or replace tissues and to ensure restoration of their impaired function by combining tissue engineering with the self-healing ability of humans. In vitro engineering of tissues and organs involves the emerging field of biotechnology in a multidisciplinary approach together with medicine, materials science, cell and molecular biology, bioengineering, and genetics [1].

Tissue engineering is a term associated with regenerative medicine and is distinct in its focus on aspects regarding the engineering and manufacturing of replacement tissue, but regenerative medicine and tissue engineering are often treated as a single field of interest in the literature. Tissue engineering aims to create functional tissue or even organs using patients' own cells, offering an alternative method to grafts or transplants. This approach is being increasingly used in dental and maxillofacial reconstruction medicine, providing a new option for the reconstruction of teeth, periodontium, bones, oral mucosa, conjunctiva, skin, temporomandibular joint, both bone and cartilage as well as nerves, muscles, tendons, and blood vessels of the oral and maxillofacial area [2].

Tissue engineering can be used to regenerate tissue for specific defects, which represents a major advantage compared with other current treatments which have numerous disadvantages for patients like loss of sensorial and motor functionalities of craniofacial structures due to prosthetic alloplastic materials, high risk of infection, inflammation, requirement for lifelong immunosuppression, or unpredictable compatibility with the donor in the case of autologous grafts. Additionally, the unlimited available bioengineered resources do not require immunosuppression [3]. Tissue engineering is classically based on three pillars: (a) the cells (stem cells/progenitor cells), responsible for synthesizing the new tissue matrix; (b) the signaling/growth factors necessary to promote and facilitate the functionalities; (c) the biomaterial scaffolds, necessary for cell differentiation, multiplication, and biosynthesis, that act as an extracellular matrix (ECM) (Figure 1).

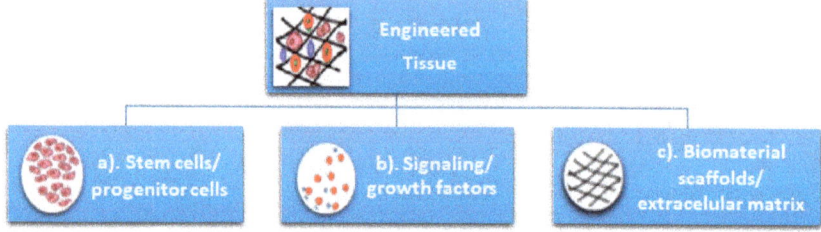

**Figure 1.** Classical pillars of tissue engineering: (**a**) the cells (stem cells/progenitor cells), (**b**) the signaling/growth factors, (**c**) the biomaterial scaffolds/extracellular matrix.

Cells communicate with their environment using different components to regenerate tissues by combining human cells with specific scaffold biomaterials. The biomaterial scaffolds provide templates for tissue regeneration and guide new tissues in their growth [4,5]. A successful approach in tissue engineering and regeneration implies that the combination of these three principles must be able to replace the damaged tissue and enable its function similarly to the original tissue or must be able to stimulate regeneration of the original tissue [6,7]. Several kinds of cells have been used in tissue engineering and regenerative medicine as reported in clinical studies, including stem cells, fibroblasts, chondrocytes, and keratinocytes originating from the same patient, another human, or animals [8].

The aim of this narrative review article is to approach this broad-spectrum subject in view of the literature from recent years specifically on the topic of potential orofacial stem cell usage in regenerative dentistry, both for hard and soft tissues. A large literature survey was performed on this topic in free-access digital archives of full-text articles (PubMed, Medline, Web of Science, and Google Scholar), with articles published between 2010–2020 being considered. More than 300 articles were referenced, with over 50% published in the last five years. The keywords used for searching were "regenerative dentistry", "tissue engineering", and "orofacial stem cells". A specific search was performed to identify clinical studies involving the application of dental stem cells for tissue regeneration in endodontics, periodontics, and maxillofacial surgery.

## 2. Stem Cells, Biomaterials, and Scaffolds for Oral Tissue Engineering and Regeneration—Types, Sources, and Technologies

### 2.1. Orofacial Stem Cells

Stem cells (SCs) are defined as primitive, unspecialized, and pluripotent cells of the human body characterized by two major properties: production of other new stem cells and multidirectional differentiation into cells with a specific functionality, such as bone cells, skin cells, and blood cells [8,9]. Their presence was first reported in bone marrow [10].

SCs have powerful potential in medicine; their study has revealed important information about the complex processes of human body development. Due to these abilities, SCs have attracted interest regarding their use in the regeneration, repair, and functionality improvement of degenerated or injured tissue using implants of engineered tissue as well as biohybrid organs. The strategies involving the use of stem cells for tissue regeneration can be optimized using bioactive scaffolds or by adding various growth factors [11].

Considering their origin, physiological stem cells include embryonic stem cells (ESCs) from embryos and adult stem cells (ASCs) from adult tissue. Other types of stem cells are the perinatal stem cells, from amniotic fluid, and induced pluripotent stem cells (iPSCs) [12], obtained by transforming regular ASCs under genetic reprogramming. iPSCs, which are generated directly from a somatic cell, were pioneered by Yamanaka, in 2006. Shinya Yamanaka's discovery was awarded with the 2012 Nobel Prize, jointly with Sir John Gurdon, who, in 1962, demonstrated that the specialization of cells is reversible. The immature cell nucleus in an egg cell of a frog was replaced with the nucleus from a mature intestinal cell. This modified egg cell developed into a normal tadpole, proving that the DNA of the mature cell still had all the information needed to develop all cells in the frog [13]. More than 40 years later, Shinya Yamanaka discovered how intact mature cells in mice could be reprogrammed to become PSCs, able to develop into all types of cells in the body, by introducing only a few genes [14–16].

The ESCs are present in the blastocyst and can be differentiated into all types of cells, and are therefore pluripotent. Various postnatal tissues present ASCs for their normal renewal as well as regeneration or injury healing. Recent research in tissue engineering and regenerative medicine has demonstrated that SCs can be widely used in dentistry, more so than synthetic materials because teeth are a rich source of SCs [17]. Mesenchymal stem cells (MSCs) are a type of ASC of great importance in regenerative medicine due to their responsibilities in tissue repair and growth, cell substitution, and wound healing due to physiological or pathological causes. MSCs can be isolated especially from bone marrow and adipose tissue, but also from other various human tissues like the placenta, amniotic fluid, liver, umbilical cord, synovial membrane, skin, muscle, and dental tissues [18].

Different types of SCs obtained from oral and maxillofacial tissues, with similar in vitro properties as bone marrow-derived MSCs, are being defined as multipotent stromal cells. They are able to differentiate into different types of cells like chondrocytes, myocytes, osteoblasts, and adipocytes. Recently, the immunomodulatory properties of MSCs have been reported, which enable their clinical use in the treatment of inflammatory conditions [19]. Considering their location in the oral and maxillofacial region, the ASCs are grouped in two major categories: dental and non-dental [20] (Figure 2).

The easy access, proliferation capacity, and multidirectional in vivo/in vitro differentiation makes orofacial SCs an important source of SCs for use in regenerative dentistry and medicine. Therefore, their potential clinical application in dentistry or other medical fields is diverse.

- Dental pulp stem cells (DPSCs), the first human dental MSCs found inside teeth, are considered a significant source for future regenerative procedures both in dental and general medical applications [21]. DPSCs are isolated from the dental pulp of primary or permanent teeth. Their high capacity for in vitro differentiation includes odontoblast, osteoblast, myoblast, adipocyte, dentin–pulp, cardiomyocyte, neuron-like cell, and hepatocyte-like cells, whereas in vivo, they are limited to only adipocytes, endotheliocytes, and myofibers [8,22,23].

- Periodontal ligament stem cells (PDLSCs), present on alveolar bone surfaces and the root, play a specific role in cementum or periodontal ligament (PDL) tissue regeneration. They are capable of giving rise to mesenchymal cell lineages to produce in vitro osteoblast-like cells, cementum tissue, Sharpey's fibers, adipocytes, and collagen-forming cells [17,24].
- Stem cells from apical papilla (SCAPs) are mesenchymal formations. They can be found within immature roots and isolated from the immature permanent apical papilla. SCAPs are good sources of and cause apexogenesis. They have a higher capacity to proliferate than DPSCs, being the first option for tissue regeneration. SCAPs represent a promising source of SCs, as they can differentiate into various lineages of cells, such as odontogenic, chondrogenic, osteogenic, adipogenic, neurogenic, and hepatogenic cells [25].
- Dental follicle stem cells (DFCs) are sourced from the dental follicle, which is loose connective tissue surrounding the developing tooth germ [17]. DFCs can differentiate osteoblast, cementoblast, alveolar bone, dentin-like tissues, PDL, cementum, adipocyte, chondrocyte, cardiomyocyte, and neuron-like cell. Their regenerative potential is highlighted by clinical applications in periodontal and neural tissue regeneration, tooth root regeneration, and bone defects [17,20,26,27].
- Tooth germ progenitor cells (TGPCs) are obtained from the dental mesenchyme of the human third molar germ in the late bell stage of tooth development. Studies on TGPCs have demonstrated their high proliferation activity and capacity to differentiation into adipogenic, chondrogenic, osteogenic, odontogenic, and neurogenic tissue [28,29]. In addition, TGPCs can differentiate into hepatocytes in vitro [25,30] and are able to form tube-like structures, possibly evidence of vascularization [31].
- Stem cells of human exfoliated deciduous teeth (SHEDs), obtained from exfoliated deciduous teeth, have higher proliferation capacity than DPSCs and the capability to differentiate into many more different body tissues than other types of SCs, including into adipocytes, osteoblasts, odontoblasts, neural cells, hepatocytes, and endothelial cells. SHEDs have a high proliferation capacity, high multipotency, immunosuppressive ability, and minimal risk of oncogenesis [32]. The major disadvantage of SHEDs is that an incomplete pulp-dentin-like complex is formed in vivo [17].
- Alveolar bone-derived mesenchymal stem cells (ABMSCs), isolated from the human alveolar bone, are a more convenient tissue source of MSCs and have the ability of multipotent differentiation into osteoblasts, adipocytes, and chondroblasts. In addition, they can induce ectopic bone formation in vivo [19].
- Salivary gland-derived stem cells (SGDSCs) are isolated from human salivary glands. The regeneration of salivary gland function with SGDSCs is still being investigated, though certain studies have already concluded that progenitor cells isolated from stromal tissue can be guided to differentiate into osteoblasts, chondrocytes, and adipocytes [33].
- Oral mucosa-derived mesenchymal stem cells (OMSCs), include oral epithelial stem cells (OESCs), gingiva-derived mesenchymal stem cells (GMSCs), and periosteum-derived stem cells (PSCs). SCs within the mucosa lining the oral cavity can be isolated from normal or inflamed gingiva, from attached and free gingiva, and from hyperplastic gingiva. OMSCs can differentiate into different mesenchymal lineages and have immunomodulatory properties [33].

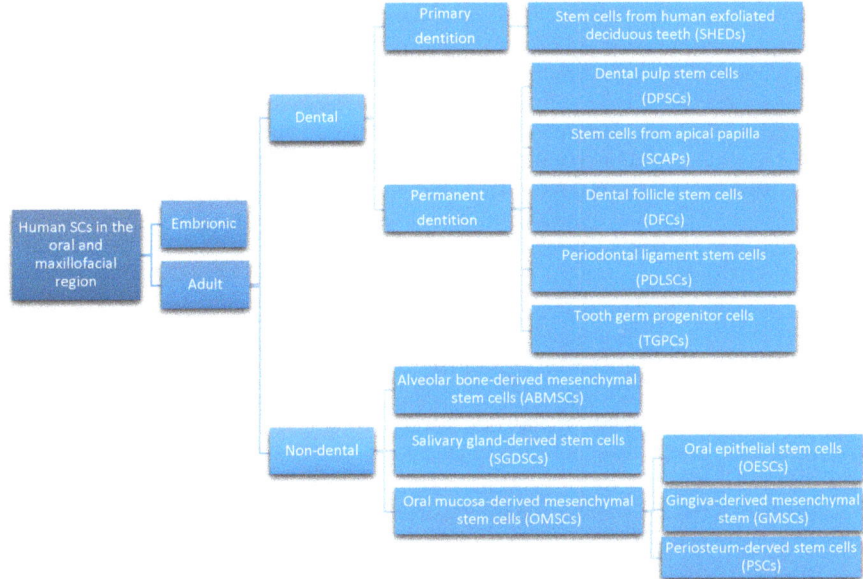

**Figure 2.** Types of human SCs in the oral and maxillofacial region.

## 2.2. Biomaterials and Scaffolds for Oral Tissue Engineering

In dental tissue regeneration, scaffolds and biomaterials are essential elements. They are used as attachment sites for regenerative cells from the surrounding tissues, as a template for tissue regeneration, as a source of implantable odontogenic cells with the capability to differentiate required cell type, and as bioactive molecules, especially growth factors that intensify the regenerative capability [34,35].

Biomaterials, natural or synthetic, alive or lifeless, are being defined as materials that interact with biological systems. They are often used in medical applications to augment or replace a natural function. Based on their biocompatibility, biomaterials are classified as bioactive, biotolerant, biodegradable, and bioinert [36].

Bioactive materials, by stimulating the biological response, may lead to osteogenesis by making strong chemical bonds. They are being classified into osteoconductive (hydroxyapatite and β-tricalcium phosphate), which stimulate bone growth along the surface, and osteoproductive (bioactive glasses), which are capable of stimulating the growth of new bone away from the bone/implant interface [36].

Biotolerant materials (polymers and most metals) are being well accepted by the host, but separated from the host tissue by the formation of a fibrous tissue, which is induced by the release of ions, corrosion products, and chemical compounds from the implant.

Biodegradable materials (polymers, such as polyglycolic and polylactic acids, and their co-polymers [37], ceramics as calcium phosphates [38], and magnesium) as biodegradable metal dissolve in contact with body fluids, the dissolution products being eliminated via the kidneys, without noticeable effects to the host. Biodegradable materials are used commonly used for surgical sutures, tissues in growth materials, and controlled drug release [36].

Bioinert materials (titanium and its alloys) are stable in the human body, and do not react with body fluids or tissues. Generally, bioinert materials are encapsulated by fibrous tissues, similar to biotolerant materials; however, in certain situations, they can develop structural and functional connection with the adjacent bone [39].

The most common approach in tissue engineering involves seeding cells onto a biomaterial matrix using a scaffold.

A wide variety of biomaterials, such as natural organic, synthetic organic, or even inorganic materials, is used for regeneration in oral and maxillofacial area, each of them having advantages and disadvantages. The natural organic materials include peptides (collagen or gelatin) and polysaccharides (alginate, chitosan, agarose). Frequently used synthetic organic materials include poly(lactic acid) (PLA), poly(caprolactone) (PCL), poly(lactic-co-glycolic acid) (PLGA), and poly(glycolic acid) (PGA) [36].

The most commonly used inorganic materials are bioactive ceramics which include glasses or calcium phosphates (hydroxyapatite, β-tricalciumphosphate), which have been extensively studied as bone replacement materials, and cementitious systems of calcium phosphate or calcium silicate [40].

Bioactive ceramics are strongly chemically bonded with bone tissues via chemical reactions [40]. Hydroxyapatite (HA), bioactive and non-degradable, is characterized by chemical and structural similarity to bone minerals. β-tricalcium phosphate also has a chemical composition similar to bone, and has higher in vivo rates of biodegradation compared to hydroxyapatite. The degradable bioactive ceramics are characterized by gradually degradation, in order to assist as scaffolds or replace the host tissue [40].

Polymers have been widely studied for medical applications, including bone tissue engineering [41]. From a biomedical perspective, polymers and co-polymers can be divided into two classes, biodegradable and biotolerant.

Biodegradable polymers, synthetic and natural, are suitable for additive manufacturing of scaffolds for tissue engineering [42]. The degradation of polymers, enzymatical or hydrolytical, is of most importance for this application. Natural polymers (chitosan, alginate, collagen, gelatin), frequently used as bioinks, are subject to enzymatic degradation, due to the microorganisms present in the biological environment [43].

The rate of enzymatic degradation varies upon the availability and concentration of respective enzymes. Hydrolytical degradation is related to synthetic polymers, and involves cleavage of hydrolytically sensitive bonds in the polymer, with consequent bulk or surface erosion, important in determining the best choice for a certain application [44].

Surface erosion offers several benefits for bone tissue engineering, such as retention of mechanical integrity, enhanced bone ingrowth, and ensures that the scaffold is gradually replaced by bone tissue [45].

PGA, PLA, PLGA, and PCL are hydrolytically degradable polymers [46].

PGA is usually used for short-term tissue engineering scaffolds and as fillers, because its rapid degradation and insolubility [47].

PLA, when mixed with glycolic acid, forms the copolymer PLGA, which is one of the most investigated degradable polymer for biomedical applications. Its great cell adhesion and proliferation properties recommend it as an excellent choice for tissue engineering [48,49].

Polymers can be processed to offer porous structures capable of facilitating the transportation of growth factors (nutrients as well as anabolites and catabolites) and are of interest due to their controllable degradation [41].

Recently, composite materials are being increasingly used due to their properties that result from the combination of both organic and inorganic elements. The most recent studies on this subject have considered the targeted and scaffold-assisted regeneration of enamel, dentin, and cementum [35].

An essential factor in tissue engineering is the scaffold. It offers a surface upon which cells adhere, multiply, thrive, and produce the ECM of proteins and saccharides that create the living tissue. Cells are expanded in culture and then transferred to the scaffold. The composition of the scaffold material and its internal architecture (dimensions of the struts, walls, pores, or channels) modulate and control the biological properties of the cells [50].

Generally, the scaffold materials must be biocompatible, biodegradable, porous, and without toxic metabolites. In particular, in dental regeneration, biomaterials must be suitable for the specific environment characteristics of the oral cavity considering pH, temperature, the presence of microorganisms, and the effect of mastication forces. To achieve these properties, most designed scaffolds deliberately mimic the structure of the natural ECM [36].

The number of suitable materials for fabricating scaffolds is limited by their biocompatibility, as they must accommodate the encapsulated cells and the recipient's body. Because of poor biocompatibility, scaffolds can generate aggressive in vivo foreign-body reactions, necessitating the development of smart immunomodulatory biomaterials that ensure the tolerance of foreign scaffolds by the host or regulating the immunological microenvironments to ensure cell survival [49].

The behavior of cells after adhesion to the scaffold is affected by pore shape, volume, size, and geometry. Different pore sizes can affect the extracellular matrix. Porosity and interconnectivity are important for the ingrowth of surrounding tissues [51]. Open and interconnected pores allow oxygen and nutrients to be transported into the interior and eliminate the waste generated by cellular metabolism [52].

A wide range of advanced smart biomaterials and constructs with intelligent properties and functions have recently been developed to improve tissue repair and regeneration processes [5]. Smart scaffolds incorporate bioactive molecules and nanoparticles and their physical and chemical properties are tailored as needed [53,54]. Their role is to improve the interactions with cells by enhancing the osteogenic differentiation for bone repair and to generate a better response to the surrounding environment [55] and include [5]:

a. Smart scaffold constructs with stem cells for bone tissue engineering

- Biomimetic and bionic smart scaffolds, such as biomimetic porous PLGA microspheres coupled with peptides prepared to mimic the composition and structure of natural tissues [56].
- Immune-sensitive smart scaffolds, such as an amino-functionalized bioactive glass scaffold developed to investigate its effects on MSCs, bone marrow, and macrophages [57]. β-tricalcium phosphate has been used to coat Mg scaffolds, and modulate its detrimental osteoimmunomodulatory properties [58].
- Shape-memory smart scaffolds, such as bone morphogenetic protein2-loaded shape-memory porous nanocomposite scaffold, consisting of chemically crosslinked poly(ε-caprolactone) and hydroxyapatite nanoparticles, used for the repair of bone defects, displayed shape-memory recovery [59].
- Electromechanical-stimulus smart scaffolds. Piezoelectric poly(vinylidene fluoride-trifluoroethylene) (PVDF-TrFE) was fabricated into flexible, 3D fibrous scaffolds. These have the ability to stimulate MSCs differentiation and tissue formation [60]. An electrospun PVDF-TrFE fiber scaffold containing zinc oxide nanoparticles was able to promote the adhesion and proliferation of human MSCs and also enhance the blood vessel formation [61].

b. Smart drug delivery for bone tissue engineering

- Stimuli-responsiveness tunable drug delivery systems. These materials can change their properties as response to an endogenous and/or exogenous stimulus; thus, delivering the required amount of drug on-demand [62]. Polymers and hydrogels are used [63,64]. A highly porous, pH-responsive bacterial cellulose-g-poly(acrylic acidco-acrylamide) hydrogel was developed as an oral controlled-release drug delivery carrier [64]. A poly(ethylene glycol) hydrogel, loaded with drugs by β-eliminative linkers, demonstrated tunable capability in drug release [65]. Farnesol-loaded nanoparticles, composed of 2-(dimethylamino)ethyl methacrylate, butyl methacrylate, and 2-propylacrylic acid are characterized by a pH-responsive drug release capability [66].

- Smart multifunctional nanoparticle-based drug delivery systems: mesoporous silica nanoparticles, bone-forming peptide-1-laden MSNs encapsulated into arginine-glycine-aspartic acid-treated alginate hydrogel [67].
- Biomimetic drug delivery systems: hydrogels, liposomes, micelles, dendrimers, polymeric carriers, and nanostructures [68,69].

c. Smart biomaterials and constructs to promote dental and periodontal regeneration, such as bilayered PLGA/calcium phosphate constructs [70] and tri-layered nanocomposite hydrogel scaffold: alveolar bone phase of chitin-PLGA/nanobioactive glass ceramic (nBGC)/platelet-rich plasma derived growth factors, PDL phase of chitin-PLGA/fibroblast growth factor, and cementum phase of chitin-PLGA/nBGC/cementum protein 1 [71].
d. Smart dental resins that respond to pH to protect tooth structures, such as dental composites containing nanoparticles of amorphous calcium phosphate and tetracalcium phosphate [72].
e. Smart pH-sensitive materials selectively inhibit acid-producing bacteria, and include cationic poly(phenylene vinylene) derivative, pH-sensitive quaternary pyridinium salts, for which the antibacterial potency can be controlled by varying the pH [73,74].
f. Smart resins that modulate the oral biofilm composition: quaternary ammonium methacrylates such as 12-methacryloyloxy dodecyl pyridinium bromide, methacryloxyethyl cetyl dimethyl ammonium chloride, quaternary ammonium polyethylenimine, and dimethylaminododecyl methacrylate [75,76].
g. Smart tailoring of alkyl chain length in quaternary ammonium methacrylates to avoid drug resistance [5,77].

SCs are capable to differentiate into various cell phenotypes based on their lineage and exposure to different environmental stimuli, such as ECM, growth factors, hypoxia, etc. [78]. The growth factor, usually a secreted protein or a steroid hormone, stimulates wound healing, cell proliferation, and occasionally cellular differentiation, and regulates various cellular processes. Cytokines and hormones bind to specific receptors on the surface of the target cells. Growth factors typically act as signaling molecules between cells, thus promoting cell differentiation and maturation [79,80].

The authors experience related to the subject includes tetracycline loaded collagen-carboxymethylcellulose/hydroxyapatite ternary composite materials [81], antiseptic composite materials containing silver nanoparticles, based on collagen, hydroxyapatite, and collagen/hydroxyapatite [82], collagen matrices with lidocaine [83], bone regeneration using synthetic HA, with high porosity and surface area for osteointegration [84–87].

### 2.3. Additive Manufacturing Technologies for Oral Tissue Engineering

Continuous development of manufacturing technologies enable printing of biofunctional scaffolds similar to the ECM, acting as a microenvironment for cell adhesion, proliferation, and differentiation [88,89].

The additive manufacturing (3D printing) of biomaterials offers promising future perspectives for the field of biomedical engineering [90], especially in regard to patient-specific clinical applications.

Additive manufacturing techniques for medical and tissue engineering purposes can be classified as: techniques which involve printing of live cells along with other materials (3D bioprinting) [91], and non-cellular fabrication techniques.

3D bioprinting, based on the layer-by-layer precise positioning of biological constituents, biochemicals and living cells, facilitates on-demand "printing" of cells, tissues and organs [92,93] for regenerative medicine purposes [94]. Utilizing diverse bioprinting techniques, tissue-engineered constructs can be tailored to obtain desired structures and properties [95,96].

Inkjet bioprinting functions by depositing small ink droplets into a predetermined location. It can be driven by thermal or piezoelectric actuation [97]. In thermal technology, heat-generated, the inflated bubble forces the ink out of the narrow nozzle and onto the substrates. In piezoelectric technology, drops are generated in absence of heat, by the transient pressure from the piezoelectric actuator. The droplets remain directional with regular and equal size [98], but, if used too frequently, this technology can cause damage to the cell membrane and cell lysis.

Laser-based bioprinting consists of a pulsed laser source, a ribbon, and a receiving substrate. The biological material, in liquid form, is irradiated by the laser, evaporates, and reaches the receiving substrate as droplets. Laser-based bioprinting enables high-resolution printing of biological material such as cells, DNA, and peptides [99]. Its drawback is that the use of the pulsed laser source may result in compromised cell viability [100].

Stereolithography bioprinting uses a photo-crosslinking light source to obtain desired patterns. It is highly tunable and prints in a layer-by-layer manner, the bioink from the reservoir being transferred to a movable platform [101].

Pressure-assisted bioprinting uses biomaterials in form of solutions, pastes or dispersions. The material, in form of a filament, is extruded by pressure through a microneedle or a microscale nozzle orifice [102].

Bioink printability has an important role in the fabrication process [103,104]. Besides being biocompatible and biodegradable, bioinks should be deformable and flowable [102]. After printing, the bioink should be stable in order to maintain shape and architecture of the design model [105].

The components of the bioink are polymers, ceramics, hydrogels, and composites, currently used in tissue engineering [106]. Hydrogel inks are much more attractive as bioprinting materials, compared to polymers and ceramics have received much more attention, and novel ink formulations have been designed [107]. Complex, functional, and biocompatible hydrogels can be fabricated using bioprinting technology. Adding different amounts of HA was attempted to a tunable alginate-gelatin hydrogel composite [108], human MSCs being subsequently mixed. Adding HA to the hydrogel resulted in enhanced mechanical properties, recommending it hard tissue reconstruction. No reduction in cell viability was detected [109]. The freeform reversible embedding of suspended hydrogels, a 3D bioprinting technique which deposits and crosslinks different kind of hydrogel inks, has been proven successfully [110].

An important concern when printing SCs—including ESCs, MSCs, and ASCs—is that their activity, including proliferation and pluripotency, may change during the process [111,112]. MSCs were successfully laser-printed for the construction of scaffold-free autologous grafts. The seed cells survived and maintained their ability to proliferate and continue differentiating into the osteogenic lineage [113].

Non-cellular additive manufacturing techniques include (Table 1):

The powder bed fusion methods which use either electron beam or laser to selectively consolidate material powder. The techniques involve spreading material powder over the previous layers, melting and fusing it [114].

The binder jetting technique is similar to the powder bed fusion technique and utilizes material powder that is spread over previous layers. Unlike powder bed fusion, this technique uses a binder as an adhesive for its consolidation [115,116].

The fused deposition modeling technique is based on the extrusion of heated polymer wires through a nozzle tip. The polymer rods are deposited and arranged in a layer by layer fashion [117].

The material jetting technique uses a liquid photopolymer resin that is light-cured. Similar to the material extrusion technique, the material is deposited from a nozzle and cured, defining a cross section. Individual cross sections are consolidated in a layer by layer fashion as the building platform moves in the vertical direction [118].

The vat polymerization technique uses a vat of liquid photopolymer resin, deposited in a layer by layer fashion. The build platform moves (depending on the position of the light source) to create additional layers on top of the previous [119].

These techniques all have their pros and cons and can process different types of biomaterials [120] (Table 1).

Table 1. Additive manufacturing methods of biomaterials for oral tissue engineering.

| Biomaterial | Type | Fabrication Method | Application | Reference |
|---|---|---|---|---|
| Hydroxyapatite | Bioactive/non-degradable ceramic | Vat polymerization; powder bed fusion; fused deposition; binder jetting | Bone tissue engineering | [121–125] |
| Bio glass | Bioactive ceramic | Vat polymerization | Bone tissue engineering | [126] |
| Calcium silicate | Bioactive ceramic | Powder bed fusion | Tissue engineering | [127] |
| β-tricalcium phosphate | Bioactive/biodegradable ceramic | Binder jetting; vat polymerization; fused deposition | Bone tissue engineering | [128–132] |
| Polycaprolactone | Biodegradable polymer | Powder bed fusion; fused deposition | Bone tissue engineering; cartilage tissue engineering | [133–136] |
| Poly(lactic acid) | Biodegradable polymer | Fused deposition | Bone regeneration | [137] |
| Poly(lactic acid-co-glycolic acid) | Biodegradable polymer | Material jetting; fused deposition | Tissue engineering | [138–141] |

## 3. Regenerative Therapies in Dentistry—Potential Clinical Applications of Dental Stem Cells

Four main groups of defects in the oral area represent the main targets of soft or hard tissue regeneration: maxillofacial defects, periodontal diseases (gingiva inflammation, PDL, alveolar bone, and cementum loss), dental pulpal diseases, and hard tissue defects of the tooth [142]. In addition, tissue engineering and regeneration are oriented toward several applications of dental SCs with the aim of accelerating the healing of oral injury without scar formation [143]. Table 2 lists the potential clinical applications of dental SCs in regenerative dentistry.

Table 2. Potential clinical applications of dental SCs in regenerative dentistry.

| Type of SCs | Regenerative Dental Applications | References |
|---|---|---|
| DPSCs | Mandibular bone defects regeneration, scaffold-based dentin–pulp repair, dentin–pulp tissue regeneration with inflamed pulp, periodontal regeneration, neural tissue regeneration, muscle regeneration, angiogenesis induction, craniofacial skeletal repair | Zhou et al. [11] Zakrzewski et al. [17] Berebichez-Fridman et al. [18] Hollands et al. [22] Tsutsui [23] Sharpe [24] Khazaei et al. [28] Chalisserry et al. [30] Somani et al. [31] Yang et al. [142] Chatzistavrou et al. [144] Bakopoulou et al. [145] Tatullo et al. [146] Potdar et al. [147] Davila et al. [148] Gronthos et al. [149] Beltrão-Braga et al. [150] Verma et al. [151] Almushayt et al. [152] Yoshida et al. [153] Aydin et al. [154] Graziano et al. [155] |
| PDLSCs | Tooth root regeneration, periodontal tissue regeneration (cementum, PDL), bone regeneration | Zhou et al. [11] Zakrzewski et al. [17] Liu et al. [20] Somani et al. [31] Verma et al. [151] Aydin et al. [154] Kitagaki et al. [156] Hynes et al. [157] Han et al. [158] Maeda et al. [159] Gay et al. [160] Kim et al. [161] |

Table 2. Cont.

| Type of SCs | Regenerative Dental Applications | References |
|---|---|---|
| SCAPs | Bone regeneration, tooth root regeneration, dentin–pulp repair, neural regeneration and repair, periodontal regeneration, angiogenesis, tooth regeneration | Zhou et al. [11]<br>Liu et al. [20]<br>Kang et al. [25]<br>Khazaei et al. [28]<br>Somani et al. [31]<br>Bakopoulou et al. [145]<br>Verma et al. [151]<br>Aydin et al. [154]<br>Schneider et al. [162]<br>Nada et al. [163]<br>Miller et al. [164]<br>Wongwatanasanti et al. [165] |
| DFCs | Bone defects, tooth root regeneration, periodontal tissue regeneration, neural tissue regeneration, enhancement of bone regeneration on titanium implant surfaces in humans | Zhou et al. [11]<br>Zakrzewski et al. [17]<br>Liu et al. [20]<br>Chalisserry et al. [30]<br>Somani et al. [31]<br>Yang et al. [142]<br>Verma et al. [151]<br>Aydin et al. [154]<br>Zhang et al. [166]<br>Shoi et al. [167]<br>Rezai-Rad et al. [168]<br>Honda et al. [169] |
| TGSCs | Bone repair and cartilage regeneration | Zhou et al. [11]<br>Chalisserry et al. [30]<br>Verma et al. [151]<br>Aydin et al. [154]<br>Caracappa et al. [170]<br>Yalvaç et al. [171]<br>Yalvaç et al. [172]<br>Doğan et al. [173] |
| SHEDs | Critical-sized craniofacial bone defect regeneration, scaffold-based dentin–pulp regeneration, neural and blood vessel regeneration, tooth root regeneration, tubular dentin | Zhou et al. [11]<br>Liu et al. [20]<br>Sharpe [24]<br>Somani et al. [31]<br>Verma et al. [151]<br>Aydin et al. [154]<br>Jeon et al. [174]<br>Araújo et al. [175]<br>Ma et al. [176]<br>Kunimatsu et al. [177]<br>Ching et al. [178]<br>Miura et al. [179]<br>Martinez Saez et al. [180]<br>Annibali et al. [181]<br>Arora et al. [182] |
| ABMSCs | Bone defects, periodontal regeneration | Zhou et al. [11]<br>Liu et al. [20]<br>Verma et al. [151]<br>Aydin et al. [154]<br>Caracappa et al. [170]<br>Mason et al. [183]<br>Liu et al. [184]<br>Pekovits et al. [185]<br>Matsubara et al. [186]<br>Park et al. [187]<br>Lim et al. [188]<br>Khazaei et al. [189] |

Table 2. *Cont.*

| Type of SCs | Regenerative Dental Applications | References |
|---|---|---|
| GMSCs | Neural regeneration, periodontal regeneration, cartilage, bone, muscle, oral mucositis, improving the regeneration of craniofacial bone | Liu et al. [20]<br>Chalisserry et al. [30]<br>Grawish [33]<br>Verma et al. [151]<br>Aydin et al. [154]<br>Caracappa et al. [170]<br>Zhang et al. [190]<br>Tomar et al. [191]<br>Tang et al. [192]<br>Wang et al. [193]<br>Marynka-Kalmani et al. [194]<br>Zhang et al. [195] |

*3.1. Regenerative Endodontics*

Regenerative endodontic therapy (RET) is defined as "biologically based procedures designed to replace damaged tooth structures, including dentin and root structures, as well as cells of the pulp–dentin complex" [196]. Regenerative endodontics aims to restore normal function of the pulp, by regenerating the dentin–pulp complex damaged by infection, trauma, or developmental anomalies of immature permanent teeth with necrotic pulp. The benefits of regenerative endodontics not only stand in revitalization of the tooth, but also continued root development and, potentially, increasing fracture resistance [197].

Apexification and apexogenesis are clinical procedures closely related to regenerative endodontics [198]. Pulp necrosis in young permanent teeth poses a challenge to clinicians due to the open and underdeveloped apex [199]. The purpose of endodontic treatment, or hermetic sealing of the foramina, can be easily achieved in mature permanent teeth where there is an apical constriction. Because the young permanent teeth do not have an apical constriction, a hermetic seal of the foramina is almost impossible. It traditionally consists of the apexification procedure with calcium hydroxide or a mineral trioxide aggregate (MTA) plug, which stimulates the periapical cells to form a dentin-like substance in the apex region. This process, even if it seals the foramina, does not add to the thickness and strength of the dentin walls, making the root prone to fractures and resulting in a weakened apical barrier [200–202]. Apexogenesis, used in case of injured but not necrotic pulp, leaves the apical one-third of the dental pulp in place, to allow complete formation of the root [198].

The first studies on pulp regeneration were conducted by Nygaard-Otsby et al. [203,204]. Intentionally, overinstrumentation was used to induce bleeding from the periapical tissues into the root canal, followed by a short obturation to allow tissue growth into the canal space. The histological examination of the extracted teeth revealed that fibrous connective tissue and cellular cementum formed in the canal space [203]. Later on, Banchs and Trope [205] proposed a revascularization protocol based on the experiments of Kling et al. [206] on implanted teeth, Hoshino et al. [207] on root canal disinfection, and Nygaard-Otsby et al. [204] on blood clots in the canal space.

Regenerative endodontics originates from the revascularization literature, which focuses only on the delivery of blood into the root canal space. It aims to allow its filling with vital tissue as a result of wound healing, but does not include a source of SCs within the apical tissues, their delivery into root canals, and the intentional release and use of local growth factors embedded into the dentin [208].

The American Association of Endodontists' (AAE) clinical considerations RET define success by three measures [209]: the primary/essential goal, which is the elimination of symptoms and the evidence of bony healing and is the objective of all endodontic treatments; the secondary/desirable goal, which is increased root wall thickness and/or increased root length and, thus, the continuation of root maturation leading to a smaller incidence in root fracture; and the tertiary goal, which is a positive response to vitality testing.

RET represents an extension of root canal therapy, aiming to heal apical periodontitis. Conventional root canal therapy only cleans and fills the pulp chamber with biologically inert material. RET aims to replace live tissue in the pulp chamber and regenerate its normal function, by stimulating its regrowth or by inserting bioactive substances in the pulp chamber [210].

Previous studies evaluated combinations of SCs, growth factors, and scaffolds that result in histological regeneration of pulp tissues [211] (Figure 3).

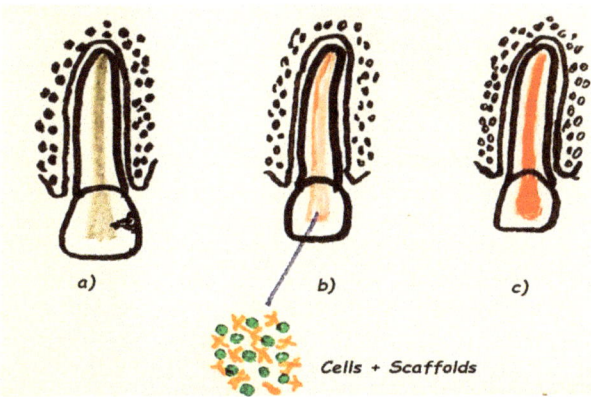

**Figure 3.** Regeneration of functional pulpal tissue: (**a**) non-vital pulp, (**b**) transplantation of stem cells, (**c**) regenerated pulp.

ASCs, especially MSCs (DPSCs, SCAPs) are used in RET. Lacerating the apical papilla and subsequently delivering a high local concentration of SCs into the root canal space does not necessarily result in their differentiation into cells of the pulp-dentin complex. Growth factors act as important adjuncts in RET. Histologic signs of tissue repair rather than regeneration may be due to lack of control of endogenous growth factors [212].

SCs are capable of differentiating into odontoblasts, pulp fibroblasts, and other niche cells characteristic of dentin–pulp complex. To ensure the success of RET in the adult, exogenously delivered and/or endogenous growth factors must induce the sprouting of neural fibrils and endothelial cells along with other blood vessel resident cells [213].

Regenerative endodontics is based on adequate disinfection of the root canal system, induction of bleeding through overinstrumentation to create a scaffold for stem cells, and coronal sealing of the blood clot with a biocompatible material, such as MTA [214].

However, certain variables related to patient age, apex diameter, canal instrumentation, disinfection, medication, and coronal seal have to be considered when evaluating RET success.

Even though RET has been used on mature teeth, most of the reported cases are on young patients where pulp necrosis has halted the root maturation process. According to Estefans et al. [215] younger age groups are better candidates for revascularization procedures than older age groups.

In immature permanent teeth, apical diameter is of importance for RET. In cases of a preoperative apical diameter wider than 1 mm, greater root maturation was observed [215]. Nevertheless, apical diameters of 0.5–1.0 mm demonstrated the highest clinical success rate [216]. The pulp tissue regeneration is influenced by the presence of prior infection, which negatively affects the tissue-forming cells as well as SCs in the periapical tissues [217].

The removal of pulp necrotic tissue is vital to the success of pulp regeneration but mechanical removal may be contraindicated because it weakens the already affected dentinal walls [20] and could damage vital tissue remnants in the apical part of the canal [218,219]. According to Lin et al. [220] most of the bacteria are hosted in the apical portion and the biofilm formed on the canal walls penetrates the dentinal tubules. They concluded that, to some degree, mechanical debridement might be necessary to disrupt the biofilm for better chances of root maturation to continue [220], as root-canal-irrigating solutions and intracanal medicaments are not able to completely eliminate bacteria biofilms in infected root canals during root canal therapy [221,222].

Infection prevents regeneration, repair, and SCs activity, so disinfecting the root canal system is crucial to the success of RET [223]. Strategies for optimal disinfection of the pulp space with minimal disruption of the necessary biological factors from dentin, the progenitor cells in periapical vital tissues, and the vascularity, to promote periapical healing as well as soft and hard tissue development after an infectious process are being currently available [214].

After an infection, new tissues cannot form inside the canal space. Only if osteoblasts, cementoblasts, periodontal ligament cells, and endothelial cells can migrate inside the canal is there a chance of developing new tissues.

The chemicals used to disinfect the root canal system have bacteriostatic or bactericidal properties and should not damage healthy tissues, thus lowering the chances of RET success [214,224].

NaOCl is a potent antimicrobial agent that effectively dissolves necrotic and organic tissue [225], which is very effective against biofilm [226,227]. Based on the cytotoxic effect of NaOCl on in vitro survival of SCAPs, a concentration of 1.5% NaOCl is recommended [58,228]. Other studies [229] reported that the SCAPs survival rate is 74% after being exposed to 6% NaOCl followed by 17% ethylenediaminetetraacetic acid (EDTA) and 6% NaOCl once more. The AAE suggests irrigation with NaOCl for 5 min and then with saline or EDTA for 5 min, using a system that lowers the possibility of irrigant extrusion into the periapical space, at about 1 mm shorter than the working length, to maximize the survival rate of SCAPs [230]. Hence, the NaOCl concentrations could be adjusted with some precautions and the SCAP survival rate is not significantly affected [205,218,219,231].

EDTA is a chelating agent used to remove smear layer in conventional root canal therapy [232] and to cause the release of growth factors from dentin matrix in RET [233], resulting in dentin demineralization and its exposure to the released growth factors [230,234]. The use of 17% EDTA resulted in an increased SCAP survival rate as well as partial reversal of the deleterious effects of NaOCl [229]. EDTA conditioning of dentin promoted the adhesion, migration, and differentiation of DPSCs toward or onto dentin [230]. Therefore, a final rinse with EDTA before creation of a blood clot is advised. Release of growth factors from dentin matrix after EDTA treatment was reported in non-infected root canals [233,234]. A residual biofilm may significantly diminish the bioavailability or bioactivity of dentin-matrix-associated growth factors [235]. Dentin-matrix-derived growth factors released after EDTA treatment may signal SCAPs to differentiate into odontoblast-like cells [236].

The use of chlorhexidine (CHX) as canal disinfectant is based on its antimicrobial activity that extends by interacting with the dentin. CHX cannot dissolve tissues and it is not advisable to use it as the only irrigation solution [225,237]. Haapasalo et al. [225] suggested that the initial NaOCl irrigation should be followed by sterile saline and 2% CHX, the role of saline solution being to stop any interactions between NaOCl and CHX.

Intracanal medication between endodontic treatment sessions assists with the control of microbial infection by using different substances as calcium-hydroxide-based and polyantibiotic pastes. It aims to stop microbial proliferation in the root canal system and combine antibacterial and anti-inflammatory properties with the capacity to induce mineralized tissue formation, having beneficial effects on repairing the apical tissues [238].

Traumatized immature permanent teeth with infected necrotic pulp have similar microbial ecology as mature permanent teeth [239], including biofilms formation on the radicular canal walls and bacteria penetration into the canal dentinal tubules [240].

Antibiotics have been used as intracanal medication in root canal treatment since the 1950s [241], but local application of antibiotics in endodontics has been restricted because of the risks of adverse effects. The interest in using a combination of antibiotics has reemerged with the introduction of the triple antibiotic paste (TAP) [238]. The ciprofloxacin, metronidazole, and minocycline TAP [207] is sufficiently potent to eradicate bacteria from the root canal. A double antibiotic paste of metronidazole and ciprofloxacin [218] has also proven its efficacy. Studies have shown that TAP is biocompatible [239] but, unfortunately, antimicrobial combinations can prove to be cytotoxic and increase the risk of adverse effects, and bacterial resistance [239,240]. Augmentin has been shown to kill 100% of the microorganisms isolated from the infected root canal associated with in vitro apical abscess [241]. It acts by inhibiting bacterial cell wall synthesis, only affecting bacterial cells and not human cells, as the latter do not have a cell wall.

Calcium hydroxide is considered the first choice for intracanal medication in RET. It offers good antimicrobial properties, anti-inflammatory activity, consequent stimulation of apical repair, and participation in mineralized tissue formation, inducing differentiation of periodontal ligament cementoblasts and cementogenesis by increasing extracellular calcium levels and tissue compatibility [242]. According to prior studies, dentin is capable of inactivating root canal medication [243,244], thereby limiting the efficacy of calcium hydroxide as an intracanal dressing [245]. Because of its high pH, it can damage the cells that have regenerative capacity [246]. When treated with calcium hydroxide rather than TAP, human apical cells attach to the root dentin walls at a higher rate [247].

Various other materials have been used to induce apexification, such as tricalcium phosphate [248], collagen calcium phosphate [248], osteogenic protein-1 [246], and MTA [246] without affecting root elongation or maturation [246]. The apical plug of MTA and gutta-percha filling has several advantages over calcium hydroxide-induced apexification. MTA is biocompatible, has osteoinductive properties, sets in the presence of moisture, and the treatment can be completed in a single appointment, though it does not strengthen the remaining tooth structure [249].

After disinfection of the canal and resolution of symptoms, RET usually involves lacerating of the periapical tissues to initiate bleeding or the use of platelet-rich plasma (PRP) [250], platelet-rich fibrin (PRF) unmineralized tissue matrices, and synthetic materials like polyglycol or collagen [251,252].

Studies have shown that inducing bleeding into the disinfected canal is an important step in regenerative procedures; a stable blood clot (BC) not only serves as a scaffold but triggers significant accumulation of undifferentiated STCs into the canal space [253] and stimulates cell growth and the differentiation of STCs into odontoblast-like cells [228,253–255].

A common problem is the failure to induce apical bleeding or to achieve adequate blood volume in the canal [202,256,257]. In pluri-rooted teeth, this can be achieved by transferring some blood from other roots, but this approach cannot be used for single-rooted teeth. Because of this, researchers have searched for other scaffold options. PRP, PRF, and platelet pellet (PP) are options that have shown promising clinical and radiological results [256]. Cehreli et al. [257] reported the clinical outcomes of PRP, PRF, and PP used in the presence or absence of a BC. PRP, PRF, and PP, even if more expensive than the BC method, can offer a longer exposure to growth factors, and are possibly better scaffolds since they also eliminate the progressing obliteration of the root, a problem found with the BC method [257].

After the scaffold has set and stability has been confirmed, a coronal seal should be placed over the blood clot to serve as an internal matrix. The AAE recommends an MTA layer of approximately 3 mm, followed by a 3–4 mm layer of glass ionomer and a layer of reinforced composite resin [209]. The MTA, which hardens in wet conditions, acts like an antibacterial barrier, but is also associated with teeth discoloration. An alternative to MTA, such as bioceramics and tricalcium silicate cements, should be used in teeth where there are aesthetic concerns [209].

The true success of RET is being difficult to evaluate. Regardless of the presence or absence of an intracanal BC, the concentration of irrigating solution, or type of intracanal medication used, different treatment protocols were able to eliminate clinical symptoms and signs of apical periodontitis. Its potential to promote thickening of the canal walls and/or continued root development is, unfortunately, not yet predictable [224].

*3.2. Regenerative Periodontics*

Considered a distinctive tissue structure, periodontal tissue consists of a three-dimensional complex of alveolar bone, PDL, and cementum. The incidence of periodontal disease, the main cause of tooth loss, is increasing among the population, affecting about 20–50% of the global population without being influenced by age or sex [258–261].

It has a microbial cause and, in most cases, results in irreversible destructive phenomena. Chronic inflammation severely affects the periodontium, leading to the resorption of the alveolar bone, a pathological phenomenon that cannot be stopped by natural processes [257,262].

Nonsurgical periodontal therapies, such as scaling and root planning, represent the first choice methods in preventing disease progression in its first stages, but the removal of pathogens and necrotic tissues provide only partial, local regeneration of the periodontal tissue. Surgery, needed in the advanced stages, or other currently common periodontal therapies, such as growth factors [263] and grafts, could be replaced by the use of SCs as a successful method for treating periodontal diseases due to the existence of SCs in the PDL [264,265].

Since 2004, when PDLSCs were first identified and considered for periodontal tissue regeneration, many other types of stem cells have demonstrated their capacity to form periodontal tissues under certain conditions (Table 2). SC usage has become increasingly relevant in the last decade in the search for an effective solution for periodontitis treatment, despite the fact that regeneration of periodontal tissues is one of the most complex processes in the human body [266]. Thus, aiming high, the target of regenerative dentistry is to develop effective therapies and techniques to treat periodontal diseases using applied tissue engineering and regeneration on the lost or affected support tissue of the periodontium: alveolar bone, periodontal ligament, and cementum [266].

Two major strategies for periodontal regeneration have been outlined: guided tissue regeneration (GTR) and tissue engineering [267]. GTR, a regenerative surgical technique, has been extensively used for periodontium regeneration in recent decades. It aims to prevent apical migration of the epithelium in the bone defect by placing a membrane at the root surface [268,269].

Two types of barrier membranes are used in GTR: non-absorbable and absorbable membranes. The use of the non-absorbable membranes, such as cellulose acetate filters (Millipore filters), rubber dam, specifically processed expanded polytetrafluoroethylene and dense polytetrafluoroethylene has a high risk of infection because a second surgery is required to remove them [270]. Resorbable membranes—such as allogenic soft tissues, freeze-dried skin, freeze-dried duramater, and reconstituted collagen membranes, have been introduced later on—changing GTR into a single-step procedure [270]. The goal of the membrane is to prevent contact between the gingival tissue and the surface of the root, preventing gum growth in the bone space, thereby selectively guiding cells derived from the periodontal tissue onto the root surface. Thus, the periodontal tissue can be regenerated. In practice, a small piece of tissue-like material is inserted between the gingival tissue and the bone [267].

Periodontal therapy with SCs has been considered in studies performed on animals, which have reported an effective contribution to the regeneration process of the SCs implanted into periodontal defects [271]. Periodontal tissue regeneration must be viewed as an integrated healing process—a result of the coordinated interaction between stem cells, biomaterials, growth factors, and the particularities of the patient's immune system (Figure 4). In periodontal regeneration, the tissue engineering strategy may take one of two approaches: scaffold-free or scaffold-based [271]. The scaffold-free approach uses cells or cell aggregates transplanted onto the wound area with no carrier cell. Clinical studies reported that PDLSCs and DPSCs have the potential to form periodontal tissues, but problems occur with cell diffusion out of the defect zone. It has been proven to be a non-relevant regeneration strategy because of the low cell survival rate after transplantation [272]. The cell sheet technique has been developed as a scaffold-free strategy for cell delivery and has been tried in various tissue regenerations, including for periodontal tissue. Cell sheet engineering aims to prevent ECM degradation by isolating cells using enzymes and completely retaining them to ensure normal cell function. Cell sheet engineering can prevent cell migration, but only simple-structured tissues can be regenerated [272]. In conclusion, scaffold-free techniques are not suitable for the complex structure of the periodontium.

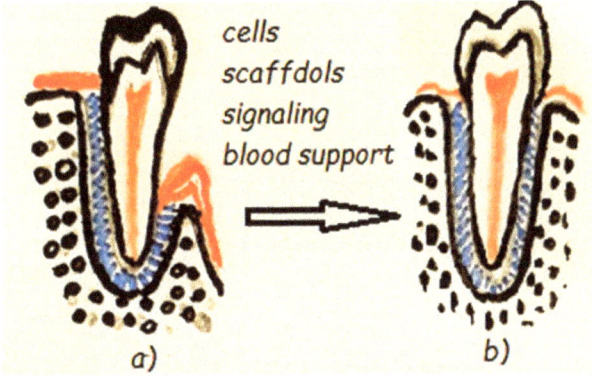

**Figure 4.** Periodontal tissue regeneration: (**a**) diseased periodontium, (**b**) regenerated periodontium.

For the periodontal ligament, cementum, and alveolar bone complex structure regeneration, the scaffold-based approach is more suitable [273].

Multiphasic scaffolds, with distinctive particularities of each layer both in architecture and chemical/biochemical composition, are required to imitate the complex structure of the periodontium. Additionally, the ECM contributes a 3D substructure for cell adhesion and movement, and contains growth factors facilitating the signal delivery needed for morphogenesis and differentiation. PDLSCs sheets demonstrated the potential of periodontal tissue regeneration in experimental deficiencies in rats, dogs, and pigs [274].

Raju et al. reported successful three-dimensional tissue regeneration of a large-scale tissue injury using bioengineered tissue to simulate the anatomical structure in which two types of cells were used for cell sheet fabrication: rat PDL cells extracted from molars and osteoblast-like cells [275]. Periodontal regeneration with autologous periodontal-ligament-derived cell sheets combined with β-tricalcium phosphate bone was reported as safe and efficacious in a study by Iwata et al. [276].

Biomaterials and controlled drug delivery for periodontal regeneration involve the use of inorganic, polymeric, or composite biomaterials. For bone and cementum repair/regeneration, inorganic biomaterials are the material of choice due to their similarities in composition and mechanical properties. For PDL regeneration, polymeric biomaterials are appropriate. By combining inorganic and polymeric biomaterials, biomimetic scaffolds for bone and cementum regeneration can be fabricated [277].

Thus, bioinspired innovative materials are needed to mimic the complex structure of periodontal tissues at the micro- and nanolevel because, at present, functional periodontal tissue regeneration has yet not been achieved. Many studies with the objective of regenerating the periodontal tissues highlighted that the actual biomaterials cannot exactly mimic the natural architecture of periodontal tissues, so the connections between their components, cementum–PDL–alveolar bone, remain unstable and cannot support teeth or bear occlusal force [278].

For periodontal tissue regeneration, to ensure an ECM-like microenvironment, biomimetic nanofibrous and multilayer scaffolds have been developed. In a recent review, Liang et al. focused on the relevance of advanced bioinspired scaffolding biomaterials and the temporospatial control of multidrug delivery in the regeneration of the cementum–periodontal ligament–alveolar bone complex [267]. A systematic review by Liu et al. [279] presents the newest regeneration developments in the case of all three types of periodontal tissues and for simultaneous regeneration the entire periodontal complex using stem cells, 3D-printing, gene therapy, and layered biostructures.

## 3.3. Regenerative Oral and Maxillofacial Surgery

Oral and maxillofacial surgeries play important roles in the treatment of traumatic and degenerative disease with tissue loss. The techniques used have been improved over time, from using growth factors and platelet concentrates to biomaterial scaffolds and autologous tissues and, currently, SCs in regenerative dentistry. In oral and maxillofacial surgery, tissue engineering and regeneration are the approaches currently available for achieving the goals of reconstruction procedures [280].

In maxillofacial reconstruction, surgeons have two main objectives: to provide the anatomic form and the function of the oromaxillofacial area. Because the facial skeleton has a complex structure, reconstruction should restore the volume, shape, bone continuity, and symmetry of the skeletal bone. Because the numerous soft and hard tissues that form this area provide important functions such as articulation, facial expressions, mastication, swallowing, and breathing, the reconstruction must restore, maintain, and stabilize these tissue functions. In addition, the reconstruction must be performed not only for reconstructive goals but also for aesthetic goals. Hence, different types of tissues must be reconstructed layer by layer [281].

Oral and maxillofacial surgery can use MSCs from the oral cavity, which are an important and easily accessible source to the surgeon. Several maxillofacial bone defects can be approached using bone tissue regeneration. Soft tissue, such as skin and oral mucosa, can also be regenerated [282]. Cartilage regeneration, salivary gland regeneration, fat, muscle, blood vessels, and nerve regeneration represent other applications of tissue engineering in oral and maxillofacial surgery [2,278]. Recent studies highlight the possibility of using GMSCs as the cellular components for 3D bioprinting of scaffold-free nerve constructs needed for peripheral nerve repair and regeneration [283] or for treating gingival defects [284].

3.3.1. Bone Regeneration

Substantial bone defects of the maxilla and mandible, in need of surgery, originate from congenital abnormalities, accidental traumatic injuries, tooth extraction, surgical resection of benign or malign tumors, and infections. The most challenging situation for the maxillofacial surgeon is the restoration of large bony defects due to trauma or post-resection.

In the standard reconstruction of maxillofacial bone defects, autologous grafting is still the gold standard technique, even if it presents many disadvantages [285].

A perfect technique and material for bone reconstruction has not yet been found, even if many clinical approaches have been attempted in recent years. Bone tissue engineering techniques provide a solution for reconstructing large size bone defects in the oral and maxillofacial region using autologous bone grafts, conditioned by adequate vascularization. Wu et al. [286] reviewed new strategies for improving vascularization of engineered bone tissue and their possible feasible clinical applications using SCs, mainly MSCs originating from bone marrow or adipose tissue as well from dental tissues. MSCs are a key element in bone regeneration due to their capacity to induce bone regeneration by mimicking biological processes [287].

After being seeded into newly regenerated tissue, MSCs can be directed to differentiate into osteoblasts which finally initiate the process of mineralization. MSCs can indirectly improve bone regeneration through the secretion of cytokines and growth factors. Two strategies are used: the MSCs are directly transplanted into the defect bone site and combined with an external scaffold; MSCs isolated from the patient and expanded ex vivo are seeded onto suitable internal 3D scaffolds which, in controlled culture conditions, proliferate and pre-differentiate [288]. The most promising is the combination of cells with scaffolds fabricated from different materials and technologies, recently summarized by Chocholata et al. [289]. Several investigations in bone tissue engineering have reported various types of MSCs combined with different scaffolds as potentially suitable for regeneration for surgical procedures in the oral and maxillofacial region [290–293]. A clinical research study reported biocomplexes fabricated from DPSCs and collagen sponges in human mandible repair with remarkable results [294].

Recently, the use of human GMSCs was considered as a strategy for accidental or trauma surgery treatment, especially for cranial bones. Three-dimensional-engineered scaffolds complexed with GMSCs could provide a new therapeutic approach to improving bone tissue regeneration [295].

Common bone defects in the maxilla and mandible after tooth loss include atrophy of hard and soft alveolar tissue, which result in reduced horizontal and vertical dimensions [296]. In some cases, bone regeneration is required in the atrophic mandible and for maxillary sinus augmentation and dorsal augmentation in rhinoplasty [282]. The atrophic mandible, characterized by a vertical height of less than 20 mm, presents hypovascularity that can determine tooth loss and alveolar processes. The atrophic resorption patterns create important anatomical changes with the risk of soft tissue breakdown and dehiscence as secondary effect of deficiency in blood supply in that area because of the lack of muscle attachments. In Gjerde et al. [297], regeneration of severe mandibular ridge resorption was performed using bone-marrow-derived MSCs, which is a less invasive approach than classical bone grafting. Aspirated from the posterior iliac crest, the bone marrow cells and the plastic adherent cells were expanded in culture medium with human platelet lysate. Afterwards, the cells were inserted into the defect together with biphasic calcium phosphate granules. A significant new regenerated bone formation was induced with a volume appropriate for dental implant installation [297]. Di Stefano et al. [298] tested the effectiveness of enzymatically deantigenated equine bone block as a scaffold during horizontal augmentation of the lower jaw for guided bone regeneration. In addition, they reported the augmentation of a partially edentulous atrophic mandible using an equine-derived block with an expanded polytetrafluoroethylene membrane. The new regenerated bone allowed for a definitive prosthesis [298].

3.3.2. Cartilage Regeneration

The temporomandibular joint (TMJ) is affected by many diseases and defects that can compromise the cartilaginous layer of the condyle. Cartilage is an avascular tissue that has a limited capacity to heal and repair because of limited supplies of nutrients and does not have the availability of blood-borne or perivascular progenitor cells. Many surgical procedures are available for TMJ disorders, but all are aggressive and dangerous for the patient. From simple arthrocentesis to joint replacement, they cannot produce integral regeneration [299].

A recent research objective is the insertion a cell source to manufacture neocartilage after displacement of the dysfunctional disc. Biocompatible scaffolds seeded with cells and biological modulators can be useful in such a process. Thus, the regeneration process of the TMJ is based on several main factors, such as scaffold design and material, stem cells, bioactive agents, biochemical compatibility between the scaffold and the surrounding environment, and the ability of the host to accept the scaffold and facilitate tissue formation [300]. Both natural and synthetic polymers were used for the regeneration of soft cartilage tissue. Collagen, gelatin, hyaluronic acid, fibrin, silk, agarose, polylactic acid, or poly vinyl alcohol are only some of the materials that can be used in cartilage tissue engineering, as reviewed by Jazayeri et al. [300]. Extracting SCs from the synovial capsule surrounding the joint holds has been proven to be a promising choice for generating neocartilage. Recently, Shetty et al. concluded that human DPSCs in porous chitosan scaffolds are useful for regenerating chondrogenic cells [301].

3.4. Tooth Regeneration

Nowadays, the regeneration of the entire tooth and its replacement represent the final objective of tooth tissue engineering (Figure 5). Even if dental tissues have no capacity for self-regeneration, the teeth are an important source of SCs, offering possible regeneration based on a patient's own SCs. This technique could be used to create replacements for dental implants and eliminate the risk of rejection, as the new tooth would not be a foreign tissue [302].

Tooth regeneration research using adult SCs has been considered. Autologous DPSCs or postnatal tooth germ cells have limited window of availability, so they can only provide a casual source for whole-tooth regeneration.

The classical tissue recombination has been improved by using collagen drops on the organic culture or by seeding the re-aggregated germ cells on biodegradable polymers. The experiments on animals have shown that tooth-like organs, with dentin and enamel, can be developed by ectopic subcutaneous grafting these cell aggregates under the renal capsule or into the anterior eye chamber [303].

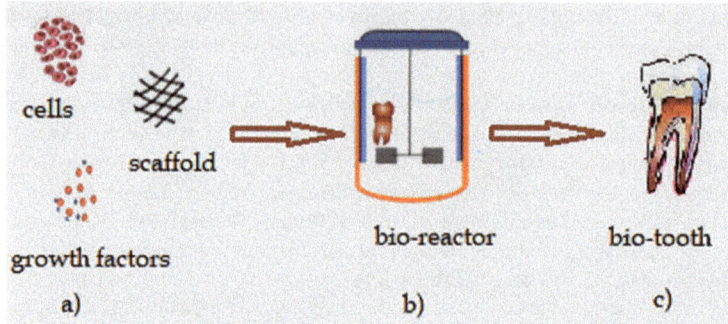

**Figure 5.** Bio-engineered tooth: (**a**) selection of dental cells sources and scaffolds, with addition of growth factors, (**b**) bio-reactor for in vitro development of bio-engineered tooth bud, (**c**) bio-tooth.

After implantation into the animal's jaw, a whole tooth could be generated. Ikeda et al. [304] reported successful tooth replacement in an adult mouse, representing an important first step for the transplantation of the bioengineered tooth germ into the alveolar bone to replace a lost tooth. Teeth represent a particular goal for regenerative medicine; they are difficult to recreate due to their complicated structure and numerous functions such as in articulation, mastication, and facial aesthetics. Thus, even if incontestable advancement can be achieved, tooth regeneration based on SCs still has uncertain applicability. Several research studies have reported similar tooth tissues regenerated using different cell types on biodegradable scaffolds, such as silk protein, chitosan [305].

SCs collected from postnatal tooth buds of animals, self-replicated and differentiated in vitro, have been seeded onto a biodegradable scaffold. Their in vivo maturation was achieved by transplanting the seeded scaffolds either into the renal capsule or the omentum, followed by their reimplantation into an extracted tooth place or the jaw [31]. However, by using non-human cells, the chance of immune rejection exists [306].

Ono et al. performed the autologous transplantation of a bioengineered tooth germ in a postnatal canine model and reported functional tooth restoration. The results of the study represented a relevant advancement in whole-organ replacement therapy as well as a practical model for future attempts [307]. Nevertheless, entire-tooth engineering or regeneration is still complicated, and the literature on the subject highlights several problems, such as how to program the stem and progenitor cells to develop into tooth-specific cell types [308,309].

Based on the proven successful applications of SCs in dental tissue regeneration, researchers realize whole-tooth regeneration could be achieved by applying one of two hybrid strategies. The first involves biological PDL and the tooth crown, obtained using stem cells, combined with a metallic or ceramic implant [310]; the second involves a biologically regenerated tooth root combined with a prosthetic crown [311].

## 4. Concluding Remarks and Future Perspectives

In recent decades, major progress has been achieved in regenerative medicine and especially in tissue engineering, which has been used in many clinical applications, but only the first steps toward these goals have been completed [312]. Tissue engineering based on stem or progenitor cells is a promising approach for restoring the integrity of dental and maxillofacial tissues. Research and clinical applications of dental SCs have proven their utility and advantages, such as the capacity for self-regeneration and multidirectional differentiation, easy accessibility, and, importantly, low autologous transplant rejection. However, for real and stable tissue regeneration in dentistry, many other theoretical and technological approaches must be applied in the future for the induction and genetic modification of orofacial SCs. Regeneration of the entire tooth is a major objective for replacing classical dental implants and overcoming their disadvantages. Such an approach would allow the reconstruction or regeneration of teeth in the near future, significantly increasing the quality of dental health.

Future studies are still necessary to identify suitable SCs for performing the physiological role of native tissue, growth factors able to support both cellular differentiation and replication, and to determine the role of microvascularization in tissue regeneration.

**Author Contributions:** Conceptualization, L.-C.R. and A.M.; software, D.C. and M.B.; validation, L.C.A. and L.-C.R.; data curation, A.M.; writing—original draft preparation, A.M., D.C., M.B., L.-C.R. and L.C.A.; writing—review and editing, L.C.A.; supervision, L.-C.R., L.C.A., E.A.B. and M.L.; funding acquisition, A.M. All authors have read and agreed to the published version of the manuscript.

**Funding:** This research received no external funding.

**Conflicts of Interest:** The authors declare no conflict of interest.

## Abbreviations

| | |
|---|---|
| ECM | Extracellular matrix |
| SCs | Stem cells |
| ESCs | Embryonic stem cells |
| ASCs | Adult stem cells |
| iPSCs | Induced pluripotent stem cells |
| MSCs | Mesenchymal stem cells |
| DPSCs | Dental pulp stem cells |
| PDLSCs | Periodontal ligament stem cells |
| PDL | Periodontal ligament |
| SCAPs | Stem cells from apical papilla |
| DFCs | Dental follicle stem cells |
| TGPCs | Tooth germ progenitor cells |
| SHEDs | Stem cells of human exfoliated deciduous teeth |
| ABMSCs | Alveolar bone-derived mesenchymal stem cells |
| SGDSCs | Salivary gland-derived stem cells |
| OMSCs | Oral mucosa-derived mesenchymal stem cells |
| OESCs | Oral epithelial stem cells |
| GMSCs | Gingiva-derived mesenchymal stem cells |
| PSCs | Periosteum-derived stem cells |
| PLA | Poly(lactic acid) |
| PGA | Poly(glycolic acid) |
| PLGA | Poly(lactic-co-glycolic acid) |
| PCL | Poly(caprolactone) |
| HA | Hydroxyapatite |
| PVDF-TrFE | Poly(vinylidene fluoride-trifluoroethylene) |
| nBGC | Nanobioactive glass ceramic |
| RET | Regenerative endodontic therapy |
| MTA | Mineral trioxide aggregate |
| AAE | American Association of Endodontists' |
| EDTA | Ethylenediaminetetraacetic acid |
| CHX | Chlorhexidine |
| TAP | Triple antibiotic paste |
| PRP | Platelet-rich plasma |
| PRF | Platelet-rich fibrin |
| BC | Blood clot |
| GTR | Guided tissue regeneration |
| TMJ | Temporomandibular joint |

## References

1. Tatullo, M.; Marrelli, M.; Paduano, F. The regenerative medicine in oral and maxillofacial surgery: The most important innovations in the clinical application of mesenchymal stem cells. *Int. J. Med. Sci.* **2015**, *12*, 72–77. [CrossRef] [PubMed]
2. Rai, R. Tissue engineering: Step ahead in maxillofacial reconstruction. *J. Int. Oral Health* **2015**, *9*, 138–142.
3. Borrelli, M.R.; Hu, M.S.; Longaker, M.T.; Lorenz, H.P. Tissue engineering and regenerative medicine in craniofacial reconstruction and facial aesthetics. *J. Craniofac. Surg.* **2020**, *31*, 15–27. [CrossRef] [PubMed]
4. Upadhyay, R.K. Role of Biological Scaffolds, Hydro Gels and Stem Cells in Tissue Regeneration Therapy. *Adv. Tissue Eng. Regen. Med. Open Access* **2017**, *2*, 121–135. [CrossRef]
5. Zhang, K.; Wang, S.; Zhou, C.; Cheng, L.; Gao, X.; Xie, X.; Sun, J.; Wang, H.; Weir, M.D.; Reynolds, M.A.; et al. Advanced smart biomaterials and constructs for hard tissue engineering and regeneration. *Bone Res.* **2018**, *6*, 31. [CrossRef]
6. Guan, X.; Avci-Adali, M.; Alarcin, E.; Cheng, H.; Kashaf, S.S.; Li, Y.; Chawla, A.; Jang, H.L.; Khademhosseini, A. Development of hydrogels for regenerative engineering. *Biotechnol. J.* **2017**, *12*, 1600394. [CrossRef]
7. Gao, Z.H.; Hu, L.; Liu, G.L.; Wei, F.L.; Liu, Y.; Liu, Z.H.; Fan, Z.P.; Zhang, C.M.; Wang, J.S.; Wang, S.L. Bio-Root and Implant-Based Restoration as a Tooth Replacement Alternative. *J. Dent. Res.* **2016**, *95*, 642–649. [CrossRef]
8. Har, A.; Park, J.C. Dental Stem Cells and Their Applications. *Chin. J. Dent. Res.* **2015**, *18*, 207–212. [CrossRef]
9. Ledesma-Martínez, E.; Mendoza-Núñez, V.M.; Santiago-Osorio, E. Mesenchymal Stem Cells Derived from Dental Pulp: A Review. *Stem Cells Int.* **2016**, 1–12. [CrossRef]
10. Drela, K.; Stanaszek, L.; Nowakowski, A.; Kuczynska, Z.; Lukomska, B. Experimental strategies of mesenchymal stem cell propagation: Adverse events and potential risk of functional changes. *Stem Cells Int.* **2019**, *2019*, 7012692. [CrossRef]
11. Zhou, T.; Pan, J.; Wu, P.; Huang, R.; Du, W.; Zhou, Y.; Wan, M.; Fan, Y.; Xu, X.; Zhou, X.; et al. Dental Follicle Cells: Roles in Development and Beyond. *Stem Cells Int.* **2019**, *2019*, 9159605. [CrossRef] [PubMed]
12. The Nobel Prize in Physiology or Medicine—2012 Press Release. Available online: www.nobelprize.org/prizes/medicine/2012/press-release/ (accessed on 12 November 2020).
13. Gurdon, J.B. The Developmental Capacity of Nuclei Taken from Intestinal Epithelium Cells of Feeding Tadpoles. *J. Embryol. Exp. Morphol.* **1962**, *10*, 622–640. [PubMed]
14. Yamanaka, S. Patient-specific pluripotent stem cells become even more accessible. *Cell Stem Cell* **2010**, *7*, 1–2. [CrossRef] [PubMed]
15. Takahashi, K.; Tanabe, K.; Ohnuki, M.; Narita, M.; Ichisaka, T.; Tomoda, K.; Yamanaka, S. Induction of pluripotent stem cells from adult human fibroblasts by defined factors. *Cell* **2007**, *131*, 861–872. [CrossRef]
16. Takahashi, K.; Yamanaka, S. Induction of pluripotent stem cells from mouse embryonic and adult fibroblast cultures by defined factors. *Cell* **2006**, *126*, 663–676. [CrossRef]
17. Zakrzewski, W.; Dobrzyński, M.; Szymonowicz, M.; Rybak, Z. Stem cells: Past, present, and future. *Stem Cell Res. Ther.* **2019**, *10*, 1–22. [CrossRef]
18. Berebichez-Fridman, R.; Pablo, R.; Montero-Olvera, P.R. Sources and Clinical Applications of Mesenchymal Stem Cells. *Sultan Qaboos Univ. Med. J.* **2018**, *18*, e264. [CrossRef]
19. Cao, C.; Tarlé, S.; Kaigler, D. Characterization of the immunomodulatory properties of alveolar bone-derived mesenchymal stem cells. *Stem Cell Res.* **2020**, *11*, 102. [CrossRef]
20. Liu, J.; Yu, F.; Sun, Y.; Jiang, B.; Zhang, W.; Yang, J.; Xu, G.T.; Liang, A.; Liu, S. Concise reviews: Characteristics and potential applications of human dental tissue-derived mesenchymal stem cells. *Stem Cells* **2015**, *33*, 627–638. [CrossRef]
21. Pisciotta, A.; Carnevale, G.; Meloni, S.; Riccio, M.; De Biasi, S.; Gibellini, L. Human dental pulp stem cells (hDPSCs): Isolation, enrichment, and comparative differentiation of two sub-populations. *BMC Dev. Biol.* **2015**, *15*, 14. [CrossRef]
22. Hollands, P.; Aboyeji, D.; Orcharton, M. Dental pulp stem cells in regenerative medicine. *Br. Dent. J.* **2018**, *224*, 747. [CrossRef]
23. Tsutsui, T.W. Dental Pulp Stem Cells: Advances to Applications. *Stem Cells Cloning Adv. Appl.* **2020**, *13*, 33–42. [CrossRef]
24. Sharpe, P.T. Dental mesenchymal stem cells. *Development* **2016**, *143*, 2273–2280. [CrossRef] [PubMed]

25. Kang, J.; Fan, W.; Deng, Q.; He, H.; Huang, F. Stem Cells from the Apical Papilla: A Promising Source for Stem Cell-Based Therapy. *BioMed Res. Int.* **2019**, *2019*, 6104738. [CrossRef]
26. Tian, Y.; Bai, D.; Guo, W.; Li, J.; Zeng, J.; Yang, L.; Jiang, Z.; Feng, L.; Yu, M.; Tian, W. Comparison of human dental follicle cells and human periodontal ligament cells for dentin tissue regeneration. *Regen. Med.* **2015**, *10*, 461–479. [CrossRef]
27. Dave, J.R.; Tomar, G.B. Dental Tissue-Derived Mesenchymal Stem Cells: Applications in Tissue Engineering. *Crit. Rev. Biomed. Eng.* **2018**, *46*, 429–468. [CrossRef]
28. Paz, A.G.; Maghaireh, H.; Mangano, F.G. Stem Cells in dentistry: Types of intra- and extraoral tissue-derived stem cells and clinical applications. *Stem Cells Int.* **2018**, *2018*, 4313610. [CrossRef]
29. Motwani, B.K.; Singh, M.; Kaur, G.; Singh, S.; Gangde, P.O. Stem cells: A new paradigm in dentistry. *Stem Cells* **2016**, *2*, 140. [CrossRef]
30. Chalisserry, E.P.; Nam, S.Y.; Park, S.H.; Anil, S. Therapeutic potential of dental stem cells. *J. Tissue Eng.* **2017**, *8*, 1–17. [CrossRef]
31. Somani, R.; Jaidka, S.; Bajaj, N.; Arora, S. Miracle cells for natural dentistry—A review. *J. Oral Biol. Craniofac. Res.* **2017**, *7*, 49–53. [CrossRef]
32. Taguchi, T.; Yanagi, Y.; Yoshimaru, K.; Zhang, X.Y.; Matsuura, T.; Nakayama, K.; Kobayashi, E.; Yamaza, H.; Nonaka, K.; Ohga, S.; et al. Regenerative medicine using stem cells from human exfoliated deciduous teeth (SHED): A promising new treatment in pediatric surgery. *Surg. Today* **2019**, *49*, 316–322. [CrossRef] [PubMed]
33. Grawish, M.E. Gingival-derived mesenchymal stem cells: An endless resource for regenerative dentistry. *World J. Stem Cells* **2018**, *10*, 116–118. [CrossRef] [PubMed]
34. Tonk, C.; Witzler, M.; Schulze, M.; Tobiasch, E. Mesenchymal Stem Cells. In *Essential Current Concepts in Stem Cell Biology*; Brand-Saberi, B., Ed.; Springer: Berlin, Germany, 2020; pp. 21–39.
35. Baranova, J.; Büchner, D.; Götz, W.; Schulze, M.; Tobiasch, E. Tooth Formation: Are the Hardest Tissues of Human Body Hard to Regenerate? *Int. J. Mol. Sci.* **2020**, *21*, 4031. [CrossRef]
36. Marin, E.; Boschetto, F.; Pezzotti, G. Biomaterials and biocompatibility: An historical overview. *J. Biomed. Mater. Res.* **2020**, *108*, 1617–1633. [CrossRef]
37. Tian, H.; Tang, Z.; Zhuang, X.; Chen, X.; Jing, X. Biodegradable synthetic polymers: Preparation, functionalization and biomedical application. *Prog. Polym. Sci.* **2012**, *37*, 237–280. [CrossRef]
38. Xie, Y.; Chen, Y.; Sun, M.; Ping, Q. A mini review of biodegradable calcium phosphate nanoparticles for gene delivery. *Curr. Pharm. Biotechnol.* **2013**, *14*, 918–925. [CrossRef]
39. Bergmann, C.P.; Stumpf, A. Biomaterials. In *Dental Ceramics: Microstructure, Properties and Degradation*; Bergmann, C., Stumpf, A., Eds.; Springer: Berlin/Heidelberg, Germany, 2013; pp. 9–13. [CrossRef]
40. Ferrage, L.; Bertrand, G.; Lenormand, P.; Grossin, D.; Ben-Nissan, B. A review of the additive manufacturing (3DP) of bioceramics: Alumina, zirconia (PSZ) and hydroxyapatite. *J. Aust. Ceram. Soc.* **2017**, *53*, 11–20. [CrossRef]
41. Liu, X.; Ma, P.X. Polymeric Scaffolds for Bone Tissue Engineering. *Ann. Biomed. Eng.* **2004**, *32*, 477–486. [CrossRef]
42. Nair, L.S.; Laurencin, C.T. Biodegradable polymers as biomaterials. *Prog. Polym. Sci.* **2007**, *32*, 762–798. [CrossRef]
43. Banerjee, A.; Chatterjee, K.; Madras, G. Enzymatic degradation of polymers: A brief review. *Mater. Sci. Technol.* **2014**, *30*, 567–573. [CrossRef]
44. Rey-Vinolas, S.; Engel, E.; Mateos-Timoneda, M. Polymers for bone repair. In *Bone Repair Biomaterials*, 2nd ed.; Pawelec, K.M., Planell, J.A., Eds.; Woodhead Publishing: Cambridge, UK, 2019; pp. 179–197. [CrossRef]
45. Rezwan, K.; Chen, Q.Z.; Blaker, J.J.; Boccaccini, A.R. Biodegradable and bioactive porous polymer/inorganic composite scaffolds for bone tissue engineering. *Biomaterials* **2006**, *27*, 3413–3431. [CrossRef] [PubMed]
46. Ulery, B.D.; Nair, L.S.; Laurencin, C.T. Biomedical Applications of Biodegradable Polymers. *J. Polym. Sci.* **2011**, *49*, 832–864. [CrossRef]
47. Maurus, P.B.; Kaeding, C.C. Bioabsorbable implant material review. *Oper. Tech. Sports Med.* **2004**, *12*, 158–160. [CrossRef]
48. Gentile, P.; Chiono, V.; Carmagnola, I.; Hatton, P.V. An Overview of Poly(lactic-co-glycolic)Acid (PLGA)-Based Biomaterials for Bone Tissue Engineering. *Int. J. Mol. Sci.* **2014**, *15*, 3640–3659. [CrossRef]

49. Elmowafy, E.M.; Tiboni, M.; Soliman, M.E. Biocompatibility, biodegradation and biomedical applications of poly(lactic acid)/poly(lactic-co-glycolic acid)micro and nanoparticles. *J. Pharm. Investig.* **2019**, *49*, 347–380. [CrossRef]
50. Derby, B. Printing and prototyping of tissues and scaffolds. *Science* **2012**, *338*, 921–926. [CrossRef]
51. Matsiko, A.; Gleeson, J.P.; O'Brien, F.J. Scaffold mean pore size influences mesenchymal stem cell chondrogenic differentiation and matrix deposition. *Tissue Eng. Part A* **2015**, *21*, 486–497. [CrossRef]
52. Domingos, M.; Intranuovo, F.; Russo, T.; De Santis, R.; Gloria, A.; Ambrosio, L.; Ciurana, J.; Bartolo, P. The first systematic analysis of 3D rapid prototyped poly(epsilon-caprolactone) scaffolds manufactured through BioCell printing: The effect of pore size and geometry on compressive mechanical behaviour and in vitro hMSC viability. *Biofabrication* **2013**, *5*, 045004. [CrossRef]
53. Motamedian, S.R.; Hosseinpour, S.; Ahsaie, M.G.; Khojasteh, A. Smart scaffolds in bone tissue engineering: A systematic review of literature. *World J. Stem Cells* **2015**, *7*, 657–668. [CrossRef]
54. Kaigler, D.; Wang, Z.; Horger, K.; Mooney, D.J.; Krebsbach, P.H. VEGF scaffolds enhance angiogenesis and bone regeneration in irradiated osseous defects. *J. Bone Min. Res.* **2006**, *21*, 735–744. [CrossRef]
55. Khan, F.; Tanaka, M. Designing smart biomaterials for tissue engineering. *Int. J. Mol. Sci.* **2018**, *19*, 17. [CrossRef]
56. Mittal, A.; Negi, P.; Garkhal, K.; Verma, S.; Kumar, N. Integration of porosity and bio-functionalization to form a 3D scaffold: Cell culture studies and in vitro degradation. *Biomed. Mater.* **2010**, *5*, 045001. [CrossRef] [PubMed]
57. Zeng, D.; Zhang, X.; Wang, X.; Huang, Q.; Wen, J.; Miao, X.; Peng, L.; Li, Y.; Jiang, X. The osteoimmunomodulatory properties of MBG scaffold coated with amino functional groups. *Artif. Cells Nanomed. Biotechnol.* **2018**, *46*, 1425–1435. [CrossRef] [PubMed]
58. Chen, Z.; Mao, X.; Tan, L.; Friis, T.; Wu, C.; Crawford, R.; Xiao, Y. Osteoimmunomodulatory properties of magnesium scaffolds coated with β-tricalcium phosphate. *Biomaterials* **2014**, *35*, 8553–8565. [CrossRef] [PubMed]
59. Liu, X.; Zhao, K.; Gong, T.; Song, J.; Bao, C.; Luo, E.; Weng, J.; Zhou, S. Delivery of growth factors using a smart porous nanocomposite scaffold to repair a mandibular bone defect. *Biomacromolecules* **2014**, *15*, 1019–1030. [CrossRef] [PubMed]
60. Damaraju, S.M.; Shen, Y.; Elele, E.; Khusid, B.; Eshghinejad, A.; Li, J.; Jaffe, M.; Arinzeh, T.L. Three-dimensional piezoelectric fibrous scaffolds selectively promote mesenchymal stem cell differentiation. *Biomaterials* **2017**, *149*, 51–62. [CrossRef] [PubMed]
61. Augustine, R.; Dan, P.; Sosnik, A.; Kalarikkal, N.; Tran, N.; Vincent, B.; Thomas, S.; Menu, P.; Rouxel, D. Electrospun poly(vinylidene fluoride-trifluoroethylene)/zinc oxide nanocomposite tissue engineering scaffolds with enhanced cell adhesion and blood vessel formation. *Nano Res.* **2017**, *10*, 3358–3376. [CrossRef]
62. Liu, D.; Yang, F.; Xiong, F.; Gu, N. The Smart Drug Delivery System and Its Clinical Potential. *Theranostics* **2016**, *6*, 1306–1323. [CrossRef]
63. Kondiah, P.J.; Choonara, Y.E.; Kondiah, P.P.D.; Marimuthu, T.; Kumar, P.; Du Toit, L.C.; Pillay, V. A Review of Injectable Polymeric Hydrogel Systems for Application in Bone Tissue Engineering. *Molecules* **2016**, *21*, 1580. [CrossRef]
64. Mohd Amin, M.C.; Ahmad, N.; Pandey, M.; Jue Xin, C. Stimuli-responsive bacterial cellulose-g-poly(acrylic acid-co-acrylamide) hydrogels for oral controlled release drug delivery. *Drug Dev. Ind. Pharm.* **2014**, *40*, 1340–1349. [CrossRef]
65. Ashley, G.W.; Henise, J.; Reid, R.; Santi, D.V. Hydrogel drug delivery system with predictable and tunable drug release and degradation rates. *Proc. Natl. Acad. Sci. USA* **2013**, *110*, 2318–2323. [CrossRef] [PubMed]
66. Horev, B.; Klein, M.I.; Hwang, G.; Li, Y.; Kim, D.; Koo, H.; Benoit, D.S. pH-activated nanoparticles for controlled topical delivery of farnesol to disrupt oral biofilm virulence. *ACS Nano* **2015**, *9*, 2390–2404. [CrossRef] [PubMed]
67. Luo, Z.; Zhang, S.; Pan, J.; Shi, R.; Liu, H.; Lyu, Y.; Han, X.; Li, Y.; Yang, Y.; Xu, Z.; et al. Time-responsive osteogenic niche of stem cells: A sequentially triggered, dual-peptide loaded, alginate hybrid system for promoting cell activity and osteo-differentiation. *Biomaterials* **2018**, *163*, 25–42. [CrossRef] [PubMed]
68. Sant, S.; Hancock, M.J.; Donnelly, J.P.; Iyer, D.; Khademhosseini, A. Biomimetic gradient hydrogels for tissue engineering. *Can. J. Chem. Eng.* **2010**, *88*, 899–911. [CrossRef] [PubMed]

69. Sheikhpour, M.; Barani, L.; Kasaeian, A. Biomimetics in drug delivery systems: A critical review. *J. Control Release* **2017**, *253*, 97–109. [CrossRef]
70. Carlo Reis, E.C.; Borges, A.P.; Araújo, M.V.; Mendes, V.C.; Guan, L.; Davies, J.E. Periodontal regeneration using a bilayered PLGA/calcium phosphate construct. *Biomaterials* **2011**, *32*, 9244–9253. [CrossRef]
71. Sowmya, S.; Mony, U.; Jayachandran, P.; Reshma, S.; Kumar, R.A.; Arzate, H.; Nair, S.V.; Jayakumar, R. Tri-layered nanocomposite hydrogel scaffold for the concurrent regeneration of cementum, periodontal ligament, and alveolar bone. *Adv. Healthc. Mater.* **2017**, *6*, 1601251. [CrossRef]
72. Weir, M.D.; Ruan, J.; Zhang, N.; Chow, L.C.; Zhang, K.; Chang, X.; Bai, Y.; Xu, H.H.K. Effect of calcium phosphate nanocomposite on in vitro remineralization of human dentin lesions. *Dent. Mater.* **2017**, *33*, 1033–1044. [CrossRef]
73. Li, L.; He, J.; Eckert, R.; Yarbrough, D.; Lux, R.; Anderson, M.; Shi, W. Design and characterization of an acid-activated antimicrobial peptide. *Chem. Biol. Drug Des.* **2010**, *75*, 127–132. [CrossRef]
74. Yang, Y.; Reipa, V.; Liu, G.; Meng, Y.; Wang, X.; Mineart, K.P.; Prabhu, V.M.; Shi, W.; Lin, N.J.; He, X.; et al. pH-sensitive compounds for selective inhibition of acid-producing bacteria. *ACS Appl. Mater. Interfaces* **2018**, *10*, 8566–8573. [CrossRef]
75. Cheng, L.; Weir, M.D.; Zhang, K.; Wu, E.J.; Xu, S.M.; Zhou, X.; Xu, H.H. Dental plaque microcosm biofilm behavior on calcium phosphate nanocomposite with quaternary ammonium. *Dent. Mater.* **2012**, *28*, 853–862. [CrossRef] [PubMed]
76. Wang, S.; Wang, H.; Ren, B.; Li, X.; Wang, L.; Zhou, H.; Weir, M.D.; Zhou, X.; Masri, R.M.; Oates, T.W.; et al. Drug resistance of oral bacteria to new antibacterial dental monomer dimethylaminohexadecyl methacrylate. *Sci. Rep.* **2018**, *8*, 5509. [CrossRef] [PubMed]
77. Li, F.; Weir, M.D.; Xu, H.H. Effects of quaternary ammonium chain length on antibacterial bonding agents. *J. Dent. Res.* **2013**, *92*, 932–938. [CrossRef] [PubMed]
78. Li, L.; Zhu, Y.Q.; Jiang, L.; Peng, W.; Ritchie, H.H. Hypoxia Promotes Mineralization of Human Dental Pulp Cells. *J. Endod.* **2011**, *37*, 799–802. [CrossRef] [PubMed]
79. Huang, G.T.J.; Shagramanova, K.; Chan, S.W. Formation of Odontoblast-Like Cells from Cultured Human Dental Pulp Cells on Dentin In Vitro. *J. Endod.* **2006**, *32*, 1066–1073. [CrossRef]
80. Del Angel-Mosqueda, C.; Gutiérrez-Puente, Y.; López-Lozano, A.P.; Romero-Zavaleta, R.E.; Mendiola-Jiménez, A.; Medina-De la Garza, C.E.; Márquez, M.M.; De la Garza-Ramos, M.A. Epidermal growth factor enhances osteogenic differentiation of dental pulp stem cells in vitro. *Head Face Med.* **2015**, *11*, 29. [CrossRef]
81. Rusu, L.C.; Nedelcu, I.V.; Albu, M.G.; Sonmez, M.; Voicu, G.; Radulescu, M.; Ficai, D.; Ficai, A.; Negrutiu, M.L.; Sinescu, C. Tetracycline Loaded Collagen/Hydroxyapatite Composite Materials for Biomedical Applications. *J. Nanomater.* **2015**, *2015*, 361969. [CrossRef]
82. Patrascu, J.M.; Nedelcu, I.A.; Sonmez, M.; Ficai, D.; Ficai, A.; Vasile, B.S.; Ungureanu, C.; Albu, M.G.; Andor, B.; Andronescu, E.; et al. Composite Scaffolds Based on Silver Nanoparticles for Biomedical Applications. *J. Nanomater.* **2015**, *2015*, 587989. [CrossRef]
83. Rusu, L.C.; Sinescu, C.; Negrutiu, M.L.; Ardelean, L.; Ogodescu, A.; Fabricky, M.; Petrescu, E.; Rominu, R.; Topala, F.; Rominu, M.; et al. Application for regenerative dentistry: The collagen matrices with lidocaine. Computational Engineering in System Applications. In Proceedings of the International Conference on Energy, Environment, Economics, Devices, Systems, Communications, Computers, Iasi, Romania, 1–3 July 2011; pp. 60–64.
84. Rusu, L.C.; Manescu, A.; Negrutiu, M.L.; Sinescu, C.; Ardelean, S.; Hoinoiu, B.; Rominu, M. The Micro CT Evaluation of Different Types of Matrices in Rats Bone Augumentation. *Key Eng. Mater.* **2013**, *587*, 338–342. [CrossRef]
85. Rusu, L.C.; Negrutiu, M.L.; Sinescu, C.; Hoinoiu, B.; Topala, F.I.; Duma, V.F.; Rominu, M.; Podoleanu, A.G. Time domain optical coherence tomography investigation of bone matrix interface in rat femurs. In Proceedings of the ISPDI 2013-Fifth International Symposium on Photoelectronic Detection and Imaging (SPIE 8914), Beijing, China, 25–27 June 2013; p. 89141H. [CrossRef]
86. Rusu, L.C.; Negrutiu, M.L.; Sinescu, C.; Hoinoiu, B.; Zaharia, C.; Ardelean, L.; Duma, V.F.; Podoleanu, A.G. Different matrix evaluation for the bone regeneration of rats' femours using time domain optical coherence tomography. In Proceedings of the Fifth International Conference on Lasers in Medicine: Biotechnologies Integrated in Daily Medicine (SPIE 8925), Timisoara, Romania, 19–21 September 2013; p. 89250V. [CrossRef]

87. Manescu, A.; Oancea, R.; Todea, C.; Rusu, L.C.; Mazzoni, S.; Negrutiu, M.L.; Sinescu, C.; Giuliani, A. On Long Term Effects of Low Power Laser Therapy on Bone Repair: A Demonstrative Study by Synchrotron Radiation-based Phase-Contrast Microtomography. *Int. J. Radiol. Imaging Technol.* **2016**, *2*, 010. [CrossRef]
88. Baumgartner, S.; Gmeiner, R.; Schönherr, J.A.; Stampfl, J. Stereolithography-based additive manufacturing of lithium disilicate glass ceramic for dental applications. *Mater. Sci. Eng. C* **2020**, *116*, 111180. [CrossRef]
89. Jasiuk, I.; Abueidda, D.W.; Kozuch, C.; Pang, S.; Su, F.Y.; McKittrick, J. An Overview on Additive Manufacturing of Polymers. *JOM* **2018**, *70*, 275–283. [CrossRef]
90. Mederle, N.; Marin, S.; Marin, M.M.; Danila, E.; Mederle, O.; Kaya, M.G.A.; Ghica, M.V. Innovative biomaterials based on collagen-hydroxyapatite and doxycycline for bone regeneration. *Adv. Mater. Sci. Eng.* **2016**, *2016*, 3452171. [CrossRef]
91. Papaioannou, T.G.; Manolesou, D.; Dimakakos, E.; Tsoucalas, G.; Vavuranakis, M.; Tousoulis, D. 3D Bioprinting Methods and Techniques: Applications on Artificial Blood Vessel Fabrication. *Acta Cardiol. Sin.* **2019**, *35*, 284–289. [CrossRef] [PubMed]
92. Zadpoor, A.A.; Malda, J. Additive manufacturing of biomaterials, tissues, and organs. *Ann. Biomed. Eng.* **2017**, *45*, 1–11. [CrossRef]
93. Ngo, T.D.; Kashani, A.; Imbalzano, G.; Nguyen, K.T.Q.; Hui, D. Additive manufacturing (3D printing): A review of materials, methods, applications and challenges. *Compos. B Eng.* **2018**, *143*, 172–196. [CrossRef]
94. Murphy, S.V.; Atala, A. 3D bioprinting of tissues and organs. *Nat. Biotechnol.* **2014**, *32*, 773–785. [CrossRef]
95. Wang, X.; Ao, Q.; Tian, X.; Fan, J.; Wei, Y.; Hou, W.; Tong, H.; Bai, S. 3D bioprinting technologies for hard tissue and organ engineering. *Materials* **2016**, *9*, 802. [CrossRef]
96. Ji, X.; Zhu, H.; Zhao, L.; Xiao, J. Recent advances in 3D bioprinting for the regeneration of functional cartilage. *Regen. Med.* **2018**, *13*, 73–87. [CrossRef]
97. Nakamura, M.; Kobayashi, A.; Takagi, F.; Watanabe, A.; Hiruma, Y.; Ohuchi, K.; Iwasaki, Y.; Horie, M.; Morita, I.; Takatani, S. Biocompatible inkjet printing technique for designed seeding of individual living cells. *Tissue Eng.* **2005**, *11*, 1658–1666. [CrossRef]
98. Saunders, R.E.; Gough, J.E.; Derby, B. Delivery of human fibroblast cells by piezoelectric drop-on-demand inkjet printing. *Biomaterials* **2008**, *29*, 193–203. [CrossRef] [PubMed]
99. Catros, S.; Fricain, J.C.; Guillotin, B.; Pippenger, B.; Bareille, R.; Remy, M.; Lebraud, E.; Desbat, B.; Amedee, J.; Guillemot, F. Laser-assisted bioprinting for creating on-demand patterns of human osteoprogenitor cells and nanohydroxyapatite. *Biofabrication* **2011**, *3*, 025001. [CrossRef] [PubMed]
100. Guillemot, F.; Souquet, A.; Catros, S.; Guillotin, B. Laser-assisted cell printing: Principle, physical parameters versus cell fate and perspectives in tissue engineering. *Nanomedicine* **2010**, *5*, 507–515. [CrossRef] [PubMed]
101. Lin, H.; Zhang, D.; Alexander, P.G.; Yang, G.; Tan, J.; Cheng, A.W.; Tuan, R.S. Application of visible light-based projection stereolithography for live cell-scaffold fabrication with designed architecture. *Biomaterials* **2013**, *34*, 331–339. [CrossRef] [PubMed]
102. Li, J.; Chen, M.; Fan, X.; Zhou, H. Recent advances in bioprinting techniques: Approaches, applications and future prospects. *J. Transl. Med.* **2016**, *14*, 271. [CrossRef]
103. Theus, A.S.; Ning, L.; Hwang, B.; Gil, C.; Chen, S.; Wombwell, A.; Mehta, R.; Serpooshan, V. Bioprintability: Physiomechanical and Biological Requirements of Materials for 3D Bioprinting Processes. *Polymers* **2020**, *12*, 2262. [CrossRef]
104. Dorishetty, P.; Dutta, N.K.; Choudhury, N.R. Bioprintable tough hydrogels for tissue engineering applications. *Adv. Colloid Interface Sci.* **2020**, *281*, 102163. [CrossRef]
105. Compaan, A.M.; Christensen, K.; Huang, Y. Inkjet Bioprinting of 3D Silk Fibroin Cellular Constructs Using Sacrificial Alginate. *ACS Biomater. Sci. Eng.* **2017**, *3*, 1519–1526. [CrossRef]
106. Jose, R.R.; Rodriguez, M.J.; Dixon, T.A.; Omenetto, F.; Kaplan, D.L. Evolution of Bioinks and Additive Manufacturing Technologies for 3D Bioprinting. *ACS Biomater. Sci. Eng.* **2016**, *2*, 1662–1678. [CrossRef]
107. Nicodemus, G.D.; Bryant, S.J. Cell encapsulation in biodegradable hydrogels for tissue engineering applications. *Tissue Eng. B Rev.* **2008**, *14*, 149–165. [CrossRef]
108. Wust, S.; Godla, M.E.; Muller, R.; Hofmann, S. Tunable hydrogel composite with two-step processing in combination with innovative hardware upgrade for cell-based three-dimensional bioprinting. *Acta Biomater.* **2014**, *10*, 630–640. [CrossRef] [PubMed]

109. Duffy, R.M.S.Y.; Feinberg, A.W. Understanding the role of ECM protein composition and geometric micropatterning for engineering human skeletal muscle. *Ann. Biomed. Eng.* **2016**, *44*, 2076–2089. [CrossRef] [PubMed]
110. Hinton, T.J.; Jallerat, Q.; Palchesko, R.N.; Park, J.H.; Grodzicki, M.S.; Shue, H.J.; Ramadan, M.H.; Hudson, A.R.; Feinberg, A.W. Three-dimensional printing of complex biological structures by freeform reversible embedding of suspended hydrogels. *Sci. Adv.* **2015**, *1*, e1500758. [CrossRef] [PubMed]
111. Levato, R.; Visser, J.; Planell, J.A.; Engel, E.; Malda, J.; Mateos-Timoneda, M.A. Biofabrication of tissue constructs by 3D bioprinting of cell-laden microcarriers. *Biofabrication* **2014**, *6*, 035020. [CrossRef] [PubMed]
112. Duarte Campos, D.F.; Blaeser, A.; Weber, M.; Jakel, J.; Neuss, S.; Jahnen-Dechent, W.; Fischer, H. Three-dimensional printing of stem cell-laden hydrogels submerged in a hydrophobic high-density fluid. *Biofabrication* **2013**, *5*, 015003. [CrossRef]
113. Gruene, M.; Deiwick, A.; Koch, L.; Schlie, S.; Unger, C.; Hofmann, N.; Bernemann, I.; Glasmacher, B.; Chichkov, B. Laser printing of stem cells for biofabrication of scaffold-free autologous grafts. *Tissue Eng. C Methods* **2011**, *17*, 79–87. [CrossRef]
114. Yan, D.; Zeng, B.; Han, Y.; Dai, H.; Liu, J.; Sun, Y.; Li, F. Preparation and laser powder bed fusion of composite microspheres consisting of poly(lactic acid) and nano-hydroxyapatite. *Addit. Manuf.* **2020**, *34*, 101305. [CrossRef]
115. Mostafaei, A.; Elliott, A.M.; Barnes, J.E.; Li, F.; Tan, W.; Cramer, C.L.; Nandwana, P.; Chmielus, M. Binder jet 3D printing—Process parameters, materials, properties, and challenges. *Prog. Mater. Sci.* **2020**, 100707. [CrossRef]
116. Gonzalez, J.; Mireles, J.; Lin, Y.; Wicker, R. Characterization of ceramic components fabricated using binder jetting additive manufacturing technology. *Ceram. Int.* **2016**, *42*, 10559–10564. [CrossRef]
117. Pu'ad, N.M.; Haq, R.A.; Noh, H.M.; Abdullah, H.Z.; Idris, M.I.; Lee, T.C. Review on the fabrication of fused deposition modelling (FDM) composite filament for biomedical applications. *Mater. Today Proc.* **2020**, *29*, 228–232. [CrossRef]
118. Yap, Y.L.; Wang, C.; Sing, S.L.; Dikshit, V.; Yeong, W.Y.; Wei, J. Material jetting additive manufacturing: An experimental study using designed metrological benchmarks. *Precis. Eng.* **2017**, *50*, 275–285. [CrossRef]
119. Davoudinejad, A.; Diaz-Perez, L.C.; Quagliotti, D.; Pedersen, D.B.; Albajez-García, J.A.; Yagüe-Fabra, J.A.; Tosello, G. Additive manufacturing with vat polymerization method for precision polymer micro components production. *Procedia CIRP* **2018**, *75*, 98–102. [CrossRef]
120. Woesz, A.; Rumpler, M.; Stampfl, J.; Varga, F.; Fratzl-Zelman, N.; Roschger, P.; Klaushofer, K.; Fratzl, P. Towards bone replacement materials from calcium phosphates via rapid prototyping and ceramic gelcasting. *Mater. Sci. Eng. C* **2005**, *25*, 181–186. [CrossRef]
121. Lakhdar, Y.; Tuck, C.; Binner, J.; Terry, A.; Goodridge, R. Additive manufacturing of advanced ceramic materials. *Prog. Mater. Sci.* **2021**, *116*, 100736. [CrossRef]
122. Shuai, C.; Gao, C.; Nie, Y.; Hu, H.; Zhou, Y.; Peng, S. Structure and properties of nano-hydroxypatite scaffolds for bone tissue engineering with a selective laser sintering system. *Nanotechnology* **2011**, *22*, 285703. [CrossRef]
123. Miranda, P.; Pajares, A.; Saiz, E.; Tomsia, A.P.; Guiberteau, F. Fracture modes under uniaxial compression in hydroxypatite scaffolds fabricated by robocasting. *J. Biomed. Mater. Res. A* **2007**, *83*, 646–655. [CrossRef]
124. Gao, Y.; Cao, W.L.; Wang, X.Y.; Gong, Y.D.; Tian, J.M.; Zhao, N.M.; Zhang, X.F. Characterization and osteoblast-like cell compatibility of porous scaffolds: Bovine hydroxyapatite and novel hydroxyapatite artificial bone. *J. Mater. Sci. Mater. Med.* **2006**, *17*, 815–823. [CrossRef]
125. Warnke, P.H.; Seitz, H.; Warnke, F.; Becker, S.T.; Sivananthan, S.; Sherry, E.; Liu, Q.; Wiltfang, J.; Douglas, T. Ceramic scaffolds produced by computer-assisted 3D printing and sintering: Characterization and biocompatibility investigations. *J. Biomed. Mater. Res. B* **2010**, *93*, 212–217. [CrossRef]
126. Gmeiner, R.; Deisinger, U.; Schonherr, J.; Lechner, B.; Detsch, R.; Boccaccini, A.; Stampfl, J. Additive manufacturing of bioactive glasses and silicate bioceramics. *J. Ceram. Sci. Technol.* **2015**, *6*, 75–86. [CrossRef]
127. Shuai, C.; Mao, Z.; Han, Z.; Peng, S.; Li, Z. Fabrication and characterization of calcium silicate scaffolds for tissue engineering. *J. Mech. Med. Biol.* **2014**, *14*, 1450049. [CrossRef]
128. Vorndran, E.; Klarner, M.; Klammert, U.; Grover, L.M.; Patel, S.; Barralet, J.E.; Gbureck, U. 3D Powder Printing of Beta-Tricalcium Phosphate Ceramics Using Different Strategies. *Adv. Eng. Mater.* **2008**, *10*, B67–B71. [CrossRef]

129. Felzmann, R.; Gruber, S.; Mitteramskogler, G.; Tesavibul, P.; Boccaccini, A.R.; Liska, R.; Stampfl, J. Lithography-Based AdditiveManufacturing of Cellular Ceramic Structures. *Adv. Eng. Mater.* **2012**, *14*, 1052–1058. [CrossRef]
130. Bian, W.; Li, D.; Lian, Q.; Zhang, W.; Zhu, L.; Li, X.; Jin, Z. Design and fabrication of a novel porous implant with pre-set channels based on ceramic stereolithography for vascular implantation. *Biofabrication* **2011**, *3*, 034103. [CrossRef] [PubMed]
131. Bose, S.; Darsell, J.; Kintner, M.; Hosick, H.; Bandyopadhyay, A. Pore size and pore volume effects on alumina and TCP ceramic scaffolds. *Mater. Sci. Eng. C* **2003**, *23*, 479–486. [CrossRef]
132. Butscher, A.; Bohner, M.; Roth, C.; Ernstberger, A.; Heuberger, R.; Doebelin, N.; von Rohr, P.R.; Müller, R. Printability of calcium phosphate powders for three-dimensional printing of tissue engineering scaffolds. *Acta Biomater.* **2012**, *8*, 373–385. [CrossRef] [PubMed]
133. Partee, B.; Hollister, S.J.; Das, S. Selective Laser Sintering Process Optimization for Layered Manufacturing of CAPA® 6501 Polycaprolactone Bone Tissue Engineering Scaffolds. *J. Manuf. Sci. Eng.* **2005**, *128*, 531–540. [CrossRef]
134. Chen, C.H.; Lee, M.Y.; Shyu, V.B.H.; Chen, Y.C.; Chen, C.T.; Chen, J.P. Surface modification of polycaprolactone scaffolds fabricated via selective laser sintering for cartilage tissue engineering. *Mater. Sci. Eng. C* **2014**, *40*, 389–397. [CrossRef]
135. Shor, L.; Güçeri, S.; Chang, R.; Gordon, J.; Kang, Q.; Hartsock, L.; An, Y.; Sun, W. Precision extruding deposition (PED) fabrication of polycaprolactone (PCL) scaffolds for bone tissue engineering. *Biofabrication* **2009**, *1*, 015003. [CrossRef]
136. Sobral, J.M.; Caridade, S.G.; Sousa, R.A.; Mano, J.F.; Reis, R.L. Three-dimensional plotted scaffolds with controlled pore size gradients: Effect of scaffold geometry on mechanical performance and cell seeding efficiency. *Acta Biomater.* **2011**, *7*, 1009–1018. [CrossRef]
137. Korpela, J.; Kokkari, A.; Korhonen, H.; Malin, M.; Närhi, T.; Seppälä, J. Biodegradable and bioactive porous scaffold structures prepared using fused deposition modeling. *J. Biomed. Mater. Res. B* **2013**, *101*, 610–619. [CrossRef]
138. Ge, Z.; Wang, L.; Heng, B.C.; Tian, X.F.; Lu, K.; Tai Weng Fan, V.; Yeo, J.F.; Cao, T.; Tan, E. Proliferation and Differentiation of Human Osteoblasts within 3D printed Poly-Lactic-co-Glycolic Acid Scaffolds. *J. Biomater. Appl.* **2009**, *23*, 533–547. [CrossRef]
139. Lee, M.; Wu, B.M.; Dunn, J.C.Y. Effect of scaffold architecture and pore size on smooth muscle cell growth. *J. Biomed. Mater. Res. A* **2008**, *87*, 1010–1016. [CrossRef] [PubMed]
140. Lee, M.; Dunn, J.C.Y.; Wu, B.M. Scaffold fabrication by indirect three-dimensional printing. *Biomaterials* **2005**, *26*, 4281–4289. [CrossRef] [PubMed]
141. Guo, T.; Holzberg, T.R.; Lim, C.G.; Gao, F.; Gargava, A.; Trachtenberg, J.E.; Mikos, A.G.; Fisher, J.P. 3D printing PLGA: A quantitative examination of the effects of polymer composition and printing parameters on print resolution. *Biofabrication* **2017**, *9*, 024101. [CrossRef]
142. Yang, B.; Qiu, Y.; Zhou, N.; Ouyang, H.; Ding, J.; Cheng, B.; Sun, J. Application of stem cells in oral disease therapy: Progresses and perspectives. *Front. Physiol.* **2017**, *8*, 197. [CrossRef]
143. Hu, M.S.; Maan, Z.N.; Wu, J.-C.; Rennert, R.C.; Hong, W.X.; Lai, T.S.; Cheung, A.T.M.; Walmsley, G.G.; Chung, M.T.; McArdle, A.; et al. Tissue Engineering and Regenerative Repair in Wound Healing. *Ann. Biomed. Eng.* **2014**, *42*, 1494–1507. [CrossRef]
144. Chatzistavrou, X.; Rao, R.R.; Caldwell, D.J.; Peterson, A.W.; McAlpin, B.; Wang, Y.Y.; Zheng, L.; Fenno, J.C.; Stegemann, J.P.; Papagerakis, P. Collagen/fibrin microbeads as a delivery system for Ag-doped bioactive glass and DPSCs for potential applications in dentistry. *J. Non-Cryst. Solids* **2016**, *432*, 143–149. [CrossRef]
145. Bakopoulou, A.; Leyhausen, G.; Volk, J.; Tsiftsoglou, A.; Garefis, P.; Koidis, P.; Geurtsen, W. Comparative analysis of in vitro osteo/odontogenic differentiation potential of human dental pulp stem cells (DPSCs) and stem cells from the apical papilla (SCAP). *Arch. Oral Biol.* **2011**, *56*, 709–721. [CrossRef]
146. Tatullo, M.; Marrelli, M.; Shakesheff, K.M.; White, L.J. Dental pulp stem cells: Function, isolation and applications in regenerative medicine. *J. Tissue Eng. Regen. Med.* **2015**, *9*, 1205–1216. [CrossRef]
147. Potdar, P.D.; Jethmalani, Y.D. Human dental pulp stem cells: Applications in future regenerative medicine. *World J. Stem Cells* **2015**, *7*, 839–851. [CrossRef]
148. Davila, J.C.; Cezar, G.G.; Thiede, M.; Strom, S.; Miki, T.; Trosko, J. Use and application of stem cells in toxicology. *Toxicol. Sci.* **2004**, *79*, 214–223. [CrossRef] [PubMed]

149. Gronthos, S.; Mankani, M.; Brahim, J.; Robey, P.G.; Shi, S. Postnatal human dental pulp stem cells (DPSCs) in vitro and in vivo. *Proc. Natl. Acad. Sci. USA* **2000**, *97*, 13625–13630. [CrossRef] [PubMed]
150. Beltrão-Braga, P.C.; Pignatari, G.C.; Maiorka, P.C.; Oliveira, N.A.; Lizier, N.F.; Wenceslau, C.V.; Miglino, M.A.; Muotri, A.R.; Kerkis, I. Feeder-free derivation of induced pluripotent stem cells from human immature dental pulp stem cells. *Cell Transplant.* **2011**, *20*, 1707–1719. [CrossRef] [PubMed]
151. Verma, K.; Bains, R.; Bains, V.K.; Rawtiya, M.; Loomba, K.; Srivastava, S.C. Therapeutic potential of dental pulp stem cells in regenerative medicine: An overview. *Dent. Res. J.* **2014**, *11*, 302–308.
152. Almushayt, A.; Narayanan, K.; Zaki, A.E.; George, A. Dentin matrix protein 1 induces cytodifferentiation of dental pulp stem cells into odontoblasts. *Gene Ther.* **2006**, *13*, 611–620. [CrossRef]
153. Yoshida, S.; Tomokiyo, A.; Hasegawa, D.; Hamano, S.; Sugii, H.; Maeda, H. Insight into the Role of Dental Pulp Stem Cells in Regenerative Therapy. *Biology* **2020**, *9*, 160. [CrossRef]
154. Aydin, S.; Şahin, F. Stem Cells Derived from Dental Tissues. *Adv. Exp. Med. Biol.* **2019**, *1144*, 123–132. [CrossRef]
155. Graziano, A.; d'Aquino, R.; Laino, G.; Papaccio, G. Dental pulp stem cells: A promising tool for bone regeneration. *Stem Cell Rev.* **2008**, *4*, 21–26. [CrossRef]
156. Kitagaki, J.; Miyauchi, S.; Xie, C.J.; Yamashita, M.; Yamada, S.; Kitamura, M.; Murakami, S. Effects of the proteasome inhibitor, bortezomib, on cytodifferentiation and mineralization of periodontal ligament cells. *J. Periodontal Res.* **2015**, *50*, 248–255. [CrossRef]
157. Hynes, K.; Menicanin, D.; Gronthos, S.; Bartold, P.M. Clinical utility of stem cells for periodontal regeneration. *Periodontol 2000* **2012**, *59*, 203–227. [CrossRef]
158. Han, J.; Menicanin, D.; Gronthos, S.; Bartold, P.M. Stem cells, tissue engineering and periodontal regeneration. *Aust. Dent. J.* **2014**, *59*, 117–130. [CrossRef] [PubMed]
159. Maeda, H.; Tomokiyo, A.; Fujii, S.; Wada, N.; Akamine, A. Promise of periodontal ligament stem cells in regeneration of periodontium. *Stem Cell Res.* **2011**, *28*, 33. [CrossRef]
160. Gay, I.C.; Chen, S.; MacDougall, M. Isolation and characterization of multipotent human periodontal ligament stem cells. *Orthod. Craniofac. Res.* **2007**, *10*, 149–160. [CrossRef] [PubMed]
161. Kim, S.S.; Kwon, D.W.; Im, I.; Kim, Y.D.; Hwang, D.S.; Holliday, L.S.; Donatelli, R.E.; Son, W.S.; Jun, E.S. Differentiation and characteristics of undifferentiated mesenchymal stem cells originating from adult premolar periodontal ligaments. *Korean J. Orthod.* **2012**, *42*, 307–317. [CrossRef] [PubMed]
162. Schneider, R.; Holland, G.R.; Chiego, D., Jr.; Hu, J.C.; Nör, J.E.; Botero, T.M. White mineral trioxide aggregate induces migration and proliferation of stem cells from the apical papilla. *J. Endod.* **2014**, *40*, 931–936. [CrossRef] [PubMed]
163. Nada, O.A.; El Backly, R.M. Stem Cells From the Apical Papilla (SCAP) as a Tool for Endogenous Tissue Regeneration. *Front. Bioeng. Biotechnol.* **2018**, *24*, 103. [CrossRef]
164. Miller, A.A.; Takimoto, K.; Wealleans, J.; Diogenes, A. Effect of 3 Bioceramic Materials on Stem Cells of the Apical Papilla Proliferation and Differentiation Using a Dentin Disk Model. *J. Endod.* **2018**, *44*, 599–603. [CrossRef]
165. Wongwatanasanti, N.; Jantarat, J.; Sritanaudomchai, H.; Hargreaves, K.M. Effect of Bioceramic Materials on Proliferation and Odontoblast Differentiation of Human Stem Cells from the Apical Papilla. *J. Endod.* **2018**, *44*, 1270–1275. [CrossRef]
166. Zhang, J.; Ding, H.; Liu, X.; Sheng, Y.; Liu, X.; Jiang, C. Dental Follicle Stem Cells: Tissue Engineering and Immunomodulation. *Stem Cells Dev.* **2019**, *28*, 986–994. [CrossRef]
167. Shoi, K.; Aoki, K.; Ohya, K.; Takagi, Y.; Shimokawa, H. Characterization of pulp and follicle stem cells from impacted supernumerary maxillary incisors. *Pediatr. Dent.* **2014**, *36*, 79–84.
168. Rezai-Rad, M.; Bova, J.F.; Orooji, M.; Pepping, J.; Qureshi, A.; Del Piero, F.; Hayes, D.; Yao, S. Evaluation of bone regeneration potential of dental follicle stem cells for treatment of craniofacial defects. *Cytotherapy* **2015**, *17*, 1572–1581. [CrossRef] [PubMed]
169. Honda, M.J.; Imaizumi, M.; Tsuchiya, S.; Morsczeck, C. Dental follicle stem cells and tissue engineering. *J. Oral Sci.* **2010**, *52*, 541–552. [CrossRef] [PubMed]
170. Caracappa, J.D.; Gallicchio, V.S. The future in dental medicine: Dental stem cells are a promising source for tooth and tissue engineering. *J. Stem Cell Res.* **2019**, *5*, 30–36. [CrossRef]

171. Yalvaç, M.E.; Ramazanoglu, M.; Tekguc, M.; Bayrak, O.F.; Shafigullina, A.K.; Salafutdinov, I.I.; Blatt, N.L.; Kiyasov, A.P.; Sahin, F.; Palotás, A.; et al. Human tooth germ stem cells preserve neuro-protective effects after long-term cryo-preservation. *Curr. Neurovasc. Res.* **2010**, *7*, 49–58. [CrossRef]
172. Yalvac, M.E.; Ramazanoglu, M.; Rizvanov, A.A.; Sahin, F.; Bayrak, O.F.; Salli, U.; Palotás, A.; Kose, G.T. Isolation and characterization of stem cells derived from human third molar tooth germs of young adults: Implications in neo-vascularization, osteo-, adipo- and neurogenesis. *Pharm. J.* **2010**, *10*, 105–113. [CrossRef]
173. Doğan, A.; Demirci, S.; Şahin, F. In vitro differentiation of human tooth germ stem cells into endothelial- and epithelial-like cells. *Cell Biol. Int.* **2015**, *39*, 94–103. [CrossRef]
174. Jeon, M.; Song, J.S.; Choi, B.J.; Choi, H.J.; Shin, D.M.; Jung, H.S.; Kim, S.O. In vitro and in vivo characteristics of stem cells from human exfoliated deciduous teeth obtained by enzymatic disaggregation and outgrowth. *Arch. Oral Biol.* **2014**, *59*, 1013–1023. [CrossRef]
175. Araújo, L.B.; Cosme-Silva, L.; Fernandes, A.P.; Oliveira, T.M.; Cavalcanti, B.D.N.; Gomes Filho, J.E.; Sakai, V.T. Effects of mineral trioxide aggregate, BiodentineTM and calcium hydroxide on viability, proliferation, migration and differentiation of stem cells from human exfoliated deciduous teeth. *J. Appl. Oral Sci.* **2018**, *26*, e20160629. [CrossRef]
176. Ma, L.; Makino, Y.; Yamaza, H.; Akiyama, K.; Hoshino, Y.; Song, G.; Kukita, T.; Nonaka, K.; Shi, S.; Yamaza, T. Cryopreserved dental pulp tissues of exfoliated deciduous teeth is a feasible stem cell resource for regenerative medicine. *PLoS ONE* **2012**, *7*, e51777. [CrossRef]
177. Kunimatsu, R.; Nakajima, K.; Awada, T.; Tsuka, Y.; Abe, T.; Ando, K.; Hiraki, T.; Kimura, A.; Tanimoto, K. Comparative characterization of stem cells from human exfoliated deciduous teeth, dental pulp, and bone marrow-derived mesenchymal stem cells. *Biochem. Biophys. Res. Commun.* **2018**, *501*, 193–198. [CrossRef]
178. Ching, H.S.; Luddin, N.; Rahman, I.A.; Ponnuraj, K.T. Expression of Odontogenic and Osteogenic Markers in DPSCs and SHED: A Review. *Curr. Stem Cell Res.* **2017**, *12*, 71–79. [CrossRef]
179. Miura, M.; Gronthos, S.; Zhao, M.; Lu, B.; Fisher, L.W.; Robey, P.G.; Shi, S. SHED: Stem cells from human exfoliated deciduous teeth. *Proc. Natl. Acad. Sci. USA* **2003**, *100*, 5807–5812. [CrossRef]
180. Martinez Saez, D.; Sasaki, R.T.; Neves, A.D.; da Silva, M.C. Stem Cells from Human Exfoliated Deciduous Teeth: A Growing Literature. *Cells Tissues Organs* **2016**, *202*, 269–280. [CrossRef] [PubMed]
181. Annibali, S.; Cristalli, M.P.; Tonoli, F.; Polimeni, A. Stem cells derived from human exfoliated deciduous teeth: A narrative synthesis of literature. *Eur. Rev. Med. Pharmacol. Sci.* **2014**, *18*, 2863–2881. [PubMed]
182. Arora, V.; Arora, P.; Munshi, A.K. Banking stem cells from human exfoliated deciduous teeth (SHED): Saving for the future. *J. Clin. Pediatr. Dent.* **2009**, *2*, 289–294. [CrossRef]
183. Mason, S.; Tarle, S.A.; Osibin, W.; Kinfu, Y.; Kaigler, D. Standardization and safety of alveolar bone-derived stem cell isolation. *J. Dent. Res.* **2014**, *93*, 55–61. [CrossRef]
184. Liu, Y.; Wang, H.; Dou, H.; Tian, B.; Li, L.; Jin, L.; Zhang, Z.; Hu, L. Bone regeneration capacities of alveolar bone mesenchymal stem cells sheet in rabbit calvarial bone defect. *J. Tissue Eng.* **2020**, *11*, 2041731420930379. [CrossRef]
185. Pekovits, K.; Kröpfl, J.M.; Stelzer, I.; Payer, M.; Hutter, H.; Dohr, G. Human mesenchymal progenitor cells derived from alveolar bone and human bone marrow stromal cells: A comparative study. *Histochem. Cell Biol.* **2013**, *140*, 611–621. [CrossRef]
186. Matsubara, T.; Suardita, K.; Ishii, M.; Sugiyama, M.; Igarashi, A.; Oda, R.; Nishimura, M.; Saito, M.; Nakagawa, K.; Yamanaka, K.; et al. Alveolar bone marrow as a cell source for regenerative medicine: Differences between alveolar and iliac bone marrow stromal cells. *J. Bone Miner. Res.* **2005**, *20*, 399–409. [CrossRef]
187. Park, J.C.; Kim, J.C.; Kim, Y.T.; Choi, S.H.; Cho, K.S.; Im, G.I.; Kim, B.S.; Kim, C.S. Acquisition of human alveolar bone-derived stromal cells using minimally irrigated implant osteotomy: In vitro and in vivo evaluations. *J. Clin. Periodontol.* **2012**, *39*, 495–505. [CrossRef]
188. Lim, K.T.; Hexiu, J.; Kim, J.; Seonwoo, H.; Choung, P.H.; Chung, J.H. Synergistic effects of orbital shear stress on in vitro growth and osteogenic differentiation of human alveolar bone-derived mesenchymal stem cells. *BioMed Res. Int.* **2014**, *2014*, 316803. [CrossRef] [PubMed]
189. Khazaei, M.; Bozorgi, A.; Khazaei, S.; Khademi, A. Stem cells in dentistry, sources, and applications. *Dent. Hypotheses* **2016**, *7*, 42–52. [CrossRef]

190. Zhang, Q.; Shi, S.; Liu, Y.; Uyanne, J.; Shi, Y.; Shi, S.; Le, A.D. Mesenchymal stem cells derived from human gingiva are capable of immunomodulatory functions and ameliorate inflammation-related tissue destruction in experimental colitis. *J. Immunol.* **2009**, *183*, 7787–7798. [CrossRef] [PubMed]
191. Tomar, G.B.; Srivastava, R.K.; Gupta, N.; Barhanpurkar, A.P.; Pote, S.T.; Jhaveri, H.M.; Mishra, G.C.; Wani, M.R. Human gingiva-derived mesenchymal stem cells are superior to bone marrow-derived mesenchymal stem cells for cell therapy in regenerative medicine. *Biochem. Biophys. Res. Commun.* **2010**, *393*, 377–383. [CrossRef]
192. Tang, L.; Li, N.; Xie, H.; Jin, Y. Characterization of mesenchymal stem cells from human normal and hyperplastic gingiva. *J. Cell. Physiol.* **2011**, *226*, 832–842. [CrossRef]
193. Wang, F.; Yu, M.; Yan, X.; Wen, Y.; Zeng, Q.; Yue, W.; Yang, P.; Pei, X. Gingiva-derived mesenchymal stem cell-mediated therapeutic approach for bone tissue regeneration. *Stem Cells Dev.* **2011**, *20*, 2093–2102. [CrossRef]
194. Marynka-Kalmani, K.; Treves, S.; Yafee, M.; Rachima, H.; Gafni, Y.; Cohen, M.A.; Pitaru, S. The lamina propria of adult human oral mucosa harbors a novel stem cell population. *Stem Cells* **2010**, *28*, 984–995. [CrossRef]
195. Zhang, Q.Z.; Su, W.R.; Shi, S.H.; Wilder-Smith, P.; Xiang, A.P.; Wong, A.; Nguyen, A.L.; Kwon, C.W.; Le, A.D. Human gingiva-derived mesenchymal stem cells elicit polarization of m2 macrophages and enhance cutaneous wound healing. *Stem Cells* **2010**, *28*, 1856–1868. [CrossRef]
196. Murray, P.E.; Garcia-Godoy, F.; Hargreaves, K.M. Regenerative endodontics: A review of current status and a call for action. *J. Endod.* **2007**, *33*, 377–390. [CrossRef]
197. Trope, M. Regenerative Potential of Dental Pulp. *J. Endod.* **2008**, *34*, S13–S17. [CrossRef]
198. Hargreaves, K.M.; Diogenes, A.; Teixeira, F.B. Treatment options: Biological basis of regenerative endodontic procedures. *Pediatr. Dent.* **2013**, *35*, 129–140. [CrossRef]
199. Ding, R.Y.; Cheung, G.S.; Chen, J.; Yin, X.Z.; Wang, Q.Q.; Zhang, C.F. Pulp revascularization of immature teeth with apical periodontitis: A clinical study. *J. Endod.* **2009**, *35*, 745–749. [CrossRef]
200. Cvek, M. Prognosis of luxated non-vital maxillary incisors treated with calcium hydroxide and filled with gutta-percha. A retrospective clinical study. *Endod. Dent. Traumatol.* **1992**, *8*, 45–55. [CrossRef]
201. Andreasen, J.O.; Farik, B.; Munksgaard, E.C. Long-term calcium hydroxide as a root canal dressing may increase risk of root fracture. *Dent. Traumatol.* **2002**, *18*, 134–137. [CrossRef] [PubMed]
202. Nosrat, A.; Seifi, A.; Asgary, S. Regenerative Endodontic Treatment (Revascularization) for Necrotic Immature Permanent Molars: A Review and Report of Two Cases with a New Case Reports in Dentistry 5 Biomaterial. *J. Endod.* **2011**, *37*, 562–567. [CrossRef] [PubMed]
203. Nygaard-Ostby, B. The role of the blood in endodontic therapy. An experimental histological study. *Acta Odontol. Scand.* **1961**, *19*, 324–353. [CrossRef]
204. Nygarrd-Ostby, B.; Hjortdal, O. Tissue formation in the root canal following pulp removal. *Scand. J. Dent. Res.* **1971**, *79*, 333–349. [CrossRef]
205. Banchs, F.; Trope, M. Revascularization of immature permanent tooth with apical periodontitis: New treatment protocol? *J. Endod.* **2004**, *30*, 196–200. [CrossRef]
206. Kling, M.; Cvek, M.; Mejare, I. Rate and predictability of pulp revascularization in therapeutically reimplanted permanent incisors. *Endod. Dent. Traumatol.* **1986**, *2*, 83–89. [CrossRef]
207. Hoshino, E.; Kurihara-Ando, N.; Sato, I.; Uematsu, H.; Sato, M.; Kota, K.; Iwaku, M. In-vitro antibacterial susceptibility of bacteria taken from infected root dentine to a mixture of ciprofloxacin, metronidazole and minocycline. *Endod. J.* **1996**, *29*, 125–130. [CrossRef]
208. Nakashima, M.; Akifumi, A. The Application of Tissue Engineering to Regeneration of Pulp and Dentin in Endodontics. *J. Endod.* **2005**, *31*, 711–718. [CrossRef] [PubMed]
209. American Association of Endodontists. AAE Clinical Considerations for a Regenerative Procedure Revised 4/1/2018. Available online: https://www.aae.org/specialty/wp-content/uploads/sites/2/2018/06/ConsiderationsForRegEndo_AsOfApril2018.pdf (accessed on 15 October 2020).
210. Hargreaves, K.M.; Cohen, S.; Berman, L.H. (Eds.) *Cohen's Pathways of the Pulp*, 10th ed.; Mosby Elsevier: St. Louis, MI, USA, 2011; pp. 602–618.
211. Jung, C.; Kim, S.; Sun, T.; Cho, Y.B.; Song, M. Pulp-dentin regeneration: Current approaches and challenges. *J. Tissue Eng.* **2019**, *10*, 2041731418819263. [CrossRef] [PubMed]

212. Prescott, R.S.; Alsanea, R.; Fayad, M.I.; Johnson, B.R.; Wenckus, C.S.; Hao, J.; John, A.S.; George, A. In Vivo Generation of Dental Pulp-like Tissue by Using Dental Pulp Stem Cells, a Collagen Scaffold, and Dentin Matrix Protein 1 after Subcutaneous Transplantation in Mice. *J. Endod.* **2008**, *34*, 421–426. [CrossRef] [PubMed]
213. Kim, J.Y.; Xin, X.; Moioli, E.K.; Chung, J.; Lee, C.H.; Chen, M.; Fu, S.Y.; Koch, P.D.; Mao, J.J. Regeneration of Dental-Pulp-like Tissue by Chemotaxis-Induced Cell Homing. *Tissue Eng. Part A* **2010**, *16*, 3023–3031. [CrossRef]
214. Fouad, A.F. Microbial factors and antimicrobial strategies in dental pulp regeneration. *J. Endod.* **2007**, *43*, 46–50. [CrossRef]
215. Estefan, B.S.; El Batouty, K.M.; Nagy, M.M.; Diogenes, A. Influence of age and apical diameter on the success of endodontic regeneration procedures. *J. Endod.* **2016**, *42*, 1620–1625. [CrossRef]
216. Fang, Y.; Wang, X.; Zhu, J.; Su, C.; Yang, Y.; Meng, L. Influence of apical diameter on the outcome of regenerative endodontic treatment in teeth with pulp necrosis: A review. *J. Endod.* **2018**, *44*, 414–431. [CrossRef]
217. Kim, S.G. Infection and pulp regeneration. *Dent. J.* **2016**, *4*, 4. [CrossRef]
218. Iwaya, S.I.; Ikawa, M.; Kubota, M. Revascularization of an immature permanent tooth with apical periodontitis and sinus tract. *Dent Traumatol.* **2001**, *17*, 185–187. [CrossRef]
219. Chen, M.Y.H.; Chen, K.L.; Chen, C.A.; Tayebaty, F.; Rosenberg, P.A.; Lin, L.M. Responses of immature permanent teeth with infected necrotic pulp tissue and apical periodontitis/abscess to revascularization procedures. *Int. Endod. J.* **2012**, *45*, 294–305. [CrossRef]
220. Lin, L.M.; Shimizu, E.; Gibbs, J.L.; Loghin, S.; Ricucci, D. Histologic and histobacteriologic observations of failed revascularization/revitalization therapy: A case report. *J. Endod.* **2014**, *40*, 291–295. [CrossRef] [PubMed]
221. Haapasalo, M.; Shen, Y. Current therapeutic options for endodontic biofilms. *Endod. Top.* **2010**, *22*, 79–98. [CrossRef]
222. Haapasalo, M.; Endal, U.; Zandi, H.; Coil, J.M. Eradication of endodontic infection by instrumentation and irrigation solutions. *Endod. Top.* **2005**, *10*, 77–102. [CrossRef]
223. Fouad, A.F.; Nosrat, A. Pulp regeneration in previously infected root canal space. *Endod. Top.* **2013**, *28*, 24–37. [CrossRef]
224. Diogenes, A.; Henry, M.A.; Teixeira, F.B.; Hargreaves, K.M. An update on clinical regenerative endodontics. *Endod. Top.* **2013**, *28*, 2–23. [CrossRef]
225. Haapasalo, M.; Shen, Y.; Qian, W.; Gao, Y. Irrigation in endodontics. *Dent. Clin. N. Am.* **2010**, *54*, 291–312. [CrossRef]
226. Spratt, D.A.; Pratten, J.; Wilson, M.; Gulabivala, K. An in vitro evaluation of antimicrobial efficacy of irrigants on biofilm of root canal isolates. *Int. Endod. J.* **2001**, *34*, 300–307. [CrossRef]
227. Sena, N.T.; Gomes, B.P.F.A.; Vianna, M.E.; Berber, V.B.; Zaia, A.A.; Ferraz, C.C.R.; Souza-Filho, F.J. In vitro antimicrobial activity of sodium hypochlorite and chlorhexidine against selected single-species biofilms. *Int. Endod. J.* **2006**, *39*, 878–885. [CrossRef]
228. Trevino, E.G.; Patwardhan, A.N.; Henry, M.A.; Perry, G.; Dybdal-Hargreaves, N.; Hargreaves, K.M.; Diogenes, A. Effect of irrigants on the survival of human stem cells of the apical papilla in a platelet-rich plasma scaffold in human root tips. *J. Endod.* **2011**, *37*, 1109–1115. [CrossRef]
229. Martin, D.E.; De Almeida, J.F.A.; Henry, M.A.; Khaing, Z.Z.; Schmidt, C.E.; Teixeira, F.B.; Diogenes, A. Concentration-dependent effect of sodium hypochlorite on stem cells of apical papilla survival and differentiation. *J. Endod.* **2014**, *40*, 51–55. [CrossRef]
230. Galler, K.M.; Widbiller, M.; Buchalla, W.; Eidt, A.; Hiller, K.-A.; Hoffer, P.C.; Schmalz, G. EDTA conditioning of dentine promotes adhesion, migration and differentiation of dental pulp stem cells. *Int. Endod. J.* **2016**, *49*, 581–590. [CrossRef] [PubMed]
231. Neha, K.; Kansal, R.; Garg, P.; Joshi, R.; Garg, D.; Grover, H.S. Management of immature teeth by dentin-pulp regeneration: A recent approach. *Med. Oral Patol. Oral Cir. Bucal.* **2011**, *16*, 997–1004. [CrossRef]
232. Mohammad, Z.; Shalav, S.; Jafarzadeh, H. Ethyleneaminetetraacetic in endodontics. *Eur. J. Dent.* **2013**, *7* (Suppl. 1), 135–142. [CrossRef]
233. Galler, K.M.; Buchalla, W.; Hiller, K.-A.; Federlin, M.; Eidt, A.; Schiefersteiner, M.; Schmalz, G. Influence of root canal disinfectants on growth factor release from dentin. *J. Endod.* **2015**, *41*, 363–368. [CrossRef]

234. Galler, K.M.; D'Souza, R.N.; Federlin, M.; Cavender, A.C.; Hartgerink, J.D.; Hecker, S.; Schmalz, G. Dentin conditioning codetermines cell fate in regenerative endodontics. *J. Endod.* **2011**, *37*, 1536–1541. [CrossRef]
235. Vishwanat, L.; Duong, R.; Takimoto, K.; Phillips, L.; Espitia, C.O.; Diogenes, A.; Ruparel, S.B.; Kolodrubetz, D.; Ruparel, N.B. Effect of bacterial biofilm on the osteogenic differentiation of stem cells of apical papilla. *J. Endod.* **2017**, *43*, 916–922. [CrossRef]
236. Sonoyama, W.; Liu, Y.; Yamaza, T.; Tuan, R.S.; Wang, S.; Shi, S.; Huang, G.T.J. Characterization of apical papilla and its residing stem cells from human immature permanent teeth—A pilot study. *J. Endod.* **2008**, *34*, 166–171. [CrossRef]
237. Reynolds, K.; Johnson, J.D.; Cohenca, N. Pulp revascularization of necrotic bilateral bicuspids using a modified novel technique to eliminate potential coronal discolouration: A case report. *Int. Endod. J.* **2009**, *42*, 84–92. [CrossRef]
238. Assed Bezerra da Silva, L.; Assed Bezerra da Silva, R.; Nelson-Filho, P. Intracanal Medication in Root Canal Disinfection. Available online: https://pocketdentistry.com/13-intracanal-medication-in-root-canal-disinfection/ (accessed on 15 October 2020).
239. Wang, X.; Thibodeau, B.; Trope, M.; Lin, L.M.; Huang, G.T.J. Histologic characterization of regenerated tissues in canal space after the revitalization/revascularization procedure of immature dog teeth with apical periodontitis. *J. Endod.* **2010**, *36*, 56–63. [CrossRef]
240. Rybak, M.J.; McGrath, B.J. Combination Antimicrobial Therapy for Bacterial Infections. *Drugs* **1996**, *52*, 390–405. [CrossRef]
241. Baumgartner, J.C.; Xia, T. Antibiotic susceptibility of bacteria associated with endodontic abscesses. *J. Endod.* **2003**, *29*, 44–47. [CrossRef] [PubMed]
242. Mohammad, Z.; Dummer, P.M.H. Properties and application of calcium hydroxide in endodontics and dental traumatology. *Int. Endod. J.* **2011**, *44*, 697–730. [CrossRef]
243. Haapasalo, M.K.; Siren, E.K.; Waltimo, T.M.T.; Orstavik, D.; Haapasalo, M.P. Inactivation of local root canal medicaments by dentin: An in vitro study. *Int. Endod. J.* **2000**, *33*, 126–131. [CrossRef] [PubMed]
244. Haapasalo, M.K.; Qian, W.; Portnier, I.; Waltimo, T. Effect of dentin on antimicrobial properties of endodontic medicaments. *J. Endod.* **2007**, *33*, 917–925. [CrossRef]
245. Sathorn, C.; Parashos, P.; Messer, M. Antimicrobial efficacy of calcium hydroxide intracanal dressing: A systematic review and meta-analysis. *Int. Endod. J.* **2007**, *40*, 2–10. [CrossRef]
246. Aggarwal, V.; Miglani, S.; Singla, M. Conventional apexification and revascularization induced maturogenesis of two non-vital, immature teeth in same patient: 24 months follow up of a case. *J. Conserv. Dent.* **2012**, *15*, 68–72. [CrossRef]
247. Kitikuson, P.; Srisuwan, T. Attachment ability of human apical papilla cells to root dentin surfaces treated with either 3Mix or calcium hydroxide. *J. Endod.* **2016**, *42*, 89–94. [CrossRef]
248. Nevins, A.J.; Finkelstein, F.; Borden, B.G.; Laporta, R. Revitalization of pulpless open apex teeth in rhesus monkeys, using collagen-calcium phosphate gel. *J. Endod.* **1976**, *2*, 159–165. [CrossRef]
249. Simon, S.; Rilliard, F.; Berdal, A.; Machtou, P. The use of mineral trioxide aggregate in one-visit apexification treatment: A0 prospective study. *Int. Endod. J.* **2007**, *40*, 186–197.
250. Jadhav, G.R.; Shah, N.; Logani, A. Comparative outcome of revascularization in bilateral, non-vital, immature maxillary anterior teeth supplemented with or without platelet rich plasma: A case series. *J. Conserv. Dent.* **2013**, *16*, 568–572. [CrossRef]
251. Yamauchi, N.; Yamauchi, S.; Nagaoka, H.; Duggan, D.; Zhong, S.; Lee, S.M.; Teixeira, F.B.; Yamauchi, M. Tissue engineering strategies for immature teeth with apical periodontitis. *J. Endod.* **2011**, *37*, 390–397. [CrossRef] [PubMed]
252. Jung, I.Y.; Lee, S.J.; Hargreaves, K.M. Biologically based treatment of immature permanent teeth with pulpal necrosis: A case series. *J. Endod.* **2008**, *34*, 876–887. [CrossRef] [PubMed]
253. Lovelace, T.W.; Henry, M.A.; Hargreaves, K.M.; Diogenes, A. Evaluation of the delivery of mesenchymal stem cells into the root canal space of necrotic immature teeth after clinical regenerative endodontic procedure. *J. Endod.* **2011**, *37*, 133–138. [CrossRef] [PubMed]

254. Huang, G.T.J.; Sonoyama, W.; Liu, Y.; Liu, H.; Wang, S.; Shi, S. The hidden treasure in apical papilla: The potential role in pulp/dentin regeneration and bioroot engineering. *J. Endod.* **2008**, *34*, 645–651. [CrossRef] [PubMed]
255. Miller, E.K.; Lee, J.Y.; Tawil, P.Z.; Teixeira, F.B.; Vann Jr, W.F. Emerging therapies for the management of traumatized immature permanent incisors. *Pediatr. Dent.* **2012**, *34*, 66–69. [PubMed]
256. Torabinejad, M.; Turman, M. Revitalization of tooth with necrotic pulp and open apex by using platelet-rich plasma: A case report. *J. Endod.* **2011**, *37*, 265–268. [CrossRef]
257. Cehreli, Z.C.; Isbitiren, B.; Sara, S.; Erbas, G. Regenerative endodontic treatment (revascularization) of immature necrotic molars medicated with calcium hydroxide: A case series. *J. Endod.* **2011**, *37*, 1327–1330. [CrossRef]
258. Nazir, M.A. Prevalence of periodontal disease, its association with systemic diseases and prevention. *Int. J. Health Sci.* **2017**, *11*, 72–80.
259. Galuscan, A.; Cornianu, M.; Jumanca, D.; Faur, A.; Podariu, A.; Ardelean, L.; Rusu, L.C. Evaluation of marginal periodontium adjacent to the reconstruction materials in the dental prosthetics. Study morphopathologycal and immunohistochemical. *Mater. Plast.* **2012**, *49*, 85–89.
260. Aimetti, M.; Perotto, S.; Castiglione, A.; Mariani, G.M.; Ferrarotti, F.; Romano, F. Prevalence of periodontitis in an adult population from an urban area in North Italy: Findings from a cross-sectional population-based epidemiological survey. *J. Clin. Periodontol.* **2015**, *42*, 622–631. [CrossRef]
261. Kassebaum, N.J.; Bernabé, E.; Dahiya, M.; Bhandari, B.; Murray, C.J.; Marcenes, W. Global burden of severe periodontitis in 1990–2010: A systematic review meta-regression. *J. Dent. Res.* **2014**, *93*, 1045–1053. [CrossRef] [PubMed]
262. Matuliene, G.; Pjetursson, B.E.; Salvi, G.E.; Schmidlin, K.; Bragger, U.; Zwahlen, M.; Lang, N.P. Influence of residual pockets on progression of periodontitis and tooth loss: Results after 11 years of maintenance. *J. Clin. Periodontol.* **2008**, *35*, 685–695. [CrossRef] [PubMed]
263. Nevins, M.; Giannobile, W.V.; McGuire, M.K.; Kao, R.T.; Mellonig, J.T.; Hinrichs, J.E.; McAllister, B.S.; Murphy, K.S.; McClain, P.K.; Nevins, M.L.; et al. Platelet-derived growth factor stimulates bone fill and rate of attachment level gain: Results of a large multicenter randomized controlled trial. *J. Periodontol.* **2005**, *76*, 2205–2215. [CrossRef] [PubMed]
264. Siaili, M.; Chatzopoulou, D.; Gillam, D.G. An overview of periodontal regenerative procedures for the general dental practitioner. *Saudi Dent. J.* **2018**, *30*, 26–37. [CrossRef]
265. Yamada, Y.; Nakamura-Yamada, S.; Kusano, K.; Baba, S. Clinical potential and current progress of dental pulp stem cells for various systemic diseases in regenerative medicine: A concise review. *Int. J. Mol. Sci.* **2019**, *20*, 1132. [CrossRef]
266. Xu, X.; Li, X.; Wang, J.; He, X.T.; Sun, H.H.; Chen, F.M. Concise Review: Periodontal Tissue Regeneration Using Stem Cells: Strategies and Translational Considerations. *Stem Cells Transl. Med.* **2019**, *8*, 392–403. [CrossRef]
267. Liang, Y.; Luan, X.; Liua, X. Recent advances in periodontal regeneration: A biomaterial perspective. *Bioact. Mater.* **2020**, *5*, 297–308. [CrossRef]
268. Murphy, K.G.; Gunsolley, J.C. Guided tissue regeneration for the treatment of periodontal intrabony and furcation defects. A systematic review. *Ann. Periodontol.* **2003**, *8*, 266–302. [CrossRef]
269. Needleman, I.G.; Worthington, H.V.; Giedrys-Leeper, E.; Tucker, R.J. Guided tissue regeneration for periodontal infra-bony defects. *Chocrane Database Syst. Rev.* **2006**, *19*, 1724. [CrossRef]
270. Kaushal, S.; Kumar, A.; Khan, M.A.; Lal, N. Comparative study of nonabsorbable and absorbable barrier membranes in periodontal osseous defects by guided tissue regeneration. *J. Oral Biol. Craniofac. Res.* **2016**, *6*, 111–117. [CrossRef]
271. Zhou, L.N.; Bi, C.S.; Gao, L.N. Macrophage polarization in human gingival tissue in response to periodontal disease. *Oral Dis.* **2019**, *25*, 265–273. [CrossRef] [PubMed]
272. Seciu, A.M.; Craciunescu, O.; Zarnescu, O. Advanced Regenerative Techniques Based on Dental Pulp Stem Cells for the Treatment of Periodontal Disease. In *Periodontology and Dental Implantology*; Manakil, J., Ed.; IntechOpen Limited: London, UK, 2018. [CrossRef]
273. Susin, C.; Wikesjo, U. Regenerative periodontal therapy: 30 years of lessons learned and unlearned. *Periodontology* **2000**, *2013*, 232–242. [CrossRef]

274. Zhai, Q.; Dong, Z.; Wang, W.; Li, B.; Jin, Y. Dental stem cell and dental tissue regeneration. *Front. Med.* **2019**, *13*, 152–159. [CrossRef] [PubMed]
275. Raju, R.; Oshima, M.; Inoue, M.; Morita, T.; Huijiao, Y.; Waskitho, A.; Baba, O.; Inoue, M.; Matsuka, Y. Three-dimensional periodontal tissue regeneration using a bone-ligament complex cell sheet. *Sci. Rep.* **2020**, *10*, 1–16. [CrossRef]
276. Iwata, T.; Yamato, M.; Washio, K.; Yoshida, T.; Tsumanuma, Y.; Yamada, A.; Onizuka, S.; Izumi, Y.; Ando, T.; Okano, T.; et al. Periodontal regeneration with autologous periodontal ligament-derived cell sheets–a safety and efficacy study in ten patients. *Regen. Ther.* **2018**, *9*, 38–44. [CrossRef] [PubMed]
277. Ausenda, F.; Rasperini, G.; Acunzo, R.; Gorbunkova, A.; Pagni, G. New Perspectives in the Use of Biomaterials for Periodontal Regeneration. *Materials* **2019**, *12*, 2197. [CrossRef]
278. Sheikh, Z.; Hamdan, N.; Ikeda, Y.; Grynpas, M. Natural graft tissues and synthetic biomaterials for periodontal and alveolar bone reconstructive applications: A review. *Biomater. Res.* **2017**, 21–29. [CrossRef]
279. Liu, J.; Ruan, J.; Weir, M.D.; Ren, K.; Schneider, A.; Wang, P.; Oates, T.W.; Chan, X.; Xu, H.H. Periodontal bone-ligament-cementum regeneration via scaffolds and stem cells. *Cells* **2019**, *8*, 537. [CrossRef]
280. Belinfante, L.S. The History of Oral and Maxillofacial Surgery. In *Current Therapy In Oral and Maxillofacial Surgery*; Bagheri, S.C., Bell, R.B., Ali Khan, H., Eds.; Elsevier: Amsterdam, The Netherlands, 2012; pp. 1–5.
281. Aghaloo, T.L.; Felnsfeld, A.L. Principles of Repair and Grafting of Bone and Cartilage. In *Current Therapy In Oral and Maxillofacial Surgery*; Bagheri, S.C., Bell, R.B., Ali Khan, H., Eds.; Elsevier: Amsterdam, The Netherlands, 2012; pp. 19–26.
282. Keyhan, S.O.; Fallahi, H.; Jahangirnia, A.; Masoumi, S.M.R.; Khosravi, M.H.; Amirzade-Iranaq, M.H. Tissue Engineering Applications in Maxillofacial Surgery. In *Stem Cells in Clinical Practice and Tissue Engineering*; Sharma, R., Ed.; IntechOpen: London, UK, 2017; pp. 271–291.
283. Zhang, Q.; Nguyen, P.D.; Shi, S.; Burrell, J.C.; Cullen, D.K.; Le, A.D. 3D bioprinted scaffold-free nerve constructs with human gingiva-derived mesenchymal stem cells promote rat facial nerve regeneration. *Sci. Rep.* **2018**, *8*, 6634. [CrossRef]
284. Li, J.; Xu, S.Q.; Zhang, K.; Zhang, W.J.; Liu, H.L.; Xu, Z.; Li, H.; Lou, J.N.; Ge, L.H.; Xu, B.H. Treatment of gingival defects with gingival mesenchymal stem cells derived from human fetal gingival tissue in a rat model. *Stem Cell Res.* **2018**, *9*, 27. [CrossRef]
285. Triplett, R.G.; Schow, S.R. Autologous bone grafts and endosseous implants: Complementary techniques. *J. Oral Maxillofac. Surg.* **1996**, *54*, 486–494. [CrossRef] [PubMed]
286. Wu, V.; Helder, M.N.; Bravenboer, N.; Ten Bruggenkate, C.M.; Jin, J.; Klein-Nulend, J.; Schulten, E.A. Bone tissue regeneration in the oral and maxillofacial region: A review on the application of stem cells and new strategies to improve vascularization. *Stem Cells Int.* **2019**, *2019*, 6279721. [CrossRef] [PubMed]
287. Trubiani, O.; Marconi, G.D.; Pierdomenico, S.D.; Piattelli, A.; Diomede, F.; Pizzicannella, J. Human Oral Stem Cells, Biomaterials and Extracellular Vesicles: A Promising Tool in Bone Tissue Repair. *Int. J. Mol. Sci.* **2019**, *20*, 4987. [CrossRef]
288. Iaquinta, M.R.; Mazzoni, E.; Bononi, I.; Rotondo, J.C.; Mazziotta, C.; Montesi, M.; Sprio, S.; Tampieri, A.; Martini, F. Adult stem cells for bone regeneration and repair. *Front. Cell Dev. Biol.* **2019**, *7*, 268. [CrossRef] [PubMed]
289. Chocholata, P.; Kulda, V.; Babuska, V. Fabrication of scaffolds for bone-tissue regeneration. *Materials* **2019**, *12*, 568. [CrossRef]
290. Ceccarelli, G.; Presta, R.; Benedetti, L.; Cusella De Angelis, M.G.; Lupi, S.M.; Rodriguez y Baena, R. Emerging perspectives in scaffold for tissue engineering in oral surgery. *Stem Cells Int.* **2017**, *2017*, 4585401. [CrossRef] [PubMed]
291. Rodriguez y Baena, R.; D'Aquino, R.; Graziano, A. Autologous periosteum-derived micrografts and PLGA/HA enhance the bone formation in sinus lift augmentation. *Front. Cell Dev. Biol.* **2017**, *5*, 87. [CrossRef]
292. Mohammed, E.E.A.; El-Zawahry, M.; Farrag, A.R.H.; Aziz, N.N.A.; Sharaf El-Din, W.; Abu-Shahba, N.; Mahmoud, M.; Gaber, K.; Ismail, T.; Mossaad, M.M.; et al. Osteogenic Differentiation potential of human bone marrow and amniotic fluid-derived mesenchymal stem cells in vitro & in vivo. *Maced. J. Med. Sci.* **2019**, *7*, 507–515. [CrossRef]

293. Mazzoni, E.; D'Agostino, A.; Iaquinta, M.R.; Bononi, I.; Trevisiol, L.; Rotondo, J.C.; Patergani, S.; Giorgi, C.; Gunson, M.; Arnett, G.W.; et al. Hydroxylapatite-collagen hybrid scaffold induces human adipose-derived mesenchymal stem cells (hASCs) to osteogenic differentiation in vitro and bone re-growth in patients. *Stem Cells Transl. Med.* **2019**, *9*, 377–388. [CrossRef]
294. Park, Y.J.; Cha, S.; Park, Y.S. Regenerative applications using tooth derived stem cells in other than tooth regeneration: A literature review. *Stem Cells Int.* **2016**, *2016*, 9305986. [CrossRef]
295. Diomede, F.; Gugliandolo, A.; Cardelli, P.; Merciaro, I.; Ettorre, V.; Traini, T.; Bedini, R.; Scionti, D.; Bramanti, A.; Nanci, A.; et al. Three-dimensional printed PLA scaffold and human gingival stem cell-derived extracellular vesicles: A new tool for bone defect repair. *Stem Cell Res.* **2018**, *9*, 104. [CrossRef]
296. Sakkas, A.; Wilde, F.; Heufelder, M.; Winter, K.; Schramm, A. Autogenous bone grafts in oral implantology—Is it still a "gold standard"? A consecutive review of 279 patients with 456 clinical procedures. *Int. J. Implant. Dent.* **2017**, *3*, 23. [CrossRef] [PubMed]
297. Gjerde, C.; Mustafa, K.; Hellem, S.; Rojewski, M.; Gjengedal, H.; Yassin, M.A.; Feng, X.; Skaale, S.; Berge, T.; Rosen, A.; et al. Cell therapy induced regeneration of severely atrophied mandibular bone in a clinical trial. *Stem Cell Res.* **2018**, *9*, 213. [CrossRef]
298. Di Stefano, D.A.; Greco, G.B.; Riboli, F. Guided Bone Regeneration of an Atrophic Mandible with a Heterologous Bone Block. *Craniomaxillofac. Trauma Reconstr.* **2016**, *9*, 88–93. [CrossRef] [PubMed]
299. McGuire, T.P.; Rittenberg, B.N.; Baker, G.I. Surgery for Disorders of the Temporomandibular Joint. Available online: https://www.oralhealthgroup.com/features/surgery-for-disorders-of-the-temporomandibular-joint/ (accessed on 15 October 2020).
300. Jazayeri, H.E.; Tahriri, M.; Razavi, M.; Khoshroo, K.; Fahimipour, F.; Dashtimoghadam, E.; Almeida, L.; Tayebi, L. A current overview of materials and strategies for potential use in maxillofacial tissue regeneration. *Mater. Sci. Eng.* **2017**, *70*, 913–929. [CrossRef]
301. Shetty, L.; Badhe, R.V.; Bhonde, R.; Waknis, P.; Londhe, U. Chitosan and stemcells: A synchrony for regeneration. *J. Dent. Res. Rev.* **2020**, *7*, 95–97. [CrossRef]
302. Oshima, M.; Tsuji, T. Whole Tooth Regeneration Using a Bioengineered Tooth. In *New Trends in Tissue Engineering and Regenerative Medicine—Official Book of the Japanese Society for Regenerative Medicine*; Hibi, H., Ueda, M., Eds.; IntechOpen: London, UK, 2014. [CrossRef]
303. Wu, Z.; Wang, F.; Fan, Z.; Wu, T.; He, J.; Wang, J.; Zhang, C.; Wang, S. Whole-Tooth Regeneration by Allogeneic Cell Reassociation in Pig Jawbone. *Tissue Eng. Part A* **2019**, *25*, 1202–1212. [CrossRef]
304. Ikeda, E.; Morita, R.; Nakao, K.; Ishida, K.; Nakamura, T.; Takano-Yamamoto, T.; Ogawab, M.; Mizunoa, M.; Kasugaie, S.; Tsujia, T. Fully functional bioengineered tooth replacement as an organ replacement therapy. *Proc. Natl. Acad. Sci. USA* **2009**, *106*, 13475–13480.
305. Nakao, K.; Tsuji, T. Dental regenerative therapy: Stem cell transplantation and bioengineered tooth replacement. *Jpn. Dent. Sci. Rev.* **2008**, *44*, 70–75. [CrossRef]
306. Zhang, L.; Morsi, Y.; Wang, Y.; Li, Y.; Ramakrishna, S. Review scaffold design and stem cells for tooth regeneration. *Jpn. Dent. Sci. Rev.* **2013**, *49*, 14–26. [CrossRef]
307. Ono, M.; Oshima, M.; Ogawa, M.; Sonoyama, W.; Hara, E.S.; Oida, Y.; Shinkawa, S.; Nakajima, R.; Mine, A.; Fukumoto, S. Practical whole-tooth restoration utilizing autologous bioengineered tooth germ transplantation in a postnatal canine model. *Sci. Rep.* **2017**, *7*, 44522. [CrossRef] [PubMed]
308. Thesleff, I. From understanding tooth development to bioengineering of teeth. *Eur. J. Oral Sci.* **2018**, *126*, 67–71. [CrossRef] [PubMed]
309. Yelick, P.C.; Sharpe, P.T. Tooth Bioengineering and Regenerative Dentistry. *J. Dent. Res.* **2019**, *98*, 1173–1182. [CrossRef] [PubMed]
310. Oshima, M.; Inoue, K.; Nakajima, K.; Tachikawa, T.; Yamazaki, H.; Isobe, T.; Sugawara, A.; Ogawa, M.; Tanaka, C.; Saito, M.; et al. Functional tooth restoration by next generation bio-hybrid implants a bio-hybrid artificial organ replacement therapy. *Sci. Rep.* **2014**, *4*, 6044. [CrossRef] [PubMed]
311. Wei, F.; Song, T.; Ding, G.; Xu, J.; Liu, Y.; Liu, D.; Fan, Z.; Zhang, C.; Shi, S.; Wang, S. Functional tooth restoration by allogeneic mesenchymal stem cell-based bio-root regeneration in swine. *Stem Cells Dev.* **2013**, *22*, 1752–1762. [CrossRef]

312. Rusu, L.C.; Ardelean, L.; Negrutiu, M.L.; Dragomirescu, A.O.; Albu, M.G.; Ghica, M.V.; Topala, F.I.; Podoleanu, A.; Sinescu, C. SEM for the general structural features assesing of the synthetic polymer scaffolds. *Rev. Chim.* **2011**, *62*, 841–845.

**Publisher's Note:** MDPI stays neutral with regard to jurisdictional claims in published maps and institutional affiliations.

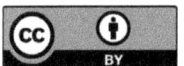

© 2020 by the authors. Licensee MDPI, Basel, Switzerland. This article is an open access article distributed under the terms and conditions of the Creative Commons Attribution (CC BY) license (http://creativecommons.org/licenses/by/4.0/).

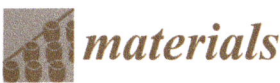

Article

# Impact of APRF+ in Combination with Autogenous Fibroblasts on Release Growth Factors, Collagen, and Proliferation and Migration of Gingival Fibroblasts: An In Vitro Study

Barbara Sterczała [1,*], Agnieszka Chwiłkowska [2,*], Urszula Szwedowicz [2], Magdalena Kobielarz [3], Bartłomiej Chwiłkowski [4] and Marzena Dominiak [1]

1. Dental Surgery Department, Wroclaw Medical University, 50-425 Wroclaw, Poland; marzena.dominiak@umed.wroc.pl
2. Department of Molecular and Cell Biology, Wroclaw Medical University, 50-556 Wroclaw, Poland; WF-26@umw.edu.pl
3. Department of Mechanics, Materials and Biomedical Engineering, Wroclaw University of Science and Technology, 50-371 Wroclaw, Poland; magdalena.kobielarz@pwr.edu.pl
4. Department of Applied Mathematics, Faculty of Pure and Applied Mathematics, Wroclaw University of Science and Technology, 50-370 Wroclaw, Poland; 249761@student.pwr.edu.pl
* Correspondence: barbara.sterczala@op.pl (B.S.); agnieszka.chwilkowska@umw.edu.pl (A.C.); Tel.: +48-502-932-269 (B.S.)

**Abstract:** The present study aimed to compare the action of advanced platelet-rich fibrin (A-PRF+) alone with the action of A-PRF+ combined with autologous gingival fibroblasts. The components released from A-PRF+ conditioned with autogenous fibroblasts that were quantified in the study were fibroblast growth factor (FGF), vascular endothelial growth factor (VEGF), trans-forming growth factor-beta1 and 2 (TGFβ1 and TGFβ2), and soluble collagen. A-PRF+ combined with fibroblasts demonstrated significantly higher values of released VEGF at every time point and, after 7 days, significantly higher values of released TGFβ2. A viability test after 72 h showed a significant increase in proliferation fibroblasts after exposition to the factors released from A-PRF+ combined with fibroblasts. Similarly, the degree of wound closure after 48 h was significantly higher for the factors released from A-RRF+ alone and the factors released from A-RRF+ combined with fibroblasts. These results imply that platelet-rich fibrin (PRF) enhanced with fibroblasts can be an alternative method of connective tissue transplantation.

**Keywords:** A-PRF+; fibroblast culture; wound healing; VEGF; TGFβ2

## 1. Introduction

Platelet-rich fibrin (PRF) contains supraphysiological concentrations of growth factors that stimulate bone and soft tissue regeneration in a natural way [1]. The protocol of obtaining PRF of the second generation, introduced by Choukroun and colleagues [2], allows one to achieve material that is completely autologous and prepared without any anticoagulants or separators. PRF contains leukocytes, as well as biochemical components, such as growth factors (GFs); platelets; immunity promoters; and cytokines, including IL-1 β, IL-4, IL-6, and TNF-α [3,4], which stimulate the healing process.

Leukocytes and fibrinogen reduce the harmfulness of the hypermetabolic phase in the first phase of healing [5]. The strong network of a PRF clot consists of polymerized fibrin and chains of structural glycoproteins [4]. Due to its biomechanical properties, the membrane is easy to use clinically. It shows flexibility and elasticity, and it is easy to form. Currently, PRF is successfully used in modern periodontal regenerative stomatology [6], among other things, due to the ease of acquirement, the activity at every stage of soft-tissue healing, and the economic aspect [2,7–9].

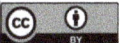

Recent advances in medical sciences have led to the development of a new procedure to obtain various products of PRF, such as APRF+ [10]. The method, speed, and time of centrifugation of the venous blood taken from the patient greatly influence the composition of the clot: the number of platelets, leukocytes, and GFs [10]. If less force and a shorter time of centrifugation are used, more leukocytes, and thus monocytes, and macrophages are obtained, which, in turn, increases the number of precursor cells at the site of application; therefore, this corresponds to improved regenerative potential. A significantly increased level of released growth factors corresponds to the increase in the number of platelets, evenly distributed in the fibrin network [8,10–13]. Transforming growth factor-beta (TGFβ), vascular endothelial growth factor (VEGF), epidermal growth factor (EGF), platelet-derived growth factor (PDGF), and insulin-like growth factor (IGF) affect intracellular and intercellular communication and, thus, stimulate cell migration, adhesion, and proliferation at the wound site [12,14,15]. In turn, the fibrin present in the network stimulates a slower degradation of the network and delays the release of growth factors for 7–10 days, which is in contrast to PRP, where the growth factors are secreted within the first hour [16,17]. In addition, sufficiently large gaps in the scaffold of the APRF+ matrix allow neutrophils to penetrate it, which affects the functionality of the transplanted and local host cells in the regenerated tissue [8,13].

Therefore, APRF+ is used as a natural polymer in tissue engineering, and the available knowledge concerning its application allows us to state the validity of the use of A-PRF+ as a carrier for isolated autogenous fibroblasts for the augmentation of keratinized gingiva. Fibroblasts play a crucial role in three stages of tissue regeneration by releasing growth factors, which regulate the processes of intra- and extra-cellular metabolism, indirectly modulating the formation of a new extracellular matrix (EMC) [14,18,19]. The advantage of autogenous cell cultures is that they provide biomaterial for augmentation in the amount of determined tissue loss.

The present study aimed to determine whether the combination of A-PRF+ with autogenous fibroblasts would change the number of released components that are important in the context of the healing processes, including fibroblast growth factor (FGF); vascular endothelial growth factor (VEGF); transforming growth factor-beta1 and 2 (TGFβ1 and TGFβ2); and collagen, the main protein of the extracellular matrix, produced by fibroblasts. The impact of the released components on the proliferation of fibroblasts and their migration was analyzed. The motivation to conduct the present study is the evolution and enhanced methods of wound healing.

## 2. Materials and Methods
### 2.1. Cell Culture and A-PRF+-Based Matrices

Primary human gingival fibroblasts (HGFs) and A-PRF+ were obtained from six systematically healthy volunteer donors, following approval by the Ethics Committee of Wroclaw Medical University, Poland (No KB-434/2017). Samples of hard palatal and gingival tissues were collected in the amount of 1–2 mm$^2$ from each donor and transported to the laboratory in the nutrient medium Dulbecco's modified Eagle's medium (DMEM, Sigma-Aldrich, Poznan, Poland) with the addition of 10% fetal calf serum (Gibco-ThermoFisher, Warsaw, Poland), penicillin (100 Ul/mL), streptomycin (0.1 mg/mL), and amphotericin B (0.1 mg/mL). Subsequently, fibroblasts were mechanically isolated and cultured according to the patented method described by Dominiak et al. [20]. The culture was carried out in a conventional DMEM culture medium in an incubator at 37 °C in a 5% $CO_2$ atmosphere. The culture medium was changed twice a week. The cells reached a full monolayer after 5–7 days. After achieving a full monolayer of cells, four tubes of blood samples were collected in the amount of 10 mL from these same six volunteer donors. Next, A-PRF+ was obtained according to the procedure developed by Choukroun [11]. The blood samples without anticoagulant were centrifuged at 1300 rpm ($200 \times g$) for 8 min in a centrifuge machine PRF DuoTM (Process for PRF, Nice, France). The A-PRF+ clots were removed from the tubes and separated from the RBC base using sterilized scissors for further investigation.

### 2.2. Assessment of Growth Factor Release from Fibroblasts Alone, A-PRF+ Alone, and A-PRF+ with Fibroblasts

Primary human fibroblasts at a concentration of $4 \times 10^5$ cells/mL were placed into a twelve-well dish with 1.5 mL of culture media (DMEM) and allowed to grow for 24 h. Then, the medium was removed, and the sterile-flattened A-PRF+ clots were placed (not less than within 1 h from production) in a well with fibroblasts and in an empty well, and there was one well that contained only fibroblasts. Fresh medium in the amount of 1.5 mL was added to each variant. At 1, 2, 3, and 7 days, 1.5 mL of culture media was collected, frozen at $-20\ °C$, and replaced with 1.5 mL of fresh culture media. The content of soluble collagen, TGFβ1, TGFβ2, FGF1, and VEGF in the collected medium was investigated. The release of growth factors was quantified using the colorimetric test for collagen quantification and ELISA for the investigation of the remaining factors.

### 2.3. The Quantification of Growth Factors with Enzyme-Linked Immunosorbent Assay (ELISA)

To determine the amount of growth factors released from A-PRF+ alone, A-PRF+ with fibroblasts, and only fibroblasts alone at days 1, 2, 3, and 7, samples were investigated using ELISA. At the desired time points, TGFβ1 (BMS249-4, Invitrogen, range = 31 to 2000 pg/mL, sensitivity: 8.6 pg/mL), TGFβ2 (BMS254, Invitrogen, Waltham, MA, USA, range = 31 to 1000 pg/mL, sensitivity: 6.6 pg/mL), FGF1 (EHFGF1, Invitrogen, range = 16.38 to 4000 pg/mL, sensitivity: 12 pg/mL), and VEGF (KHG0111, Invitrogen, range = 23.4 to 1500 pg/mL, sensitivity: 5 pg/mL) were quantified using an ELISA kit according to the manufacturer's protocol. All samples were measured twice using a Multiskan™ FC microplate photometer (Thermo Scientific, Alab, Warsaw, Poland).

### 2.4. Quantification of Soluble Collagen Using the Sircol™ Colorimetric Test

The release of soluble collagen in the culture medium incubated with A-PRF+ alone, A-PRF+ with fibroblasts, and only fibroblasts alone at days 1, 2, 3, and 7 was analyzed with the Sircol™ assay according to the manufacturer's protocol (Biocolor Ltd., Carrickfergus, UK). The collected media were incubated with Sircol™ dye, which binds to soluble collagen, and then centrifuged to form pellets. Pellets were solubilized in sodium hydroxide, and the amount of eluted dye was measured using a Multiskan™ FC microplate photometer (Thermo Scientific, Alab, Warsaw, Poland) at 540 nm. Collagen standards supplied with the kit were used as controls.

### 2.5. Preparation of the Conditioned Media

Primary human fibroblasts at a concentration of $4 \times 10^5$ cells/mL were placed into a six-well dish with 2.5 mL of culture media (DMEM) and allowed to attach. Then, the medium was replaced with a fresh one, and sterile-flattened A-PRF+ clots, obtained as described in the previous paragraph, were placed into the well and incubated for 3 days on a plate shaker at 37 °C. A-PRF+ clots without fibroblasts were also incubated for 3 days in 2.5 mL of culture media (DMEM) on a plate shaker at 37 °C. After this time, the fluid was drawn, and conditioned media containing 20% of the pooled fluid suspended in DMEM were prepared. Concurrently, fibroblasts with culture medium, as well as culture medium alone, were incubated in the same conditions and prepared as conditioned control media.

### 2.6. Cell Migration Assay

The in vitro wound healing assay for probing collective cell migration in two dimensions was performed using 2-well silicone inserts (Ibidi GmbH, Planegg, Germany) placed into a 6-well plate, which allowed the experimental variables to be standardized. To detect migration, $5 \times 10^4$ cells/well were suspended in a volume of 70 µL 10% FCS/DMEM. The cell culture inserts were removed after 24 h, leaving a defined cell-free gap of 500 µm. At this time point (0 h), the fresh medium was supplemented with medium enriched with culture fluid after a 3-day incubation with A-PRF+ alone, A-PRF+ and fibroblasts, fibroblasts alone, and DMEM alone, and then placed into each well, and images were taken.

Cell cultures were observed and photographed under the CKX41 Olympus microscope (Tokyo, Japan) after 24 and 48 h. Software ImageJ (LOCI, University of Wisconsin) was used to quantify the areas of the closing gap.

*2.7. Cell Viability Assay*

HGFs were seeded into black 96-well plates. After 24 h, the fresh medium supplemented with medium enriched with culture fluid after a 3-day incubation with A-PRF+ alone, A-PRF+ and fibroblasts, fibroblasts alone, and DMEM alone was added into each well for 24, 48, and 72 h. All experiments were performed in quadruplicate. After the incubation, a PrestoBlue assay was performed to determine cell viability. The method is based on resazurin, which functions as a cell viability indicator. Viable cells convert the dark blue oxidized form of the dye (resazurin) into a red fluorescent reduced form (resorufin; $\lambda_{Ex}$ = 570 nm; $\lambda_{Em}$ = 590 nm).

PrestoBlue reagent (Thermo Fisher Scientific, Waltham, MA, USA) was added to each well containing 100 µL of the medium. The plate was then incubated for 30 min at 37 °C, and the change in fluorescence was measured using a Multiskan™ FC microplate photometer (Thermo Scientific, Alab, Warsaw, Poland), with the excitation/emission wavelengths set at 560/590 nm. Relative cell viability was calculated as the percentage of untreated cells.

*2.8. Statistical Analysis*

The statistical analyses of collected data ($n$ = 6) were performed using Statistica version 13.3 with a significance level of $\alpha$ = 0.05. The normality of the distribution of variables was examined based on the Shapiro–Wilk test. The one-way analysis of variance (ANOVA) was performed for the comparison of groups' means. ANOVA tests' assumptions, i.e., normally distributed data, homogeneity of variance across groups, and lack of correlation between group means with variances, were controlled. In a few cases, the assumption of homogeneity of variance was found not to hold, and, therefore, for these cases, a modified ANOVA test was applied, i.e., Welch's F-test, recommended when groups have different variances. Finally, using Tukey's test, the post hoc analysis was performed to determine the significantly different groups. Results are presented as mean ± SD.

## 3. Results

*3.1. Growth Factor Release from A-PRF+ Alone, A-PRF+ with Fibroblasts, and Fibroblasts Alone*

The release of proteins, including TGFβ1, TGFβ2, FGF1, and VEGF, was quantified with ELISA, and collagen was quantified by using a spectrophotometric assay. A-PRF+ combined with fibroblasts demonstrated significantly higher values of released VEGF than both A-PRF+ alone and fibroblasts alone (Figure 1G,H), while the total release of TGFβ2 demonstrated significantly lower values for fibroblasts alone compared with A-PRF+ alone and A-PRF+ incubated with fibroblasts (Figure 1C,D). On day 7, the level of TGFβ2 was significantly higher than in the other groups (Figure 1C) and insignificantly higher after the accumulation of collected doses (Figure 1D). Moreover, the release of collagen demonstrated significantly lower values at all time points for A-PRF+ compared with A-PRF+ combined with fibroblasts and fibroblasts alone (Figure 1I,J). In comparison, no difference in the total release of TGFβ1 and FGF1 factors was observed among the three groups (Figure 1A,B,E,F).

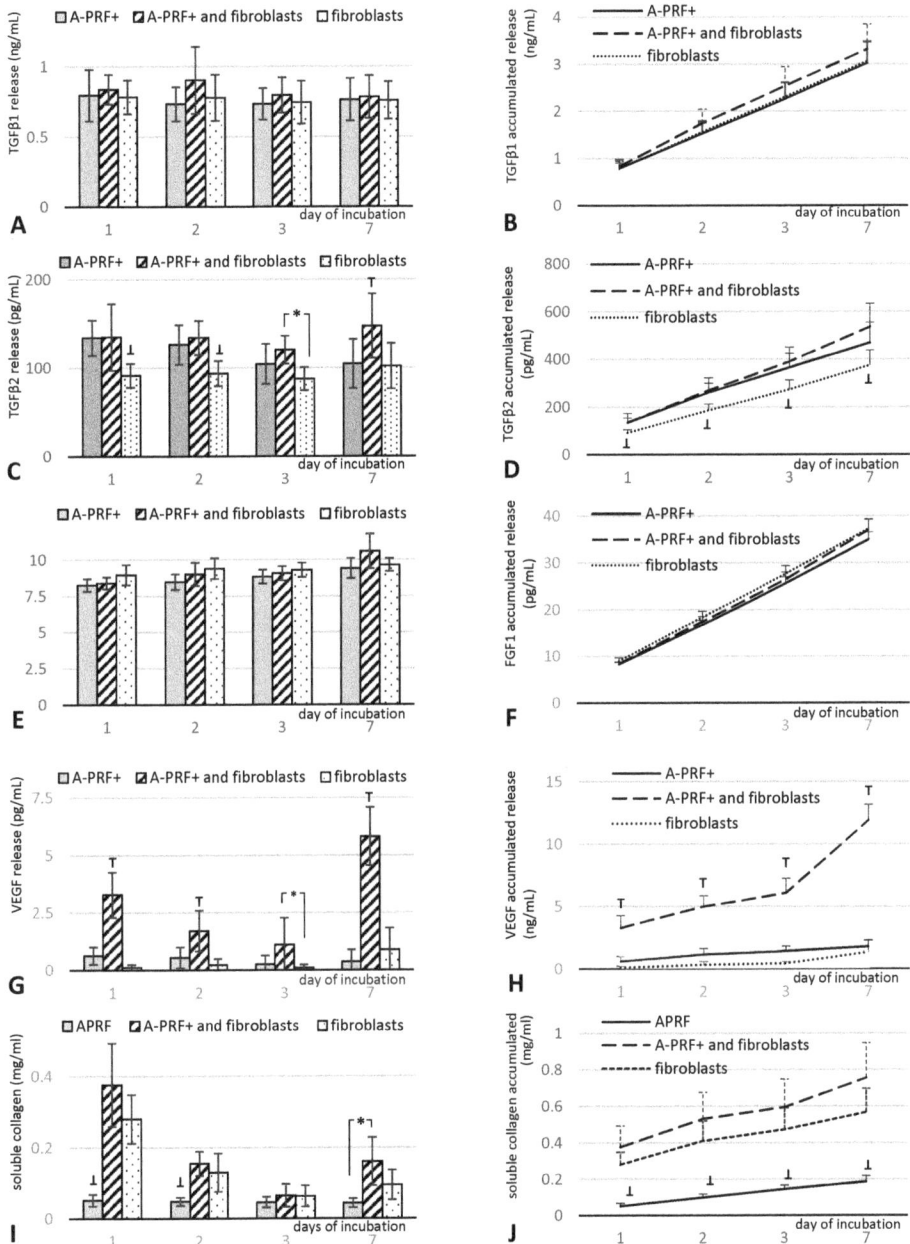

**Figure 1.** The quantification of protein released from A-PRF+ alone, A-PRF+ with fibroblasts, and fibroblasts alone at the different time points for (**A**) TGFβ1, (**C**) TGFβ2, (**E**) FGF1, (**G**) VEGF, and (**I**) soluble collagen. Total accumulated protein released over a 7-day period for (**B**) TGFβ1, (**D**) TGFβ2, (**F**) FGF1, (**H**) VEGF, and (**J**) soluble collagen. * $p < 0.05$, significant difference among groups; T $p < 0.05$, significantly higher than all other groups; ⊥ $p < 0.05$, significantly lower than all other groups. Data represent means ± SD from six different HGF donors.

## 3.2. Influence of Proteins Released from A-PRF+ Combined with Fibroblasts on Cell Viability

The results of HGF viability after stimulation by the proteins released from A-PRF+ combined with fibroblasts are shown in Figure 2. After 72 h, there was a significant increase in cell viability after exposure to the proteins released from A-PRF+ combined with fibroblasts compared to the media conditioned with the factors released from fibroblasts alone or A-PRF+ alone. A slight decrease in cell viability was observed for the control medium conditioned with the compounds released from the fibroblasts and an increase was observed for the control medium conditioned with the proteins released from A-PRF+.

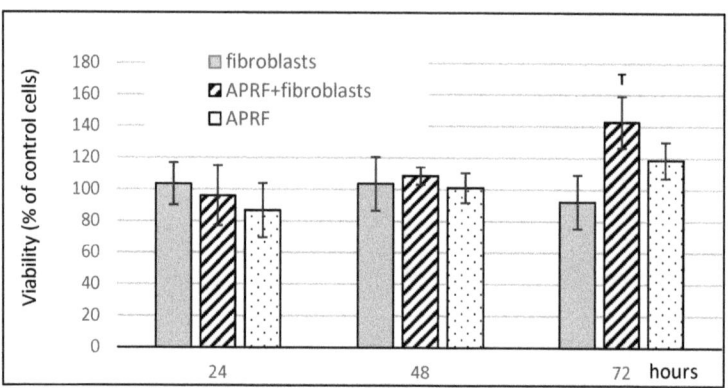

**Figure 2.** Effect of medium enriched with proteins released from A-PRF+ on fibroblast proliferation. **T** $p < 0.05$, significantly higher than all other groups. Data represent means ± SD from six different HGF donors.

## 3.3. Enhanced Wound Healing Potential of Primary Human Gingival Fibroblasts Induced with Proteins Released from A-PRF+

The effects of the factors released from fibroblasts alone, A-PRF+ alone, and fibroblasts combined with A-PRF+ on the wound healing potential of primary HGFs were analyzed by evaluating the migration of these cells using an in vitro wound healing assay. The 500 um wide gap created between the cells allowed us to analyze how the released compounds influenced the migration and invasion of cells, and the representative images of the migration of HGFs toward a wound gap are presented in Figure 3. The factors released from A-PRF+, added to the culture medium, were able to significantly increase the capacity of primary HGFs to migrate into the gap compared to controls (Figures 3 and 4).

Compared to the wound area after 24 h of 11 ± 6% and 21 ± 12% for controls, which were incubated for three days either in medium alone or in medium with fibroblasts, respectively, the compounds released from A-PRF+ caused a moderate wound closure of 27 ± 10% for the factors released from A-RRF+ alone and, significantly, 35 ± 20% for the factors released from A-RRF+ combined with fibroblasts ($p < 0.05$; Figure 4). The degrees of wound closure after 48 h were significantly higher, i.e., 66 ± 16% and 64 ± 13% for the factors released from A-RRF+ alone and the factors released from A-RRF+ combined with fibroblasts, respectively, compared to 27 +/− 13% of the control wound area ($p < 0.05$; Figure 4).

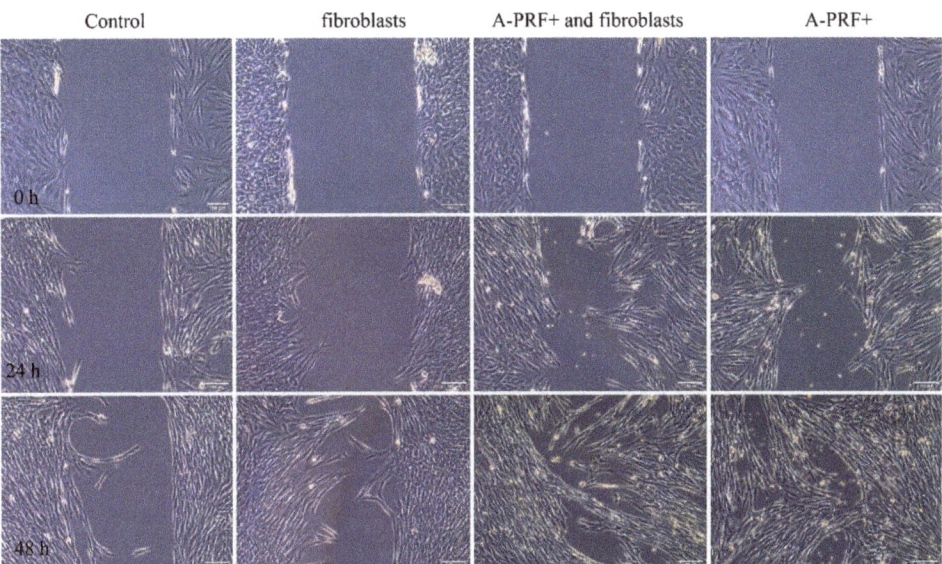

**Figure 3.** An exemplary representation of the wound healing assay under microscopic observation for control conditioned media, conditioned media with fibroblasts, with fibroblasts stimulated by A-PRF+, and with A-PRF+ alone. The scratch area is at time point 0 h, and observation time is up to 48 h.

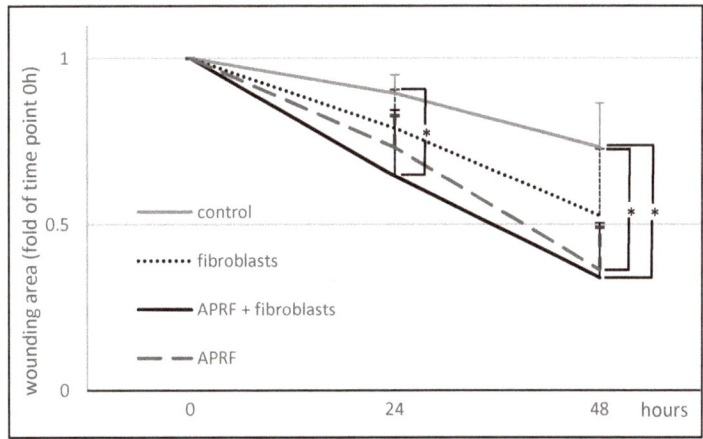

**Figure 4.** Wound closure expressed as the remaining area uncovered by the cells. The scratch area at time point 0 h was set to 48 h. * $p < 0.05$, significant difference among groups. Data represent means ± SD from six different HGF donors.

## 4. Discussion

The process of soft-tissue regeneration is a cascade of signaling reactions involving the immune system; platelets; and components of connective tissue, including fibroblasts [18]. They affect blood coagulation, activating the inflammatory process, which affects migration, the proliferation of cells to the injured site, and, consequently, the remodeling of the newly created matrix [21]. In geriatric patients or individuals with immunodeficiency conditions, such as diabetes mellitus, or patients with the inability of connective tissue to proliferate and provide recession coverage, intracellular and intercellular signaling is often disturbed, and the number of cells, including fibroblasts, is reduced. The destruction of capillaries reduces ion transport. The resulting inhibition of the migration of fibroblasts from the circumferential rifer of the wound slows down the regeneration process [17,22,23]. Therefore, it is important to use biomaterials that can stimulate the host cells and, at the same time, provide the optimal amount of cells to initiate the regeneration process at the wound site. Numerous studies have shown that platelet concentrates (PCs), including PRF, promote the adhesion, proliferation, and migration of HGFs [24,25]. Steller at al. showed the crucial impact of platelet concentrates (PCs) in an effort to enhance the local treatment of bisphosphonate-related osteonecrosis of the jaw [9]. The present study demonstrates the potential of A-PRF+ with autogenous human fibroblasts as a connective tissue substitute in the augmentation of keratinized gingiva. To the authors' knowledge, this is the first study concerning this issue. To date, the family of PRF matrices has been investigated alone, without the addition of fibroblasts [11].

The study presented in this paper compared the number of released growth factors in three groups: (1) human gingival fibroblasts alone, (2) A-PRF+ alone, and (3) A-PRF+ enriched with autologous fibroblasts. The obtained results showed a significant increase in the released VEGF in the group of A-PRF+ with autogenous human fibroblasts over a period of 7 days. One of the basic factors of proper tissue regeneration is providing nutrition through angiogenesis. The formation of a vascular network is required for the migration and proliferation of cells, which, by releasing modulators of the immune system, lead to the repopulation of the extracellular matrix and the formation of new tissue [26]. The result presented in this paper revealed a positive response in clinical terms, as according to Cabaro et al., as well as others, VEGF inhibits the hyperreactivity of T lymphocytes in the early stage of inflammation and stimulates the migration of macrophages and fibroblasts [27]. Fujioka-Kobayashi et al. showed a much higher release of VEGF from the A-PRF+ matrix up to day 3 compared to the tested LPRF and A-PRF [10]. However, from day 3 to day 10, the amount of the released VEGF was constant. Our results show that A-PRF+ enriched with autologous fibroblasts releases a statistically significantly higher amount of VEGF than that of the other groups at all points of time. It is likely that it could be the effect of stimulation by both the carrier, i.e., A-PRF+, and the fibroblasts implemented on it. In healthy patients, the formation of a wound triggers a cascade of signaling reactions involving various cells, including components of connective tissue, such as fibroblasts [18–28]. The activation of the inflammatory process affects the migration and proliferation of cells to the injured site and, consequently, leads to the remodeling of the newly formed extracellular matrix [21].

TGFβ is a cytokine activated by platelets in the fibrin network of the A-PRF+ matrix. It includes, among others, the TGFβ1 and TGFβ2 isoforms. It is responsible for angiogenesis, and it stimulates the chemotaxis of fibroblasts and their differentiation into myofibroblasts, which are involved in the remodeling of the extracellular matrix [29]. In the present study, an insignificant increase in TGFβ1 was obtained in the group of A-PRF+ with fibroblasts compared to the other two groups, and a significant increase in TGFβ2 in comparison to the group with fibroblasts alone. However, on day 7, the level of TGFβ2 was significantly higher than in the other groups. The described results indicate the stimulating nature of A-PRF+ on the secretion of both VEGF and TGFβ2 by fibroblasts.

Otherwise, the steady increase in the released FGF at all time points was the same in all treatment groups. FGF affects vascularization and accelerates wound healing [30,31], but not in its early stages [32]. Therefore, the results obtained in this study do not show differences between the three groups. Fibroblasts synthesize the main structural protein of type III collagen, which is replaced in the remodeling phase with type I collagen [18]. This affects the restoration of the functionality of the extracellular matrix, creating increased cross-linking of collagen fibers and, thus, increasing the stability and extensibility of collagen fibers [33]. Significantly higher values of collagen released at all time points were also observed for A-PRF+ with implanted fibroblasts compared to the A-PRF+ matrix alone.

Unfortunately, the comparison with the control group of fibroblasts shows an increase but without statistical significance. This discovery confirms the reports by Masuki H. et al. in terms of the ability of the A-PRF+ matrix to induce angiogenesis and to act as a scaffold into which inter alia fibroblasts can be implemented and contribute to the acceleration of healing and subsequent regeneration of the damaged tissue [34].

Fujioka-Kobayashi et al. observed an increase in cell proliferation after exposure to A-PRF+ [10]. The present study also determined how the released components from A-PRF+ with inoculated fibroblasts affect autogenous fibroblasts. The observations up to 72 h showed a significant increase in cell viability compared to the other two test groups. The degrees of wound closure after 48 h were significant higher for the medium with the factors released from A-RRF+ alone and the factors released from A-RRF+ combined with fibroblasts in comparison to the medium with the factors released from the fibroblasts alone and from the control medium. The bioactive scaffold of the A-PRF+ matrix promotes the implementation of cells; the presented research study also shows that fibroblasts are responsible for the increased release of growth factors. Ghanaati S. et al. showed that the acquisition parameters of the A-PRF matrix are conducive to increasing its porosity [8,12]. The porosity of the carrier is important in the ability to deliver signaling cells, especially hematopoietic stem cells, for the tissue healing process [35]. This structure allows for a deeper implantation of neutrophils and, thus, their longer release. As a result, they also influence the host's immune response at later stages of tissue healing. The finding of this study confirms the assumption that the implementation of the A-PRF+ matrix with autogenous fibroblasts could increase its clinical application.

The available data show that both the time from collection to centrifugation and the age and sex of the patient have an impact on the quality and quantity of the PRF matrix [8]. Therefore, this study aimed to show that the connection of the biomaterial with autologous cells is possible via the involvement of APRF+ with fibroblasts in wound healing, which could support recovery, especially in people whose matrix alone would be insufficient for adequate healing, e.g., in diabetic patients and in the elderly. An ideal carrier should not affect the host's immunogenicity, and it should exhibit biocompatible properties. In turn, biodegradability should be associated with the vascularization of the recipient site and the implementation of cells, which will affect the reconstruction of the tissue defect. The used carriers with embedded signaling molecules stimulated the migration and proliferation of stem cells, thus supporting the regeneration of the target tissue. However, apart from stimulating the regeneration process, the authors would like to administer a finished product in place of a tissue deficit. Such a solution would also accelerate regeneration in immunodeficient patients by creating bipolarity.

## 5. Conclusions

To summarize, the conducted experimental study showed a significantly increased release of VEGF and an increased viability of conditioned fibroblasts after 72 h, resulting from the combination of APRF+ and autologous human gingival fibroblasts. The obtained results indicate that the tested product, i.e., APRF+ with cultured fibroblasts, may considerably enhance the healing of surgical wounds, which is especially important in patients for whom the healing process is more problematic.

**Limitations:** Our study was carried out on a group of six patients, which was not homogeneous in terms of sex, age, and the degree of immunodeficiency. However, a group of six objects is minimal for parametric statistical evaluation. The tests performed for the starting data showed a lack of outliers at the adopted level of statistical significance. The research will be continued, considering the purposeful selection of patients for homogeneous groups. However, in the present study, despite the heterogeneity of the research group, statistically significant trends and relationships were identified, indicating improvement in fibroblast proliferation.

**Author Contributions:** Conceptualization, B.S.; methodology, A.C., B.S., U.S., B.C. and M.K.; investigation, B.S. and A.C.; writing—original draft preparation, B.S.; writing—review and editing, A.C.,

B.S. and M.D.; visualization, A.C. and U.S.; supervision, M.D. All authors have read and agreed to the published version of the manuscript.

**Funding:** This research was funded by Wroclaw Medical University, Poland, project no. STM.B040.20.078; PI: B. Sterczała. The publication was prepared under the project financed from the funds granted by the Ministry of Science and Higher Education in the "Regional Initiative of Excellence" programme for the years 2019–2022, project number 016/RID/2018/19; the amount of funding: PLN 11 998 121.30.

**Institutional Review Board Statement:** Ethics Committee of Wroclaw Medical University, Poland (No. KB-434/2017).

**Informed Consent Statement:** Informed consent was obtained from all subjects involved in the study.

**Data Availability Statement:** The authors are familiar with MDPI Research Data Policies. The data that support the findings of this study are available from the corresponding author upon reasonable request.

**Acknowledgments:** The authors are very grateful to Jolanta Saczko and Julita Kulbacka from Wroclaw Medical University for their scientific input and assistance with this manuscript.

**Conflicts of Interest:** The authors declare no conflict of interest.

## References

1. Miron, R.J.; Bishara, M.; Choukroun, J. Basics of Platelet-Rich Fibrin Therapy. *Dent. Today* **2017**, *36*, 74–76. [PubMed]
2. Dohan, D.M.; Choukroun, J.; Diss, A.; Dohan, S.L.; Dohan, A.J.J.; Mouhyi, J.; Gogly, B. Platelet-Rich Fibrin (PRF): A Second-Generation Platelet Concentrate. Part I: Technological Concepts and Evolution. *Oral Surg. Oral Med. Oral Pathol. Oral Radiol. Endodontology* **2006**, *101*, e37–e44. [CrossRef]
3. Karimi, K.; Rockwell, H. The Benefits of Platelet-Rich Fibrin. *Facial Plast. Surg. Clin. N. Am.* **2019**, *27*, 331–340. [CrossRef]
4. Dohan, D.M.; Choukroun, J.; Diss, A.; Dohan, S.L.; Dohan, A.J.J.; Mouhyi, J.; Gogly, B. Platelet-Rich Fibrin (PRF): A Second-Generation Platelet Concentrate. Part II: Platelet-Related Biologic Features. *Oral Surg. Oral Med. Oral Pathol. Oral Radiol. Endod.* **2006**, *101*, e45–e50. [CrossRef]
5. Demling, R.H. The Role of Anabolic Hormones for Wound Healing in Catabolic States. *J. Burn. Wounds* **2005**, *4*, e2.
6. Miron, R.J.; Zucchelli, G.; Pikos, M.A.; Salama, M.; Lee, S.; Guillemette, V.; Fujioka-Kobayashi, M.; Bishara, M.; Zhang, Y.; Wang, H.L.; et al. Use of Platelet-Rich Fibrin in Regenerative Dentistry: A Systematic Review. *Clin. Oral Investig.* **2017**, *21*, 1913–1927. [CrossRef] [PubMed]
7. Marrelli, M.; Tatullo, M. Influence of PRF in the Healing of Bone and Gingival Tissues. Clinical and Histological Evaluations. *Eur. Rev. Med. Pharmacol. Sci.* **2013**, *17*, 1958–1962.
8. Ghanaati, S.; Booms, P.; Orlowska, A.; Kubesch, A.; Lorenz, J.; Rutkowski, J.; Les, C.; Sader, R.; Kirkpatrick, C.J.; Choukroun, J. Advanced Platelet-Rich Fibrin: A New Concept for Cell-Based Tissue Engineering by Means of Inflammatory Cells. *J. Oral Implantol.* **2014**, *40*, 679–689. [CrossRef]
9. Steller, D.; Herbst, N.; Pries, R.; Juhl, D.; Hakim, S.G. Positive Impact of Platelet-Rich Plasma and Platelet-Rich Fibrin on Viability, Migration and Proliferation of Osteoblasts and Fibroblasts Treated with Zoledronic Acid. *Sci. Rep.* **2019**, *9*, 8310. [CrossRef] [PubMed]
10. Fujioka-Kobayashi, M.; Miron, R.J.; Hernandez, M.; Kandalam, U.; Zhang, Y.; Choukroun, J. Optimized Platelet-Rich Fibrin With the Low-Speed Concept: Growth Factor Release, Biocompatibility, and Cellular Response. *J. Periodontol.* **2017**, *88*, 112–121. [CrossRef]
11. Choukroun, J.; Ghanaati, S. Reduction of Relative Centrifugation Force within Injectable Platelet-Rich-Fibrin (PRF) Concentrates Advances Patients' Own Inflammatory Cells, Platelets and Growth Factors: The First Introduction to the Low Speed Centrifugation Concept. *Eur. J. Trauma Emerg. Surg.* **2018**, *44*, 87–95. [CrossRef]
12. el Bagdadi, K.; Kubesch, A.; Yu, X.; Al-Maawi, S.; Orlowska, A.; Dias, A.; Booms, P.; Dohle, E.; Sader, R.; Kirkpatrick, C.J.; et al. Reduction of Relative Centrifugal Forces Increases Growth Factor Release within Solid Platelet-Rich-Fibrin (PRF)-Based Matrices: A Proof of Concept of LSCC (Low Speed Centrifugation Concept). *Eur. J. Trauma Emerg. Surg.* **2019**, *45*, 467–479. [CrossRef]
13. Dohan Ehrenfest, D.M.; de Peppo, G.M.; Doglioli, P.; Sammartino, G. Slow Release of Growth Factors and Thrombospondin-1 in Choukroun's Platelet-Rich Fibrin (PRF): A Gold Standard to Achieve for All Surgical Platelet Concentrates Technologies. *Growth Factors* **2009**, *27*, 63–69. [CrossRef] [PubMed]
14. Xie, J.; Bian, H.; Qi, S.; Xu, Y.; Tang, J.; Li, T.; Liu, X. Effects of Basic Fibroblast Growth Factor on the Expression of Extracellular Matrix and Matrix Metalloproteinase-1 in Wound Healing. *Clin. Exp. Dermatol.* **2008**, *33*, 176–182. [CrossRef] [PubMed]
15. Pitzurra, L.; Jansen, I.D.C.; Vries, T.J.; Hoogenkamp, M.A.; Loos, B.G. Effects of L-PRF and A-PRF+ on Periodontal Fibroblasts in in Vitro Wound Healing Experiments. *J. Periodontal Res.* **2020**, *55*, 287–295. [CrossRef] [PubMed]
16. Marx, R.E. Platelet-Rich Plasma (PRP): What Is PRP and What Is Not PRP? *Implant Dent.* **2001**, *10*, 225–228. [CrossRef]
17. Li, J.; Chen, J.; Kirsner, R. Pathophysiology of Acute Wound Healing. *Clin. Dermatol.* **2007**, *25*, 9–18. [CrossRef] [PubMed]
18. Gurtner, G.C.; Werner, S.; Barrandon, Y.; Longaker, M.T. Wound Repair and Regeneration. *Nature* **2008**, *453*, 314–321. [CrossRef]

19. Chaussain, C.; Septier, D.; Bonnefoix, M.; Lecolle, S.; Lebreton-Decoster, C.; Coulomb, B.; Pellat, B.; Godeau, G. Human Dermal and Gingival Fibroblasts in a Three-Dimensional Culture: A Comparative Study on Matrix Remodeling. *Clin. Oral Investig.* **2002**, *6*, 39–50. [CrossRef] [PubMed]
20. Dominiak, M.; Łysiak-Drwal, K.; Saczko, J.; Kunert-Keil, C.; Gedrange, T. The Clinical Efficacy of Primary Culture of Human Fibroblasts in Gingival Augmentation Procedures-A Preliminary Report. *Ann. Anat.* **2012**, *194*, 502–507. [CrossRef]
21. Rognoni, E.; Pisco, A.O.; Hiratsuka, T.; Sipilä, K.H.; Belmonte, J.M.; Mobasseri, S.A.; Philippeos, C.; Dilão, R.; Watt, F.M. Fibroblast State Switching Orchestrates Dermal Maturation and Wound Healing. *Mol. Syst. Biol.* **2018**, *14*, e8174. [CrossRef] [PubMed]
22. Jones, R.E.; Foster, D.S.; Longaker, M.T. Management of Chronic Wounds—2018. *JAMA—J. Am. Med. Assoc.* **2018**, *320*, 1481–1482. [CrossRef] [PubMed]
23. Knychalska-Karwan, Z. Anatomia i fizjologia narządu żucia u ludzi w podeszłym wieku. In *Stomatologia wieku podeszłego*, 1st ed.; Knychalska-Karwan, Z., Ed.; Czelej: Lublin, Polska, 2005; pp. 1–21.
24. Pham, T.A.V.; Nguyen, H.T.; Nguyen, M.T.; Trinh, V.N.; Tran, N.Y.; Ngo, L.T.; Tran, H.L. Platelet-Rich Fibrin Influences on Proliferation and Migration of Human Gingival Fibroblasts. *Int. J. Exp. Dent. Sci.* **2016**, *5*, 83–88. [CrossRef]
25. Mudalal, M.; Wang, Z.; Mustafa, S.; Liu, Y.; Wang, Y.; Yu, J.; Wang, S.; Sun, X.; Zhou, Y. Effect of Leukocyte-Platelet Rich Fibrin (L-PRF) on Tissue Regeneration and Proliferation of Human Gingival Fibroblast Cells Cultured Using a Modified Method. *Tissue Eng. Regen. Med.* **2021**, *18*, 895–904. [CrossRef]
26. Dor, Y.; Djonov, V.; Keshet, E. Induction of Vascular Networks in Adult Organs: Implications to Proangiogenic Therapy. *Ann. N. Y. Acad. Sci.* **2003**, *995*, 208–216. [CrossRef]
27. Cabaro, S.; D'Esposito, V.; Gasparro, R.; Borriello, F.; Granata, F.; Mosca, G.; Passaretti, F.; Sammartino, J.C.; Beguinot, F.; Sammartino, G.; et al. White Cell and Platelet Content Affects the Release of Bioactive Factors in Different Blood-Derived Scaffolds. *Platelets* **2018**, *29*, 463–467. [CrossRef] [PubMed]
28. Hinz, B. The Role of Myofibroblasts in Wound Healing. *Curr. Res. Transl. Med.* **2016**, *64*, 171–177. [CrossRef]
29. Arora, P.D.; Narani, N.; McCulloch, C.A.G. The Compliance of Collagen Gels Regulates Transforming Growth Factor-β Induction of α-Smooth Muscle Actin in Fibroblasts. *Am. J. Pathol.* **1999**, *154*, 871–882. [CrossRef]
30. Hata, Y.; Kawanabe, H.; Hisanaga, Y.; Taniguchi, K.; Ishikawa, H. Effects of Basic Fibroblast Growth Factor Administration on Vascular Changes in Wound Healing of Rat Palates. *Cleft Palate-Craniofac. J.* **2008**, *45*, 63–72. [CrossRef]
31. Oda, Y.; Kagami, H.; Ueda, M. Accelerating Effects of Basic Fibroblast Growth Factor on Wound Healing of Rat Palatal Mucosa. *J. Oral Maxillofac. Surg.* **2004**, *62*, 73–80. [CrossRef]
32. Lin, Z.; Nica, C.; Sculean, A.; Asparuhova, M.B. Enhanced Wound Healing Potential of Primary Human Oral Fibroblasts and Periodontal Ligament Cells Cultured on Four Different Porcine-Derived Collagen Matrices. *Materials* **2020**, *13*, 3819. [CrossRef]
33. Coelho, N.M.; Arora, P.D.; van Putten, S.; Boo, S.; Petrovic, P.; Lin, A.X.; Hinz, B.; McCulloch, C.A. Discoidin Domain Receptor 1 Mediates Myosin-Dependent Collagen Contraction. *Cell Rep.* **2017**, *18*, 1774–1790. [CrossRef] [PubMed]
34. Masuki, H.; Okudera, T.; Watanebe, T.; Suzuki, M.; Nishiyama, K.; Okudera, H.; Nakata, K.; Uematsu, K.; Su, C.-Y.; Kawase, T. Growth Factor and Pro-Inflammatory Cytokine Contents in Platelet-Rich Plasma (PRP), Plasma Rich in Growth Factors (PRGF), Advanced Platelet-Rich Fibrin (A-PRF), and Concentrated Growth Factors (CGF). *Int. J. Implant Dent.* **2016**, *2*, 19. [CrossRef] [PubMed]
35. Lim, W.F.; Inoue-Yokoo, T.; Tan, K.S.; Lai, M.I.; Sugiyama, D. Hematopoietic Cell Differentiation from Embryonic and Induced Pluripotent Stem Cells. *Stem Cell Res. Ther.* **2013**, *4*, 71. [CrossRef] [PubMed]

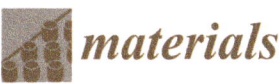

Article

# A New Anorganic Equine Bone Substitute for Oral Surgery: Structural Characterization and Regenerative Potential

Alessandro Addis [1], Elena Canciani [2], Marino Campagnol [1], Matteo Colombo [3], Christian Frigerio [3], Daniele Recupero [3], Claudia Dellavia [2] and Marco Morroni [3,*]

1. CRABCC Animal Lab, Biotechnology Research Center for Cardiothoracic Applications, Rivolta d'Adda, 26027 Cremona, Italy; alessandro.addis@crabcc.com (A.A.); marino.campagnol@unimi.it (M.C.)
2. Department of Biomedical Surgical and Dental Sciences, Università degli Studi di Milano, 20122 Milan, Italy; elena.canciani@unimi.it (E.C.); claudia.dellavia@unimi.it (C.D.)
3. Bioteck S.p.A., Arcugnano, 36057 Vicenza, Italy; m.colombo@bioteck.com (M.C.); c.frigerio@bioteck.biz (C.F.); d.recupero@bioteck.biz (D.R.)
* Correspondence: m.morroni@bioteck.com

**Abstract:** Different xenogeneic inorganic bone substitutes are currently used as bone grafting materials in oral and maxillo-facial surgery. The aim of the present study was to determine the physicochemical properties and the in vivo performance of an anorganic equine bone (AEB) substitute. AEB is manufactured by applying a process involving heating at >300 °C with the aim of removing all the antigens and the organic components. AEB was structurally characterized by scanning electron microscopy (SEM), X-ray diffraction (XRD), X-ray fluorescence (XRF), and Fourier-transformed infrared (FT-IR) spectroscopy and compared to the anorganic bovine bone (ABB). In order to provide a preliminary evaluation of the in vivo performance of AEB, 18 bone defects were prepared and grafted with AEB (nine sites), or ABB (nine sites) used as a control, in nine Yucatan Minipigs. De novo bone formation, residual bone substitute, as well as local inflammatory and tissue effects were histologically evaluated at 30 and 90 days after implantation. The structural characterization showed that the surface morphology, particle size, chemical composition, and crystalline structure of AEB were similar to cancellous human bone. The histological examination of AEB showed a comparable pattern of newly formed bone and residual biomaterial to that of ABB. Overall, the structural data and pre-clinical evidence reported in the present study suggests that AEB can be effectively used as bone grafting material in oral surgery procedures.

**Keywords:** equine bone substitute; bone formation; xenograft; anorganic bone

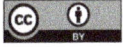

## 1. Introduction

Presently, bone grafting is a major treatment modality in oral surgery for bone volume preservation as well as for augmentation procedures [1].

An ideal bone graft should foster natural healing through osteoconductive, osteoinductive, and osteogenic mechanisms, be biocompatible, and not evoke any inflammatory response. In addition, it should be sterilizable and readily available at a reasonable cost [2]. It has been widely described in the literature that materials that feature slow resorption kinetics, without disturbing the natural bone remodeling process occurring around them, are able to obtain positive clinical results and a long-term volume stability [3,4]. Morphology, particle size, and chemical composition of a bone graft material (as largely determined by its production process) significantly influence its resorption rate [4]. Therefore, a better and more comprehensive understanding of its physicochemical properties seems necessary to achieve predictable biological and clinical response. Among the different available augmentation materials, autologous bone still represents the gold standard for bone regeneration [2,5] but has several disadvantages, including limited availability, the need for an additional surgery, and potential donor site morbidity [6,7]. Its limitations have stimulated the search for alternative solutions, and currently many alternative bone substitutes, either natural or synthetic, are available in clinical practice [8]. Among natural materials, xenogeneic bone grafts (derived from mammals' species) are the most common bone substitutes utilized clinically, due to their ready availability and their similarity to human bone regarding chemical composition and structure [9]. Indeed, among mammals, bovine bone was the first considered due to its high availability. To avoid unwanted immunological reactions and any risk of cross-infections, xenogeneic bone grafts undergo specific treatments of deantigenation and sterilization [7,8].

Among these processes, thermal treatment is one of the most used, and it is often applied on bovine bone, but also on porcine bone [10–12]. The elevated temperature applied (between 300 and 1200 °C depending on the different processes) [13] neutralizes the antigenic components while maintaining the natural architecture of the bone [7,8]. The output is an anorganic bone hydroxyapatite with physicochemical properties favorably associated with bone repairing osteogenesis and osseous growth [14–18].

One of the best-characterized xenogeneic bone substitutes obtained through thermal treatment is anorganic bovine bone (ABB). Indeed, ABB is characterized by a macro- and micro-porous structure similar to human cancellous bone [19,20], which serves as physical scaffold for the migration of bone-forming cells and provides an optimal microenvironment for bone ingrowth [21]. It is resorbed slowly, supporting the process of natural bone remodeling around it [15,22,23]. Clinically, its biocompatibility, stability, and long-term efficacy have been widely demonstrated in most varied indications, including ridge preservation, bone augmentation, and periodontal regeneration [14–18,24].

As with bovine bone, equine bone displays high similarity with human bone [25,26]. Moreover, equine bone has some additional advantages such as the absence of ethical issues and the intrinsic stability of its proteins that exclude the equine from the prion transmitting species as stated by the European Commission Regulation N. 722/2012 of 8 August 2012 [27]. Recently, an anorganic equine bone (AEB) that is subject to similar manufacturing process has been introduced in the market. AEB is produced by treating the cancellous equine bone with a very high temperature to eliminate all the organic components (including bone collagen) and to achieve a controlled decarbonation of the apatite crystals. So far, no studies investigating the chemical and biological properties of this novel biomaterial have been published.

The aim of the present study was to assess the physicochemical and structural properties of AEB, as well as its in vivo performance in an animal model of mandibular bony defects.

## 2. Materials and Methods

### 2.1. Materials

Anorganic equine bone (AEB, Calcitos®—Bioteck S.p.A., Arcugnano, Vicenza, Italy) particles are derived from cancellous bone of equine origin. The product is sterilized by beta-irradiation at 25 kGy.

Anorganic bovine bone (ABB, Bio-Oss®—Geistlich Pharma AG, Wolhusen, Switzerland) is bovine-derived and its sterilization takes place with the application of gamma-irradiation [22]. Both AEB and ABB particles are obtained through a proprietary extraction process that involves treatment with strong alkalis and solvents under high-temperature processing of >350 °C [13].

Because of the large number of publications describing the properties and the clinical performances of ABB, it has been used as benchmark in the different test performed in the present study.

### 2.2. Physicochemical and Morphological Characterization

Morphological characterization and measurement of the particle size of the materials were carried out through scanning electron microscopy (SEM; Phenom XL, Phenom-World, Eindhoven, The Netherlands) operating at a range of 4.8 kV to 20.5 kV or at 5 kV of electron acceleration, respectively. The sample was placed in a holder composed of conductive carbon and golden surface, and the image was obtained by backscattering radiation. Morphological analysis was performed using Scanning Electron Microscope XL Phenom combined with software 3D Roughness Reconstruction (Phenom-World, Eindhoven, The Netherlands). The diameters of the particles acquired from each SEM image were measured using the embedded image analysis software (Phenom Pro Suite/Fibermetric). Every particle was measured using the approach of the medium diameter, intended as the dimension visually equivalent at the diameter of the particle if its visible surface is a circle. To ensure the representativeness of the particle distribution, the counting was done on all the particles attached, during the preparation procedures, on two different conductive carbon supports, each one with a diameter of 20 mm. The number of particles on each filter is random and, for this sample type, not directly connected with the particle size.

X-ray diffraction experiments were performed in order to identify the crystalline phases in the xenografts by using ARL X'TRA X-ray diffraction (Thermo Fisher Scientific, Waltham, USA) with Cu–K$\alpha$ ray (45 kV, 40 mA). Spectra were recorded in the 2$\theta$ range of 4°–60° at a step size of 0.010° and a step time of 0.40 min.

An X-ray fluorescence (XRF) spectrometer (SPECTRO XEPOS 3, AMETEK, Berwyn, Germany) was used to quantify the elemental chemical composition of the biomaterials. The data were acquired with an axial wavelength dispersive XRF unit.

Both ABB and AEB were analyzed via infrared spectroscopy using a Cary 630 FT-IR (Agilent Technologies, Santa Clara, CA, USA) instrument with an ATR module. Spectrum window was collected from 800 to 3800 cm$^{-1}$ with a resolution of 2 cm$^{-1}$. A qualitative analysis of the spectra was then performed by comparing the wavenumber of the most significant peaks with that of a reference wavenumber library, in order to identify the main functional molecular groups.

### 2.3. Animals

Nine adult (20–24 months) Yucatan Minipigs, belonging to the same progeny, were used in the study. Animal experimentation was conducted in compliance with ISO 10993-2, European Directive 2010/63 EU, and D.Lg 26/2014, the Italian Law on the protection of animals used for scientific purposes.

### 2.4. Study Protocol and Randomization

The present study was designed as a randomized-controlled experimental study. In order to provide a preliminary evaluation of the performance of AEB and ABB, a total of 18 mandibular bone defects were prepared and grafted with AEB (nine sites), or ABB (nine sites) in nine Yucatan Minipigs. Each animal provided two grafting sites; one site was grafted with ABB, the other with AEB. Animals were divided into two groups to allow the subsequent evaluation of device resorption time, amount of newly formed bone, and local inflammation effects at two different time-points (30 and 90 days after surgery). At each time-point, animals were sacrificed (four animals at 30 days and five animals at 90 days), and bioptic samples at each grafting site were collected and histologically evaluated.

### 2.5. Grafting Surgical Procedure

The surgical procedure was performed under sterile conditions. General anesthesia was induced by intramuscular injection of ketamine (10 mg/kg) and midazolam (0.5 mg/kg), followed by administration of an oxygen and isoflurane mixture through a mechanical respirator. Anesthesia was maintained with a mixture of isoflurane 3.5% and oxygen 100%.

Through subangular incisions, the lateral portion of the mandibular body and ramus were exposed enough to allow the preparation of two standardized intraosseous defects. Defects measuring 5 mm in diameter and 5 mm in depth were prepared using a trephine with copious saline irrigation. Each defect was filled with AEB or ABB and covered with a pericardium membrane (Heart®, Bioteck S.p.A., Arcugnano, Vicenza, Italy). Finally, surgical sites were closed in multiple layers using a resorbable suture. Each step of the surgical procedure was documented by a complete set of images (Supplemental Figure S1).

All the animals were constantly monitored for 72 h after the surgery in order to assess their correct physiological recovery.

*2.6. Sampling and Histological Preparation*

Animals were sacrificed by intra-venous administration of potassium chloride saturated solution, and the samples were collected at 30 and 90 days after surgery. Biopsies of each grafting site were harvested using a 10 × 4 mm diameter trephine bur, placing the trephine at the center of the defect and collecting a bone core including basal bone and the grafting tissue for the entire depth of the defect. Each sample was fixed in buffered 10% formalin, decalcified by Osteodec (Bio Optica, Milano, Italy), dehydrated in ascending alcohol scale infiltrated, and finally embedded in paraffin (Bio-Plast, Bio Optica, Milano, Italy). Three serial longitudinal sections of 6 μm were obtained in the central portion of the block with a microtome (Leica Biosystems, Milano, Italy) and stained with Carazzi's Hematoxylin and Eosin in order to perform morphological and histomorphometric analysis.

Images of the samples were captured using high-resolution digital scanner Aperio CS2 (Leica Biosystems, Milano, Italy) and analyzed with Image Scope software (Leica Biosystems, Milano, Italy).

*2.7. Histological Measurements*

On each section, a counting grid was used to evaluate the intersection points that fall down on each kind of tissue (regenerated bone, biomaterial, and soft tissue) using the software ImageScope (Leica Biosystems, Milano, Italy). The volume fractions percentage was obtained by the ratio between the intersection points that fall down on each type of tissue and the total intersection points. Implant sites were examined for cell type/response in terms of typing of inflammatory cells and inflammatory infiltrate, in the grafted area (polymorphonuclear cells, lymphocytes, macrophages, plasma cells, giant cells, and necrosis), and tissue response observing neovascularization, fibrosis, and fatty infiltrate in the grafted area. In brief, following ISO 10993-6:2007, Annex E, an experienced pathologist examined 10 photos for each slide at a magnification of 400× in order to evaluate all parameters by using an objective score system in the microscopic field. In each section, a global score between 0 (absence of cells/absence of tissues response) and 4 (packed cells/extensive presence of tissue response) was given to each parameter at all time-points, and the mean value for each sample was given [28].

*2.8. Statistical Analysis of Cellular Content of Histological Samples*

Quantitative variables were summarized as mean ± standard errors for each biomaterial at every time point, considering all histomorphometrical parameters. The characteristics were compared at every time point between biomaterials with the Mann–Whitney test for paired data and then a non-parametric longitudinal analysis was processed using the nparLD R package [29]. The p-values were adjusted for multiple comparisons with the Bonferroni method. All p-values were 2-tailed, with statistical significance set at <0.05. Analyses were performed using R software (version 3.3.2) for Windows.

### 3. Results

*3.1. Physicochemical and Morphological Characterization of AEB*

Optical microscopy observations showed that AEB consisted of particles with similar shape, having some portions rounded and others derived by fragmentation. Some particles had circular holes of variable size (Figure 1). The SEM analysis of AEB showed that the particles had irregular shape and fragmented surfaces (Figure 2A,B). At higher magnifications, bone surfaces presented areas with generally visible stratification, with some inner portions appearing more compact and apparently without stratification (Figure 2C–F). ABB was characterized by a regular arrangement of fibers of the same height, and vacuoles of different diameters but comparable depths (Figure 2H,J). AEB showed a less regular fibrous pattern, with fibers of variable size and orientation, but equal height (Figure 2G,I). Vacuoles were also observed on AEB particles.

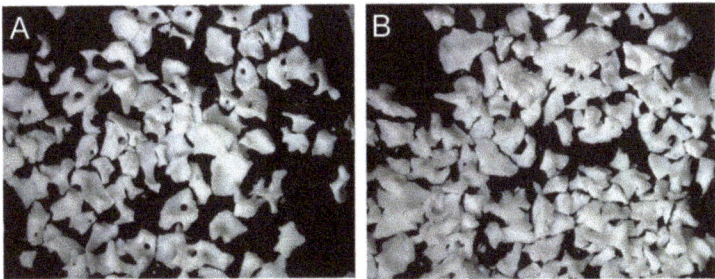

**Figure 1.** AEB (**A**) and ABB (**B**) particles observed with a stereo microscope.

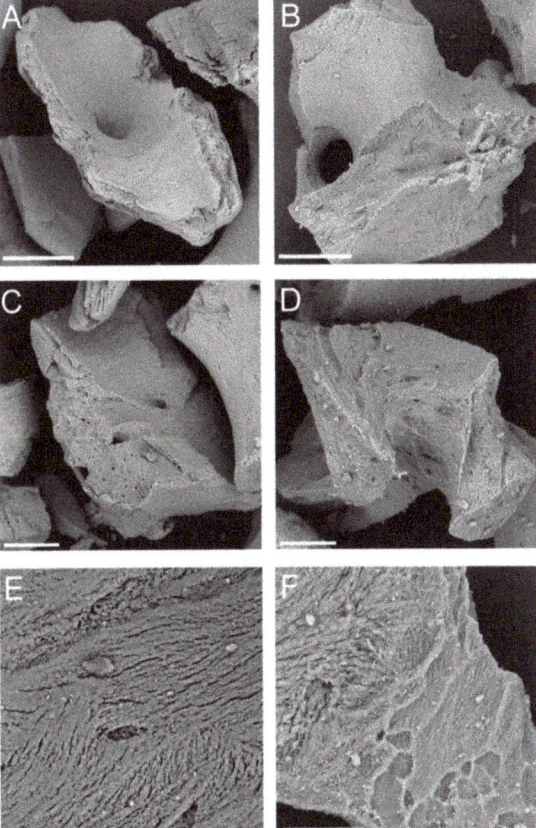

**Figure 2.** *Cont.*

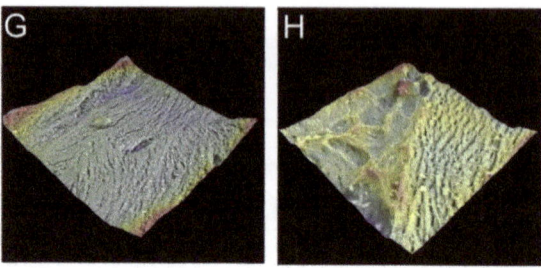

**Figure 2.** SEM images (**A–F**) and 3D surface reconstruction (**G,H**) of AEB (**A,C,E,G**) and ABB (**B,D,F,H**). Scale bars: (**A,B**): 200 µm; (**C,D**): 100 µm; (**E,F**): 30 µm.

For particles size analysis, a total of 777 and 1240 particles were analyzed for AEB and ABB, respectively. The prevalent particle size of AEB was 0.60 mm (range, 0.120–1.64 mm), which was similar to that of ABB (prevalent diameter, 0.58 mm; range, 0.11–1.54 mm) (Figure 3). The 90% of particle size of both AEB and ABB was between 0.2 mm and 1.0 mm.

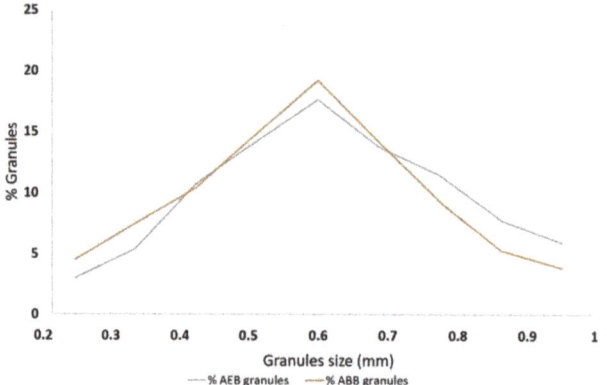

**Figure 3.** Graphical representation of the granule size distribution of AEB and ABB measured with SEM. On the $x$-axis the granules size in shown in millimeters, whereas on $y$-axis is shown the percentage of granules for each size.

X-ray diffractometry was qualitatively used to compare the crystalline structure of the biomaterials. The XRD spectra of AEB and ABB were almost superimposable and they showed the characteristics peaks of hydroxyapatite three-dimensional structure (Figure 4).

The determination of elements constituting the bone grafts was then carried out by X-ray fluorescence elemental analysis of the particles. The XRF analysis showed no substantial differences in the chemical composition of the two samples (Table 1). In both biomaterials, the most abundant elements were calcium and phosphorus (Table 1).

Sample characterization was complemented by Fourier transform infrared spectroscopy. Figure 5 presents the FT-IR spectra. Symmetric vibration bending or stretching of the absorption bands can be observed for the C-O bond at wavenumbers of 1450, 1415, and 874 cm$^{-1}$, which can be attributed to $CO_3^{2-}$ (carbonate ions type B). The band at 962 cm$^{-1}$ is part of the symmetric and asymmetric deformation modes of ν 4 O-OP, whereas the absorption bands in the range of 1020–1087 cm$^{-1}$ correspond to the ν 3 P-O [30–32].

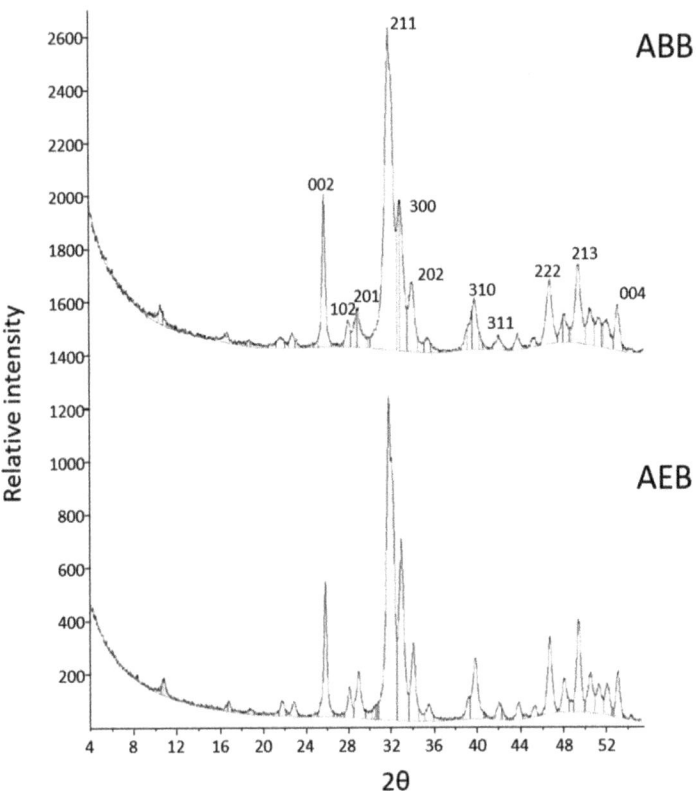

**Figure 4.** The XRD spectra obtained for ABB (**top**) and AEB (**bottom**). Both biomaterials show the typical peaks of hydroxyapatite.

**Table 1.** Abundance of the elements detected by XRF in the two samples. Limit of quantification (<LoQ) was 0.01 g/100 g.

| Element | Abundance in AEB (g/100 g) | Abundance in ABB (g/100 g) |
| --- | --- | --- |
| Aluminium | 0.14 | 0.12 |
| Barium | <LoQ | 0.03 |
| Calcium | 34.95 | 34.99 |
| Phosphorus | 13.15 | 12.48 |
| Magnesium | 0.82 | 0.71 |
| Strontium | 0.04 | 0.04 |
| Zinc | 0.02 | <LoQ |
| Sulphur | 0.02 | <LoQ |

Not detected in both samples (<LoQ): antimony, silver, arsenic, bromine, cadmium, cobalt, chrome, iron, iodine, manganese, mercury, molybdenum, nickel, lead, potassium, copper, selenium, silicon, sodium, tin, thallium, tellurium, titanium, tungsten, vanadium, zirconium.

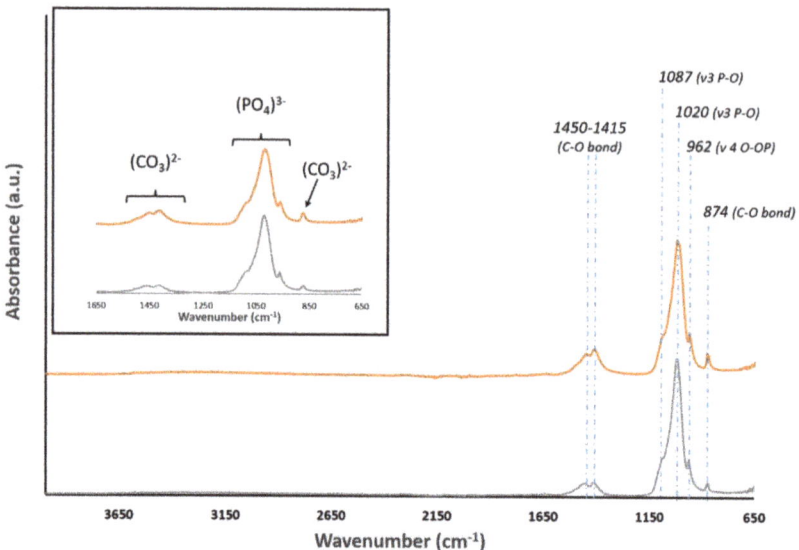

**Figure 5.** FTIR spectra of ABB (orange) and AEB (gray). Samples of both biomaterials exhibit main peaks around 1450–1415, 1020, 962, and 874 cm$^{-1}$.

*3.2. Resorption, New Bone Formation, and Local Effects after Implantation of AEB and ABB in an Animal Model*

In order to evaluate the performance of the two biomaterials, a total amount of 18 bone defects were prepared and grafted with AEB (nine sites), or ABB (nine sites). Device resorption time, amount of newly formed bone, and local inflammation effects were evaluated at 30 and 90 days after surgery.

At the histological examination, with both types of grafts, the biomaterial granules appeared surrounded by a considerable quantity of mineralized matrix at different stages of mineralization (Figure 6). At 30 days, both ABB and AEB particles seemed to be included in a thin layer of osteoid or woven bone (Figure 6). At 90 days several areas of regenerated lamellar bone appeared in both groups (Figure 6), even if a large variability was found between specimens, thus indicating a still ongoing remodeling/regeneration process. In all sites the grafted particles were still present after 90 days from application.

In both groups the regenerated bone significantly increased over time from 30 to 90 days after surgery ($p < 0.001$) with no significant differences ($p > 0.05$) between ABB and AEB for all time points considered (Figure 7A, top). When considering the residual particles, the percentage of remnants decreased significantly with time (Figure 7B; $p < 0.0001$); a similar trend was found in the two groups. No statistical differences in the percentage of residual particles between groups were observed at the time points considered (Figure 7B; $p > 0.05$).

The assessment of the host response after implantation of biomaterials showed similar local effects in the two experimental groups. In all sites a small inflammatory infiltrate was observed, especially at 30 days, and then diminished at the second time-point (Table 2). The infiltrate was mainly characterized by rare polymorphonuclear cells and rare lymphocytes. Only in some specimens a few plasma cells and macrophages were detected, and no giant cells were seen. At each time point, no significant difference was observed in the number of inflammatory cells in samples grafted with either ABB or AEB (Table 2). Also, no necrotic areas were observed. The tissue response demonstrated a complete absence of fatty infiltrate in all sites of both groups (Table 3). A fibrotic reaction consisting of a moderately thick band was detected in two sites at 30 days, one in ABB and one in AEB.

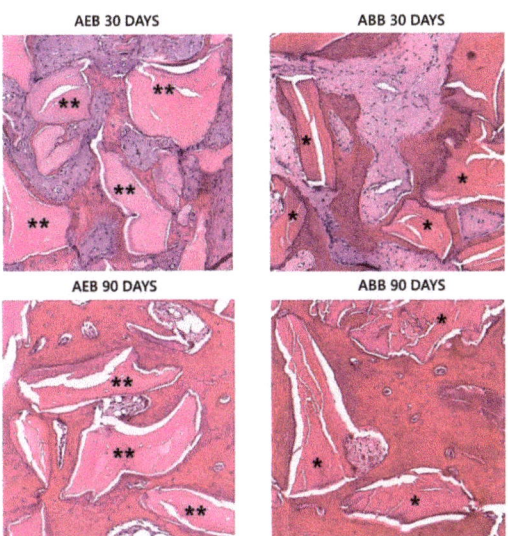

**Figure 6.** Histological examination of grafted particles at 30 and 90 days from regenerative procedure. At 30 days AEB (\*\*) and ABB (\*) particles were surrounded by a thin layer of newly formed bone. At 90 days AEB (\*\*) and ABB (\*) particles appeared integrated in extended bony islands.

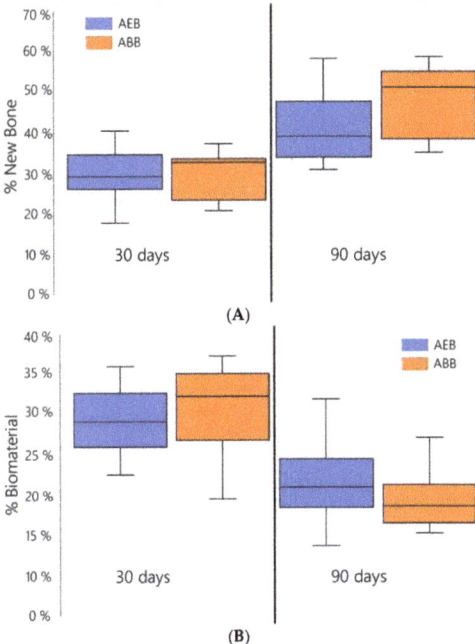

**Figure 7.** Box plot representation of the percentage of newly formed bone ((**A**) top panel) and of residual biomaterial ((**B**) bottom panel) in samples that were grafted with AEB or with ABB. No statistical differences are present between the two biomaterials.

Table 2. Average histological scores of inflammatory data in AEB and ABB specimens.

| Time Points | AEB | ABB |
|---|---|---|
| | Polymorphonuclear cells | |
| 30 days | 1.25 ± 0.5 | 1 ± 0 |
| 90 days | 0.89 ± 0.3 | 0.66 ± 0.2 |
| | Lymphocytes | |
| 30 days | 1 ± 0.5 | 0.75 ± 0.5 |
| 90 days | 0.44 ± 0.5 | 0.5 ± 0.5 |
| | Macrophages | |
| 30 days | 0.63 ± 0.5 | 0.25 ± 0.5 |
| 90 days | 0.44 ± 0.5 | 0.17 ± 0.4 |
| | Plasma cells | |
| 30 days | 0 ± 0 | 0.25 ± 0.25 |
| 90 days | 0 ± 0 | 0 ± 0 |
| | Giant cells | |
| 30 days | 0 ± 0 | 0 ± 0 |
| 90 days | 0 ± 0 | 0 ± 0 |
| | Necrosis | |
| 30 days | 0 ± 0 | 0 ± 0 |
| 90 days | 0 ± 0 | 0 ± 0 |

Scores were assigned to each specimen on a scale of 0–5 according to ISO 10993-6:2007(E). Shown are the means ± SD. All comparisons between groups at 30 and 90 days are not significant ($p > 0.05$; Wilcoxon signed rank test with continuity correction).

Table 3. Average histological scores of soft tissue response in AEB and ABB specimens.

| Time Points | AEB | ABB |
|---|---|---|
| | Adipose tissue | |
| 30 days | 0 ± 0 | 0 ± 0 |
| 90 days | 0 ± 0 | 0 ± 0 |
| | Fibrosis | |
| 30 days | 0.25 ± 0.70 | 0.5 ± 1 |
| 90 days | 0 ± 0 | 0 ± 0 |
| | Neovascularization | |
| 30 days | 1 ± 0 | 1.5 ± 0.6 |
| 90 days | 1 ± 0 | 1 ± 0 |

Scores were assigned to each specimen on a scale of 0–5 according to ISO 10993-6:2007(E). Shown are the means ± SD. Adipose tissue, fibrosis, and neovascularization scores are not significantly different between groups at 30 and 90 days ($p > 0.05$; Wilcoxon signed rank test with continuity correction).

Considering the neovascularization, both groups showed a minimal proliferation with focal buds of capillaries, and only in a few cases larger vessels with supporting fibroblastic structures were observed, with no statistical differences between groups.

## 4. Discussion

Bone availability is the main prerequisite for safe and predictable outcomes in oral-maxillofacial procedures. However, it can be hindered by bone resorption, which is commonly observed following tooth extraction or tooth loss or can be the result of trauma, pathologies, inflammatory conditions, or chronic/acute infections [33]. Bone grafting may therefore be required in order to either preserve or achieve adequate bone levels. Among xenogeneic bone grafts, mammal species are becoming more and more relevant in regenerative dentistry. They are highly osteoconductive as the three-dimensional structure is similar to that of the human bone and present the advantages that are readily available at reduced costs, are easy to handle, and are slowly resorbed and replaced by the patient's bone [5,6]. In order to eliminate immunological problems, the bone origin tissue is made non-antigenic using different kind of treatments, namely chemical, enzyme-based, or thermal. Depending on the deantigenation method employed, the resulting bone substitute has different physicochemical and biological features. Whereas the chemical and enzyme-based deantigenation methods generate collagenic bone substitutes showing a high ratio of remodeling with the patient's bone [34,35], the bone substitutes obtained with a thermal treatment (commonly known as anorganic bone) feature a slower replacement with patient's bone [36–38]. This seems to be related to a non-physiological recognition by the osteoclasts due to the absence of collagen and/or to physical alteration of the natural bone hydroxyapatite [3] due to the extremely high temperatures applied.

From a clinical point of view, several studies have shown that the anorganic bovine bone (ABB) integrates well with newly formed tissue and can be successfully used in different clinical applications, including ridge preservation, bone augmentation, and periodontal regeneration [7,8,14–16,23].

Recently, an anorganic equine bone (AEB) graft prepared by a high-temperature deproteinizing technique was introduced on the market. Since materials of equine origins may offer protection against iatrogenic prion disease transmission, there are no safety or ethical concerns regarding the use of AEB [39]. The purpose of this study concerns the determination of the morphological and physicochemical features of AEB, as well as its in vivo performance in an animal model of mandibular bony defects. As a control, the same types of analyses were performed on ABB, which has been present on the market for a long time, and its biophysical and clinical features are well documented in the literature [10,12].

The findings of the present study showed that AEB and ABB granules have an average diameter of 0.6–0.58 mm, with the majority of particles between 0.2 mm and 1.0 These data are in agreement with the data provided by the respective manufacturers (0.25–1 mm granule size). The electron microscopy images clearly identify the typical features of xenogeneic bone graft obtained by heat treatment. In particular, Figure 2 shows similar macropores and micropores in AEB and ABB, which may support new blood vessels colonization. The pore structure serves as physical scaffold for the migration of bone-forming cells [40,41]. Interestingly, it was previously reported that ABB exhibits a porosity of 70–75%, which promotes osteoconduction, enabling bone ingrowth into the inner part of the graft [19].

The crystallinity grade of AEB and ABB was assessed with XRD, which showed the typical peaks of hydroxyapatite [19]. To confirm the chemical composition of AEB, FT-IR analysis was performed, showing the bands associated with the chemical group of hydroxyapatite. The data analyzed showed the presence of phosphate ions at 1019 $cm^{-1}$ and of the carbonate group at 1418 $cm^{-1}$ and 875 $cm^{-1}$, in agreement with the literature describing the heat treatment output of xenogeneic bone substitutes [42]. The same bands were detected for ABB. As expected, elemental chemical analysis through XRF revealed calcium and phosphorus as the main components of both AEB and ABB, with magnesium as a minor impurity. It is worth noting that both AEB and ABB showed a Ca/P ratio above 2, where the theoretical value of Ca/P ratio of hydroxyapatite is 1.67 [43]. This result is not surprising, as it was already reported that an exchange of phosphate groups with carbonate groups can occur during the heating procedure [31]. This is shown by the carbonate peaks observed in the FT-IR spectra for both samples. A slight discrepancy emerged in the composition of trace elements between AEB and ABB. This is not surprising, as ion exchange can take place in the apatite component of the bone. Therefore, the composition of trace element varies considerably depending on some biological factors, such as nutrition and the turnover rate of the mineral [44].

Altogether, these findings confirm that the biophysical features of AEB are in agreement with that of the xenogeneic bone substitutes treated with high temperature and already described in literature [42]. Thus, one can expect a similar effectiveness in the repair of bone defects.

As proof of concept, the in vivo performance of AEB and ABB were evaluated in Yucatan mini-pigs. A randomized-controlled experimental study was conducted to measure the proportion of newly formed bone and remaining particles in standardized mandibular bony defects at 30 and 90 days after implantation. Even if the results must be considered as preliminary, due to the number of defects analyzed, a significant increase amount of newly formed bone was observed during time with both biomaterials. Considering the resorption rate, sites grafted with both materials showed a comparable progressive degradation pattern at the two time points considered. Local effects assessment showed a slight inflammatory and a minimal tissue response in all sites and at both time points, with no statistical differences between AEB and ABB, suggesting a neutral interaction of the grafted particles with the newly generated bone tissue.

This study, consistent with other works [37,45,46], confirmed that the use of ABB as a grafting material yielded a bone formation with no presence of inflammatory cell infiltrate. As the physicochemical structure affects the biological performance of the material [47,48], it is worthwhile considering that the similar manufacturing process could have an impact on the in vivo biomaterial behavior. In this respect, both materials exhibited a slow resorption rate as demonstrated by the observation of residual particles 90 days after surgery. In the literature there are several clinical studies showing a slower degradation of heat-treated xenogeneic bone substitutes, with the residual particles persisting in the grafted sites even years after biomaterial application [36,38,49]. As already noted, the interaction between osteoclasts and bone substitutes seems to be one central part of bone resorption. Solubility, microscopic structure, surface morphology, and physicochemical features have been proposed as regulators of osteoclastic adhesion and activity [3]. Based on these data, a better understanding of in vitro human osteoclasts behaviour when in contact with AEB would strengthen the correlation of the manufacturing process with the biological performance of the bone substitute.

## 5. Conclusions

In conclusion, the overall structural and physicochemical properties and pre-clinical evidence reported in the present study indicates that AEB has the typical features of heat-treated xenogeneic bone substitutes. Thus, it is reasonable to expect that AEB would yield similar results as other heat-treated xenogeneic bone substitutes in oral surgery procedures, and that it can be effectively used as bone grafting material. Further clinical studies are required to confirm this.

**Supplementary Materials:** The following are available online at https://www.mdpi.com/article/10.3390/ma15031031/s1, Figure S1: Example of surgical pictures taken during the surgery: performing of surgical defects (A), grafting with the devices under investigation and protection of the grafting with pericardium membrane (B), suturing (C), opening of the surgical sites after specific time points (D), collection of bone samples (E), and storing of bone cores in 10% formalin (F).

**Author Contributions:** Conceptualization, M.M.; Methodology, A.A., C.D., M.M., C.F. and D.R.; software, A.A., C.D., E.C., C.F., M.C. (Matteo Colombo); Formal Analysis, A.A., C.D., E.C., M.M., M.C. (Matteo Colombo) and C.F.; Validation, M.M., C.D., M.C. (Matteo Colombo) and C.F.; Investigation, M.M., M.C. (Matteo Colombo), C.F., D.R.; Resources, none; Data curation, C.D., E.C., C.F., D.R., M.M. and M.C. (Matteo Colombo); writing—Original draft preparation, A.A., C.D., M.M.; Writing—review and editing, M.M., C.F., C.D., E.C. and M.C. (Matteo Colombo); Visualization, M.C. (Matteo Colombo); supervision, M.M.; Project administration, M.M.; Funding acquisition, M.M. All authors have read and agreed to the published version of the manuscript.

**Funding:** This research was funded by Bioteck SPA.

**Institutional Review Board Statement:** The animal experiments were conducted in 2013 according to the guidelines of the Declaration of Helsinki, and approved by the applicable Italian Law for animal studies of the 27th of January of 1992, n° 116.

**Data Availability Statement:** Data sharing is not applicable for this article.

**Conflicts of Interest:** Matteo Colombo, Daniele Recupero, Christian Frigerio, and Marco Morroni work for Bioteck S.p.A..

## References

1. Zizzari, V.L.; Zara, S.; Tete, G.; Vinci, R.; Gherlone, E.; Cataldi, A. Biologic and clinical aspects of integration of different bone substitutes in oral surgery: A literature review. *Oral Surg. Oral Med. Oral Pathol. Oral Radiol.* **2016**, *122*, 392–402. [CrossRef] [PubMed]
2. Misch, C.M. Maxillary autogenous bone grafting. *Oral Maxillofac. Surg. Clin. N. Am.* **2011**, *23*, 229–238. [CrossRef] [PubMed]
3. Perrotti, V.; Nicholls, B.M.; Horton, M.A.; Piattelli, A. Human osteoclast formation and activity on a xenogenous bone mineral. *J. Biomed. Mater. Res. Part A* **2009**, *90*, 238–246. [CrossRef] [PubMed]
4. Russmueller, G.; Winkler, L.; Lieber, R.; Seemann, R.; Pirklbauer, K.; Perisanidis, C.; Kapeller, B.; Spassova, E.; Halwax, E.; Poeschl, W.P.; et al. In Vitro effects of particulate bone substitute materials on the resorption activity of human osteoclasts. *Eur. Cells Mater.* **2017**, *34*, 291–306. [CrossRef] [PubMed]
5. Sakkas, A.; Wilde, F.; Heufelder, M.; Winter, K.; Schramm, A. Autogenous bone grafts in oral implantology-is it still a "gold standard"? A consecutive review of 279 patients with 456 clinical procedures. *Int. J. Implant Dent.* **2017**, *3*, 23. [CrossRef]
6. Nkenke, E.; Weisbach, V.; Winckler, E.; Kessler, P.; Schultze-Mosgau, S.; Wiltfang, J.; Neukam, F.W. Morbidity of harvesting of bone grafts from the iliac crest for preprosthetic augmentation procedures: A prospective study. *Int. J. Oral Maxillofac. Surg.* **2004**, *33*, 157–163. [CrossRef]
7. Baldini, N.; De Sanctis, M.; Ferrari, M. Deproteinized bovine bone in periodontal and implant surgery. *Dent. Mater.* **2011**, *27*, 61–70. [CrossRef]
8. Thompson, T.J.U.; Gauthier, M.; Islam, M. Bone augmentation procedures in localized defects in the alveolar ridge: Clinical results with different bone grafts and bone-substitute materials. *Int. J. Oral Maxillofac. Implant.* **2009**, *24*, 218–236.
9. Wozney, J.M. The bone morphogenetic protein family and osteogenesis. *Mol. Reprod. Dev.* **1992**, *32*, 160–167. [CrossRef]
10. Richardson, C.R.; Mellonig, J.T.; Brunsvold, M.A.; McDonnell, H.T.; Cochran, D.L. Clinical evaluation of Bio-Oss: A bovine-derived xenograft for the treatment of periodontal osseous defects in humans. *J. Clin. Periodontol.* **1999**, *26*, 421–428. [CrossRef]
11. Lee, J.H.; Yi, G.S.; Lee, J.W.; Kim, D.J. Physicochemical characterization of porcine bone-derived grafting material and comparison with bovine xenografts for dental applications. *J. Periodontal Implant Sci.* **2017**, *47*, 388–401. [CrossRef] [PubMed]
12. Valentini, P.; Abensur, D. Maxillary sinus floor elevation for implant placement with demineralized freeze-dried bone and bovine bone (Bio-Oss): A clinical study of 20 patients. *Int. J. Periodontics Restor. Dent.* **1997**, *17*, 232–241.
13. Peric Kacarevic, Z.; Kavehei, F.; Houshmand, A.; Franke, J.; Smeets, R.; Rimashevskiy, D.; Wenisch, S.; Schnettler, R.; Jung, O.; Barbeck, M. Purification processes of xenogeneic bone substitutes and their impact on tissue reactions and regeneration. *Int. J. Artif. Organs* **2018**, *41*, 789–800. [CrossRef] [PubMed]
14. Carmagnola, D.; Adriaens, P.; Berglundh, T. Healing of human extraction sockets filled with Bio-Oss. *Clin. Oral Implant. Res.* **2003**, *14*, 137–143. [CrossRef] [PubMed]
15. Duda, M.; Pajak, J. The issue of bioresorption of the Bio-Oss xenogeneic bone substitute in bone defects. *Ann. Univ. Mariae Curie Sklodowska Med.* **2004**, *59*, 269–277. [PubMed]
16. Stavropoulos, A.; Karring, T. Guided tissue regeneration combined with a deproteinized bovine bone mineral (Bio-Oss) in the treatment of intrabony periodontal defects: 6-year results from a randomized-controlled clinical trial. *J. Clin. Periodontol.* **2010**, *37*, 200–210. [CrossRef] [PubMed]
17. Aludden, H.C.; Mordenfeld, A.; Hallman, M.; Dahlin, C.; Jensen, T. Lateral ridge augmentation with Bio-Oss alone or Bio-Oss mixed with particulate autogenous bone graft: A systematic review. *Int. J. Oral Maxillofac. Surg.* **2017**, *46*, 1030–1038. [CrossRef]
18. Starch-Jensen, T.; Aludden, H.; Hallman, M.; Dahlin, C.; Christensen, A.E.; Mordenfeld, A. A systematic review and meta-analysis of long-term studies (five or more years) assessing maxillary sinus floor augmentation. *Int. J. Oral Maxillofac. Surg.* **2018**, *47*, 103–116. [CrossRef]
19. Benke, D.; Olah, A.; Mohler, H. Protein-chemical analysis of Bio-Oss bone substitute and evidence on its carbonate content. *Biomaterials* **2001**, *22*, 1005–1012. [CrossRef]
20. Orsini, G.; Traini, T.; Scarano, A.; Degidi, M.; Perrotti, V.; Piccirilli, M.; Piattelli, A. Maxillary sinus augmentation with Bio-Oss particles: A light, scanning, and transmission electron microscopy study in man. *J. Biomed. Mater. Res. Part B Appl. Biomater.* **2005**, *74*, 448–457. [CrossRef]
21. Degidi, M.; Artese, L.; Rubini, C.; Perrotti, V.; Iezzi, G.; Piattelli, A. Microvessel density and vascular endothelial growth factor expression in sinus augmentation using Bio-Oss. *Oral Dis.* **2006**, *12*, 469–475. [CrossRef] [PubMed]
22. Berglundh, T.; Lindhe, J. Healing around implants placed in bone defects treated with Bio-Oss. An experimental study in the dog. *Clin. Oral Implant. Res.* **1997**, *8*, 117–124. [CrossRef] [PubMed]
23. Skoglund, A.; Hising, P.; Young, C. A clinical and histologic examination in humans of the osseous response to implanted natural bone mineral. *Int. J. Oral Maxillofac. Implant.* **1997**, *12*, 194–199.

24. Sartori, S.; Silvestri, M.; Forni, F.; Icaro Cornaglia, A.; Tesei, P.; Cattaneo, V. Ten-year follow-up in a maxillary sinus augmentation using anorganic bovine bone (Bio-Oss). A case report with histomorphometric evaluation. *Clin. Oral Implant. Res.* **2003**, *14*, 369–372. [CrossRef]
25. Bedini, R.; Meleo, D.; Pecci, R. 3D microtomography characterization of dental implantology bone substitutes used in-vivo. *Key Eng. Mater.* **2013**, *541*, 97–113. [CrossRef]
26. Bedini, R.; Pecci, R.; Meleo, D.; Campioni, I. Bone Substitutes Scaffold in Human Bone: Comparative Evaluation by 3D Micro-CT Technique. *Appl. Sci.* **2020**, *10*, 3451. [CrossRef]
27. EU-REGULATION. COMMISSION REGULATION (EU) No 722/2012 of 8 August 2012 concerning particular requirements as regards the requirements laid down in Council Directives 90/385/EEC and 93/42/EEC with respect to active implantable medical devices and medical devices manufactured utilising tissues of animal origin (REGOLAMENTO N. 722/2012 DELLA COMMISSIONE EUROPEA dell'8 agosto 2012 relativo ai requisiti particolari per quanto riguarda i requisiti di cui alle direttive 90/385/CEE e 93/42/CEE del Consiglio per i dispositivi medici impiantabili attivi e i dispositivi medici fabbricati con tessuti d'origine animale). 2012, L 212, 3–12. Available online: https://eur-lex.europa.eu/LexUriServ/LexUriServ.do?uri=OJ:L:2012:212:0003:0012:en:PDF (accessed on 20 November 2021).
28. Lovati, A.B.; Lopa, S.; Bottagisio, M.; Talo, G.; Canciani, E.; Dellavia, C.; Alessandrino, A.; Biagiotti, M.; Freddi, G.; Segatti, F.; et al. Peptide-Enriched Silk Fibroin Sponge and Trabecular Titanium Composites to Enhance Bone Ingrowth of Prosthetic Implants in an Ovine Model of Bone Gaps. *Front. Bioeng. Biotechnol.* **2020**, *8*, 563203. [CrossRef]
29. Noguchi, K.; Gel, Y.R.; Brunner, E.; Konietschke, F. nparLD: An R Software Package for the Nonparametric Analysis of Longitudinal Data in Factorial Experiments. *J. Stat. Softw.* **2012**, *50*, 23. [CrossRef]
30. Dumitrescu, C.R.; Neacsu, I.A.; Surdu, V.A.; Nicoara, A.I.; Iordache, F.; Trusca, R.; Ciocan, L.T.; Ficai, A.; Andronescu, E. Nano-Hydroxyapatite vs. Xenografts: Synthesis, Characterization, and In Vitro Behavior. *Nanomaterials* **2021**, *11*, 2289. [CrossRef]
31. Sun, R.; Lv, Y.; Niu, Y.; Zhao, X.; Cao, D.; Tang, J.; Sun, X.; Chen, K. Physicochemical and biological properties of bovine-derived porous hydroxyapatite/collagen composite and its hydroxyapatite powders. *Ceram. Int.* **2017**, *43*, 16792–16798. [CrossRef]
32. Thompson, T.J.U.; Gauthier, M.; Islam, M. The application of a new method of Fourier Transform Infrared Spectroscopy to the analysis of burned bone. *J. Archaeol. Sci.* **2009**, *36*, 910–914. [CrossRef]
33. Canellas, J.; Ritto, F.G.; Figueredo, C.; Fischer, R.G.; de Oliveira, G.P.; Thole, A.A.; Medeiros, P.J.D. Histomorphometric evaluation of different grafting materials used for alveolar ridge preservation: A systematic review and network meta-analysis. *Int. J. Oral Maxillofac. Surg.* **2020**, *49*, 797–810. [CrossRef] [PubMed]
34. Di Stefano, D.A.; Gastaldi, G.; Vinci, R.; Cinci, L.; Pieri, L.; Gherlone, E. Histomorphometric comparison of enzyme-deantigenic equine bone and anorganic bovine bone in sinus augmentation: A randomized clinical trial with 3-year follow-up. *Int. J. Oral Maxillofac. Implant.* **2015**, *30*, 1161–1167. [CrossRef]
35. Giuliani, A.; Iezzi, G.; Mazzoni, S.; Piattelli, A.; Perrotti, V.; Barone, A. Regenerative properties of collagenated porcine bone grafts in human maxilla: Demonstrative study of the kinetics by synchrotron radiation microtomography and light microscopy. *Clin. Oral Investig.* **2018**, *22*, 505–513. [CrossRef]
36. Mordenfeld, A.; Hallman, M.; Johansson, C.B.; Albrektsson, T. Histological and histomorphometrical analyses of biopsies harvested 11 years after maxillary sinus floor augmentation with deproteinized bovine and autogenous bone. *Clin. Oral Implant. Res.* **2010**, *21*, 961–970. [CrossRef]
37. Scarano, A. Maxillary Sinus Augmentation with Decellularized Bovine Compact Particles: A Radiological, Clinical, and Histologic Report of 4 Cases. *Biomed. Res. Int.* **2017**, *2017*, 2594670. [CrossRef] [PubMed]
38. Traini, T.; Valentini, P.; Iezzi, G.; Piattelli, A. A histologic and histomorphometric evaluation of anorganic bovine bone retrieved 9 years after a sinus augmentation procedure. *J. Periodontol.* **2007**, *78*, 955–961. [CrossRef]
39. Khan, M.Q.; Sweeting, B.; Mulligan, V.K.; Arslan, P.E.; Cashman, N.R.; Pai, E.F.; Chakrabartty, A. Prion disease susceptibility is affected by beta-structure folding propensity and local side-chain interactions in PrP. *Proc. Natl. Acad. Sci. USA* **2010**, *107*, 19808–19813. [CrossRef]
40. Artzi, Z.; Tal, H.; Dayan, D. Porous bovine bone mineral in healing of human extraction sockets. Part 1: Histomorphometric evaluations at 9 months. *J. Periodontol.* **2000**, *71*, 1015–1023. [CrossRef]
41. Tapety, F.I.; Amizuka, N.; Uoshima, K.; Nomura, S.; Maeda, T. A histological evaluation of the involvement of Bio-Oss in osteoblastic differentiation and matrix synthesis. *Clin. Oral Implant. Res.* **2004**, *15*, 315–324. [CrossRef]
42. Di Stefano, D.A.; Zaniol, T.; Cinci, L.; Pieri, L. Chemical, Clinical and Histomorphometric Comparison between Equine Bone Manufactured through Enzymatic Antigen-Elimination and Bovine Bone Made Non-Antigenic Using a High-Temperature Process in Post-Extractive Socket Grafting. A Comparative Retrospective Clinical Study. *Dent. J.* **2019**, *7*, 70. [CrossRef]
43. Olszta, M.J.; Cheng, X.; Jee, S.S.; Kumar, R.; Kim, Y.Y.; Kaufman, M.J.; Douglas, E.P.; Gower, L.B. Bone structure and formation: A new perspective. *Mater. Sci. Eng. R Rep.* **2007**, *58*, 77–116. [CrossRef]
44. Joschek, S.; Nies, B.; Krotz, R.; Goferich, A. Chemical and physicochemical characterization of porous hydroxyapatite ceramics made of natural bone. *Biomaterials* **2000**, *21*, 1645–1658. [CrossRef]
45. Clergeau, L.P.; Danan, M.; Clergeau-Guerithault, S.; Brion, M. Healing response to anorganic bone implantation in periodontal intrabony defects in dogs. Part I. Bone regeneration. A microradiographic study. *J. Periodontol.* **1996**, *67*, 140–149. [CrossRef]
46. Hislop, W.S.; Finlay, P.M.; Moos, K.F. A preliminary study into the uses of anorganic bone in oral and maxillofacial surgery. *Br. J. Oral Maxillofac. Surg.* **1993**, *31*, 149–153. [CrossRef]

47. Berberi, A.; Samarani, A.; Nader, N.; Noujeim, Z.; Dagher, M.; Kanj, W.; Mearawi, R.; Salemeh, Z.; Badran, B. Physicochemical characteristics of bone substitutes used in oral surgery in comparison to autogenous bone. *Biomed. Res. Int.* **2014**, *2014*, 320790. [CrossRef]
48. do Desterro Fde, P.; Sader, M.S.; Soares, G.D.; Vidigal, G.M., Jr. Can inorganic bovine bone grafts present distinct properties? *Braz. Dent. J.* **2014**, *25*, 282–288. [CrossRef]
49. Scarano, A.; Pecora, G.; Piattelli, M.; Piattelli, A. Osseointegration in a sinus augmented with bovine porous bone mineral: Histological results in an implant retrieved 4 years after insertion. A case report. *J. Periodontol.* **2004**, *75*, 1161–1166. [CrossRef]

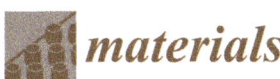 

Article

# The Role of Biomaterials in Upper Digestive Tract Transoral Reconstruction

Raluca Grigore [1,2], Bogdan Popescu [1,2,*], Şerban Vifor Gabriel Berteşteanu [1,2], Cornelia Nichita [3,4], Irina Doiniţa Oașă [1], Gloria Simona Munteanu [2,5], Alexandru Nicolaescu [2], Paula Luiza Bejenaru [2], Catrinel Beatrice Simion-Antonie [2], Dragoș Ene [6,7] and Răzvan Ene [8,9]

[1] Otorhynolaryngology Department, Colţea Clinical Hospital, 917151 Bucharest, Romania; raluca.grigore@umfcd.ro (R.G.); serban.bertesteanu@umfcd.ro (Ş.V.G.B.); irinaoasa@gmail.com (I.D.O.)
[2] Department 12-Otorhynolaryngology, Ophtalmology, Faculty of Medicine, "Carol Davila" University of Medicine and Pharmacy, 050474 Bucharest, Romania; gloriamunteanu@gmail.com (G.S.M.); alexandrunicolaescu@ymail.com (A.N.); drpaulabejenaru@gmail.com (P.L.B.); catrinel_antonie@yahoo.com (C.B.S.-A.)
[3] 3Nano-SAE Res Center, Faculty of Physics, University of Bucharest, 077125 Bucharest-Magurele, Romania; cornelia@3nanosae.org
[4] National Institute for Chemical-Pharmaceutical Research and Development, 031299 Bucharest, Romania
[5] Otorhynolaryngology Department, "Carol Davila" Emergency University Military Hospital, 010825 Bucharest, Romania
[6] General Surgery Department, Emergency Clinical Hospital, 917151 Bucharest, Romania; dragos.ene@umfcd.ro
[7] Department 10-General Surgery, Faculty of Medicine, "Carol Davila" University of Medicine and Pharmacy, 050474 Bucharest, Romania
[8] Orthopedics and Trauma Department, Emergency Clinical Hospital, 917151 Bucharest, Romania; razvan.ene@umfcd.ro
[9] Department 14-Orthopedics, Anaesthesia Intensive Care Unit, Faculty of Medicine, "Carol Davila" University of Medicine and Pharmacy, 050474 Bucharest, Romania
* Correspondence: dr.bpopescu@gmail.com; Tel.: +4072-2605443

**Abstract:** This study aims to establish whether the use of biomaterials, particularly polydimethylsiloxane (PDMS), for surgical reconstruction of the esophagus with templates, Montgomery salivary tube, after radical oncology surgery for malignant neoplasia is an optimal choice for patients' safety and for optimal function preservation and organ rehabilitation. Structural analysis by Raman spectrometry and biomechanical properties with dynamic mechanical analysis are performed for fatigue strength and toughness, essential factors in durability of a prosthesis in the reconstruction practice of the esophagus. Nanocomposites with silicone elastomers and nanoparticles used in implantable devices and in reconstruction surgery present risks of infection and fatigue strength when required to perform a mechanical effort for long periods of time. This report takes into account the effect of silver (Ag) nanoparticles on the fatigue strength using polydimethylsiloxane (PDMS) matrix, representative for silicon elastomers used in implantable devices. PDMS with 5% (wt) Ag nanoparticles of 100–150 nm during mechanical fatigue testing at shear strength loses elasticity properties after 400 loading-unloading cycles and up to 15% shear strain. The fatigue strength, toughness, maximum shear strength, as well as clinical properties are key issues in designing Montgomery salivary tube and derivates with appropriate biomechanical behavior for each patient. Prosthesis design needs to indulge both clinical outcomes as well as design methods and research in the field of biomaterials.

**Keywords:** malignant neoplasia; transoral reconstruction; polydimethyl siloxane; Ag nanoparticles; fatigue strenght; prosthesis

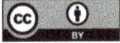

## 1. Introduction

Silicone is used for head and neck implantable devices in the form of cochlear implants [1], nose implants [2], and prosthesis of the upper respiratory and digestive tract [3,4].

The main issue of implantable prosthesis is by far related to the physical and mechanical characteristics regarding strength, shear strain and longevity. For this issue to be addressed some improvements in the structure of the silicone polymers used have been made. Nanocomposites are the result of different molecules incorporated in the structure of the polymers [5,6] The development of such composite mixtures must increase the performance, utility, productivity and product uniformity [7,8], as well as to ensure optimal blend by polymer dispersion for improved properties [9].

Depending on the polymers used to increase the strength and shear strain different results can be achieved. In the head and neck region a silicone elastomer mixed with nano alumina ceramic fiber was used by Nouri Al-qenae for facial reconstruction. However, their results established that this mixture does not have significant outcome in terms of needed properties [10]. Nonetheless, Sara M. Zayed et al. and Dhuha A. Shakir and Faiza M. Abdul-Ameer conducted a series of mechanical testing regarding $SiO_2$ nanoparticles, respectively $TiO_2$ nanoparticles. Results showed that after incorporation all mechanical properties of the polymers improved [11,12].

More recent studies concerning silicone polymers revealed that 3D printed prosthesis is likely to suffice mechanical problems like viscosity when compared to the classical indirect molding technique, as described by Eric et al. [13].

Viscosity of the polymer tends to act inversely to strain hardening effect in terms of mechanical cycles, therefore less viscosity more cycles [14].

Malignant neoplasia of the upper digestive tract is subject to oncology therapy which implies surgery. In most cases, radical resection needs to be performed and the tissue defect needs to be replaced so that function can be restored. Several techniques have been imagined and used in this type of reconstruction. In the E.N.T. Clinic of Colțea Clinical Hospital, we developed a proprietary method which resides in the use of a prosthesis by which the upper digestive tract continuity is being re-established.

Biomaterials used for reconstruction after oncology reconstruction must fulfill demands of biocompatibility ranging from simple biomechanical use to high bioaffinity with tissues and organs. In general, biocompatibility refers to implantable medical devices and organ replacements for reconstructive surgery. Multiple reviews and research focus on different types of biomaterials with specific relation to a targeted application. Hierarchically, the biomaterials must perform a main function (or more) with associated biocompatibility defined by local bioenvironment [15–17]. The esophagus may have the capacity to change its propulsive force in response to bolus size and neurohumoral agents [18]. Esophagus reconstruction surgery has a bioenvironment that is quite complex. The biomaterials used in reconstruction are in direct contact with tissues and local organs respective, food (bolus), beverages and saliva, whilst being in indirect contact with external environment. In such applications, they should fulfill several properties (Table 1).

Table 1. Properties of artificial esophagus used for reconstruction surgery.

| Properties of Artificial Esophagus | Application Requirements Fulfillment |
| --- | --- |
| Biomechanical | Related to the stress-strain mechanical response<br>Optimized storage modulus for organ biomechanics<br>Optimal dynamics for propulsive forces related to bolus size |
| Tribological (inner surface) | Self-cleaning<br>Hydrophobic compatibility with saliva and bolus dynamics |
| Thermo-physical | Low swelling related to biological fluids and water-intake<br>Chemically inert<br>Non-biodegradable |
| Bacteriostatic and antifungal | Inner lining bacteriostatic and antifungal activity |
| Connectivity to other organs | Biocompatibility with the surrounding tissues |
| Electroactivity | Responsiveness to neurohumoral agents |

Today, the most used templates for esophageal prosthesis are Montgomery salivary bypass tube [19–21], a viable alternative in reconstruction. In the tubular region, the prosthesis has two spherical zones (areas) which assure a better stability and optimal saliva leaking along of tube, independent of head and neck position (Figure 1).

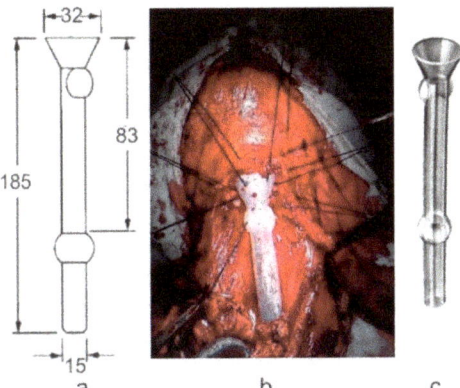

**Figure 1.** (a) Montgomery salivary tube, constructive principle (dimensions in mm) (b) A case study implemented by the Colțea Hospital ENT Team (iconography Dr. C.R Popescu [22]) (c) Montgomery tube made of silicon rubber.

In the range of silicon rubbers, polydimethylsiloxanes (PDMS) have several advantages in designing esophageal prosthesis: it can be molded in different shapes in vacuum or by centrifugation for degassing; the ratio silicon resins/hardener (curing agent) can be adjusted to elaborate a cross-linked rubber with convenient biomechanical properties: molecular weight, viscosity, elasticity related to the shear forces; the PDMS surfaces can be treated (such as plasma treatment) to obtain superhydrophobic/hydrophilic properties or to insert various antioxidants and bacteriostatic agents (addition of Ag). The biofilm represents a sessile microbial community comprising microbial cells with altered phenotype, characterized by a reduced growth rate and altered gene expression [23]. Biofilms are generally included in a protective polysaccharide matrix secreted by biofilm cells and are found attached to a surface [24–29].

In addition, by designing appropriate composites with different nanomaterials PDMS can be radio-opaque or radio-transparent for locally induced radiotherapy. Moreover, it can be designed for appropriate insertion of biopolymers containing various drugs with controlled release for local therapy.

One key issue with PDMS is biomechanical stability during working conditions, such as fatigue strength, maximum strain deformation, storage and dissipation modulus. These characteristics should be accommodated with the biomechanical properties of each patients' tissue particularities where one prosthesis replaces one organ.

This study reviews the mechanical behavior during cyclic loading-unloading by simulating the bolus dynamics (fatigue strength, toughness, shear strain) for the in vitro part of the study and reviews the parameters of clinical outcome in terms of biocompatibility, functionality and antibacterial and antifungal properties of the PDMS template with Ag addition. Ag nanoparticle PDMS templates used for surgical reconstruction of the hypopharynx and cervical esophagus help surgeons and improve the quality of life for patients, since this type of surgery is in most cases a challenge for the oncology head and neck surgeon [22,30–32].

This study aims to establish whether the use of biomaterials, particularly polydimethylsiloxane (PDMS) with Ag nanoparticles, for surgical reconstruction of the esophagus with templates, after radical oncology surgery for malignant neoplasia is an optimal choice for patients' safety and for optimal function preservation and organ rehabilitation. Esophagus prosthesis used for upper digestive tract reconstruction are prone to fungi colonization, in most cases with *Candida albicans*. One of our aims during this study was to establish whether silicone elastomers mixed with silver nanoparticles present antifungal properties.

## 2. Materials and Methods

Our design for the study encompassed: preparation of PDMS samples for testing, reference and silicone-silver nanoparticle polymers, Raman spectrometry to determine the chemical structure of the polymer, mechanical analysis of the samples and comparison analysis, and in vitro testing of prosthesis for biocompatibility and clinical surgery.

### 2.1. Sample Preparation

We designed a study to compare the use of biomaterials in hypopharynx and cervical esophagus transoral reconstruction, with or without mandible reconstruction. For this we used a reference sample, transparent Montgomery esophageal tube (Boston Medical Product, Inc, Shrewsbury, MA, USA) and PDMS recipes, described as following. There is a large class of siloxane base oligomers and associated curing agents. Similar to silicon rubber used in Montgomery salivary tube (Boston Medical Products, Inc.) there are series of other silicon rubber used in designing components for microfluidics and soft lithography such as Sylgard 182–186 (Dow Corning, Midland, MI, USA).

After curing, the elastomers are translucent and have various mechanical properties following smart design with appropriate ratio silicon oligomers/curing agent. Usually, the recommended ratio is 10:1 and the curing temperature up to 150 °C. Slight variations in silicon oligomers/curing agent ratio means that the mechanical properties are well reproduced as Montgomery salivary tube. Samples were tested in the shear stress conditions.

The S1 sample was taken from Montgomery Salivary tube (as specified in Figure 1). S1a- samples were prepared from Sylgard 184 to match the resistance properties of the S1 sample and similar mechanical properties. S2-samples were prepared with Sylgard 184 with a specific ratio oligomer/curing agent (10:1) to obtain similar mechanical properties as S1. S2 was prepared by mixing the Sylgard 184 oligomer with silver (Ag) nanopowder (transmission electron microscopy-TEM diameter ~100–150 nm, average hydrodynamic diameter ~230 nm, measured by dynamic light scattering-DLS) in 5% (wt/wt) and then adding curing agent and treated at 130 °C for 30 min. Silver nanoparticles were prepared using specific methods [33]. All samples were shaped so they could form test specimens of 10 mm diameter and 1mm thickness.

### 2.2. Raman Spectrometry

Raman spectrometry used for data spectral data analysis included Jasco, NRS-3100 (Easton, PN, USA) with dual laser beams, 532 and 785 nm, resolution 4 cm$^{-1}$, with specific configuration and backscattering.

Raman analysis is performed to acquire data from a chemical point of view. We performed the spectral analysis to quantify the number of repeatable units in PDMS—rubber, to establish PDMS network with cross-linkage on –Si–O–Si– and to verify cross-linked PDMS-network via vinyl groups.

### 2.3. Mechanical Analysis

Mechanical analysis was performed using Dynamic mechanical analyzer/Simultaneous thermal analysis DMA/SDTA861, STAR SYSTEM, produced by Mettler Toledo (Greifensee, Switzerland). The operating mode implied Shear function (shear force vs shear strain). This mode is ideal for elastomers, thermo-plastic materials and thermosets. In the shear mode, two identical samples were clamped symmetrically between two fixed outer parts (2) and a central moving part, (1) (Figure 2). The shear clamp guarantees a homogeneous temperature distribution. A thermocouple mounted directly in the clamp measures the samples' temperature so precisely that simultaneous heat flow effects could also be determined (SDTA). The shear force F ranged from 1 mN to 40 N, frequency ranged from 1 mHz to 1000 Hz. The sample diameter had a maximum ≤14 mm and the thickness had a maximum ≤6.5 mm. The experimental set-up included a sample of 10 mm in diameter, thickness of 1 mm, with 1Hz frequency, at room temperature. Maximum shear strain for the samples investigated were 100 microns, respective 150 microns. That corresponded to the increase in diameter of the Montgomery tube at around of 10%, respective 15%.

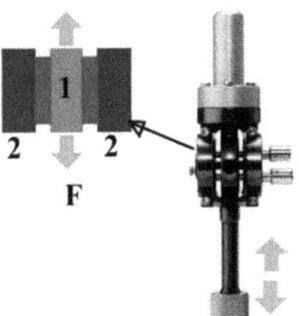

**Figure 2.** Configuration for shear operating mode in DMA/SDTA 861, STAR SYSTEM, produced by Mettler Toledo. 1-mobile plate, 2-fixed back support. F-shear force.

*2.4. Clinical Surgery*

After in vitro testing of the new biocompatible prosthesis, we performed clinical testing. Clinical testing included accurate selection of patients according to clinical inclusion criteria (age above 18 years of age, informed consent of the patient, malignant neoplasia of the upper esophagus, esophagectomy prior to esophagus reconstruction, no radiotherapy as adjuvant therapy). Exclusion criteria were the absence of one or more of the abovementioned inclusion criteria or the preference of the patient to leave the clinical study. No such aspects were encountered. The publication of surgical therapy and clinic trial results were approved by The Ethical Committee of Coltea Clinical Hospital according to decision 20911/05.11.2020. Patients have been distributed into two groups, one of 21 patients treated by using the original Montgomery tube and the second one including 18 patients treated by using PDMS Ag-nanoparticle implant.

Colțea ENT Clinic used an original implantation technique of the Montgomery prosthesis that met the criteria for optimal reconstruction: refueling facility, oral method, reduced complications and mortality, period of hospitalization with lower costs [22]. In selected cases, where mandible reconstruction was needed, a multidisciplinary team of general surgeon and orthopedic surgeon was required [34,35].

The surgical intervention was performed in all cases under general anesthesia and orotracheal intubation. The removal of the larynx, part of the hypopharynx, and the cervical esophagus was the main surgical act, and it was performed since all patients included in the clinical study were diagnosed with malignant neoplasia of the hypopharynx and cervical esophagus. The resection of the larynx is included in the surgery protocol since both the hypopharynx and the cervical esophagus cannot be removed without larynx removal for this type of cancer patients. Reconstruction was made by using the original Montgomery tube for group 1 and PDMS Ag-nanoparticle implant for group 2. The insertion of the prosthesis was performed transoral for better fitting at the base of the tongue. Surgery was completed by reconstructing the muscle, subcutaneous and skin tissues. A nasogastric feeding tube was placed through the prosthesis to ensure feeding until healing was completed.

Follow-up included the immediate postoperative period of 14 days at the end of which sutures were removed and oral feeding was restarted. Late follow-up included scheduled visits of patients for endoscopic examination every other 2 months. Cervical computer tomograph evaluation was performed at an interval of 6 months for a period of 2 years after surgery.

## 3. Results

### 3.1. Raman Spectroscopy

Raman spectrometry used for data spectral data analysis included Jasco, NRS-3100 with dual laser beams, 532 and 785 nm, resolution 4 cm$^{-1}$, with specific configuration and backscattering, averaging over 1000 spectra giving the confidence interval. Error is under 0.1%. Raman spectroscopy gives a strong information related to the structural modifications and it is not appropriate for statistical analysis. Statistical analysis should be performed only in case there are strong variations in structure. Raman spectra for samples S1 and S1a show specific features for PDMS-rubber. For exemplification, the spectrum is recorded for S1 (Figure 3).

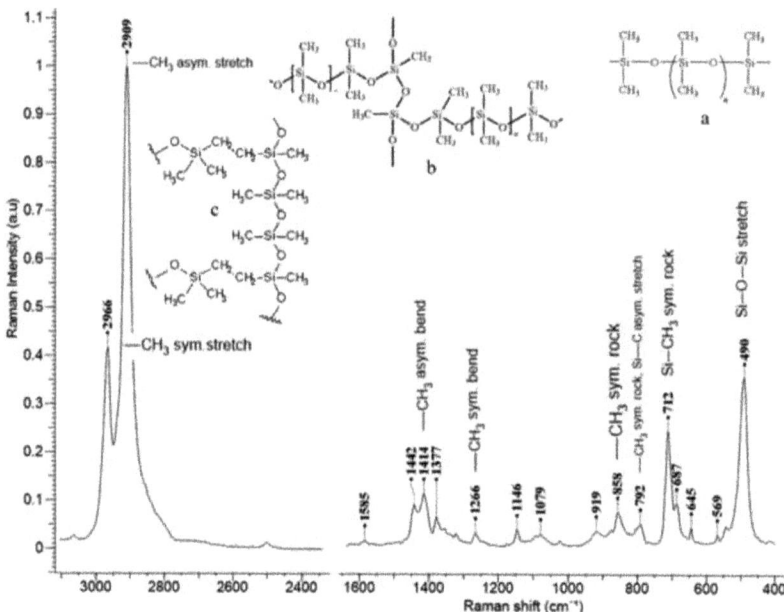

**Figure 3.** Raman spectrum recorded for S1, (a) the repeatable unit in PDMS—rubber, (b) PDMS network with cross-linkage on –Si–O–Si–, (c) PDMS-network cross-linked via vinyl groups.

The spectrum shows several features specific for simple repeatable units (Figure 3a). We identified several bands assigned to –CH$_3$ groups respective to the backbone –Si–O–Si–. They are well defined and have high intensity. The other bands with weak intensity are associated with a particular type of cross-linkage developed in PDMS network: 1585 cm$^{-1}$ (C=C, in phase-stretching), 1442 cm$^{-1}$ ($\delta$(CH$_2$) scissoring), 1377 cm$^{-1}$ (–CH$_3$, methyl rocking), 1146 cm$^{-1}$ (C–C stretching), 1079 cm$^{-1}$ (in-plan rocking for C=CH group). In conclusion, the polymer develops a network with cross-linkage on –Si–O– (Figure 3b) with low levels of cross-linking on –CH$_2$–CH$_2$– vinyl group (Figure 3c).

### 3.2. Shear Stress/Shear Strain

Mechanical analysis was performed using DMA/SDTA861, STAR SYSTEM, produced by Mettler Toledo. The mechanical properties measured in shear mode are shown in Figure 4 for samples S1 and S1a. For the same reason we show results for S1.

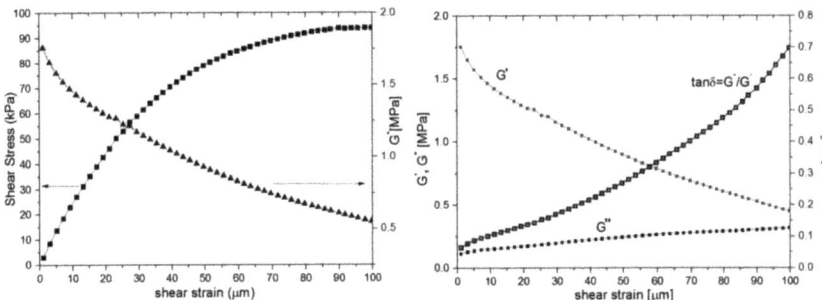

**Figure 4.** Mechanical properties measured by DMA, sample S1, maximum shear strain 100 microns: (**left**) shear stress vs shear strain and G*-shear modulus; (**right**) storage (G'), dissipative modulus (G'') and loss tangent tanδ.

The shear stress/shear strain curve has a quasilinear behavior up to 30 microns per millimeter reaching a plateau at shear strain ~100 microns (Figure 4 left). This is consistent with rubber-elastic materials and their capacity to reach a "rubbery plateau" with quasi-reversible return in an initial state [36]. The shear modulus (Figure 4, left) is dependent of shear strain, which is typical for a viscoelastic rubber material. The shear modulus (G*) varies from 1.8 to 0.5 MPa. The loss modulus (G'') increases slightly with the shear strain, therefore the dissipative energy during loading, mainly bolus transition, reaches at ~1–2 mJ. Even though the storage modulus (G') involved in elastic energy recovery decreases with the strain deformation, PDMS still has a good capacity to regain the initial state after deformation (Figure 4, right). The loss tangent continuously increases at values less than unit without any phase changes. That is consistent with the behavior of quasi-elastic materials with high flexibility.

### 3.3. Fatigue Strength

The statistical method we used is one-way analysis of variance (ANOVA) with mean, standard deviation, standard error, F-statistic value and $p$-value determinations. Each group of the S1 (Montgomery tube), S1a (Sylgard 184) and S2 (Sylgard 184 with Ag nano-powder) polymers consisted of 20 samples for testing and statistical analysis. The statistical analysis was aimed on comparing the properties of S1 and S1a samples and S1a and S2 samples. S1a sample was manufactured from Sylgard 184 to match the characteristics of the S1 sample since we used Montgomery tube as reference. S1a/S2 comparison was performed after establishing the similarities of S1a to S1 (Tables 2 and 3).

**Table 2.** Comparison of compression modulus of S1 and S1a samples as obtained by the slope of the share-strain curve in linear viscoelastic region.

| Data Summary | | | | | |
|---|---|---|---|---|---|
| | Groups | N | Mean | Std. Dev | Std. Error |
| | Group 1 | 20 | 49.8795 | 1.1082 | 0.2478 |
| | Group 2 | 20 | 49.034 | 0.7865 | 0.1759 |
| ANOVA Summary | | | | | |
| Source | Degrees of Freedom DF | Sum of Squares SS | Mean Square MS | F-Stat | $p$-Value |
| Between Groups | 1 | 7.1487 | 7.1487 | 7.7422 | 0.0084 |
| Within Groups | 38 | 35.0871 | 0.9233 | | |
| Total | 39 | 42.2358 | | | |

**Table 3.** Comparison of compression modulus of S1a and S2 samples as obtained by the slope of the share-strain curve in linear viscoelastic region.

| | Data Summary | | | | |
|---|---|---|---|---|---|
| | Groups | N | Mean | Std. Dev | Std. Error |
| | Group 1 | 20 | 51.7685 | 1.3128 | 0.2935 |
| | Group 2 | 20 | 51.036 | 1.5143 | 0.3386 |
| | ANOVA Summary | | | | |
| Source | Degrees of freedom DF | Sum of Squares SS | Mean Square MS | F-Stat | $p$-Value |
| Between Groups | 1 | 5.3656 | 5.3656 | 2.6717 | 0.1104 |
| Within Groups | 38 | 76.3144 | 2.0083 | | |
| Total | 39 | 81.68 | | | |

Samples S1, S1a and S2 are cyclically loaded and unloaded up to 150 microns, their maximum shear strain. After each 100, respective 400 cycles each sample is mechanical tested at their maximum shear strain of 100 microns. After 100 cycles samples S1 keep a rubber-elastic shear strength behavior with a rubbery plateau decreased from 90 KPa to 60 KPa (Figure 5). After 400 cycles, the sample S1 keeps elastic properties in the range of shear-strain up to 70 microns. At higher shear deformation, S1 has quite a different behavior with increased toughness. It can be hypothesized that PDMS network, during cyclic loading-unloading, reinforces by increasing self-cross-linkage between dangling bonds. Similar behavior is observed for sample S2. The elastic state reduces up to 40 microns shear strain and after this value the reinforcing increases more prominent than S1.

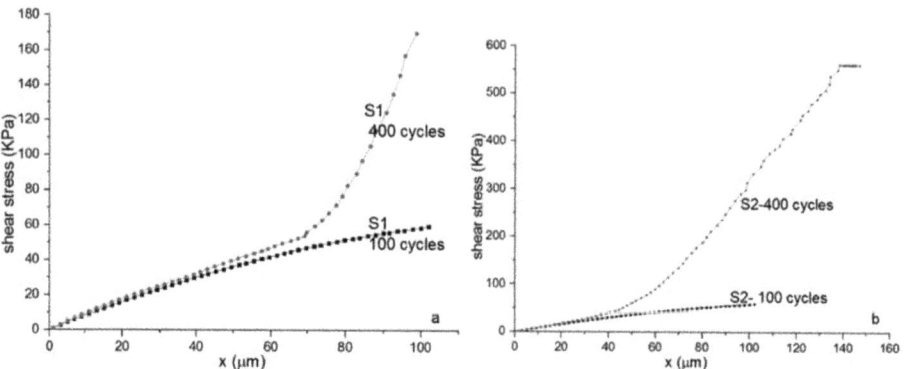

**Figure 5.** Mechanical tests: Fatigue strength in shear mode. (**a**) Sample S1, (**b**) Sample S2. Samples are loaded up to 100 µm and unloaded at shear strain rate 0.1 µm/s. Maximum shear strain 100 µm. Toughness increases with the number of cycles tested to fatigue strength. S2-Ag nanoparticles decreases toughness.

As shown in Table 2, there is no statistical difference between S1a and S1 samples which is consistent with similar properties between the two. We were looking for a Sylgard 184 sample with the closest properties to Montgomery tube. Therefore, the share-strain curve in linear viscoelastic region for both S1 and S1a samples is similar.

As shown in Figure 5 and Table 3 there is a mechanical difference between S1/S1a samples and S2 samples. However, the logarithmic regression of the share-strain curve in linear viscoelastic region for the two different type of samples is similar. Statistical analysis showed that there is no statistical differences between the two groups ($p$-value = 0.1104).

## 3.4. Clinical Testing

We compared the PDMS Ag-nanoparticle implant to the original Montgomery tube used for esophagus reconstruction. While 21 cases were treated by using the original Montgomery tube some 18 cases underwent esophagus reconstruction using PDMS Ag-nanoparticle implant. In terms of biocompatibility and functionality the results were similar with a $p$-value of 0.0012, respectively 0.0004, were as for antibacterial and antifungal purposes the PDMS Ag-nanoparticle implant performed better since only 2 *Candida albicans* included biofilms have been detected at 12 months after surgery. In comparison, the original Montgomery tube developed on the inner surface *Candida albicans*, *Staphylococcus aureus* and *Actinomyces* spp. in 17 out of 21 cases ($p$ = 0.42) (Table 4).

Table 4. Comparison of clinical parameters of original Montgomery tube and PDMS with silver-nanoparticles implant.

| Samples | Montgomery Tube Cases | PDMS Ag-Nanoparticle Implant Cases | $p$-Value |
| --- | --- | --- | --- |
| Biocompatibility | 20/21 | 18/18 | 0.048 |
| Functionality | 20/21 | 18/18 | 0.048 |
| Antibacterial/Antifungal action | 4/21 | 16/18 | 0.42 |

The microscopic examination of Gram-stained smears performed directly from the biofilm developed on the surface of the voice prosthesis revealed the presence of a frequent association between different morphological types, indicating the specific nature of microbial biofilm (Figures 6 and 7). The examination of the colonized esophageal prosthesis specimens by scanning electron microscopy (SEM) revealed the presence of a mature biofilm, with a consistent matrix and a complex three-dimensional structure (Figure 8). The microscopic examination of different regions of the prosthetic device has shown that biofilm deposits are accumulating along the entire surface of the device. The well-developed biofilm could therefore be responsible for the prosthesis dysfunction and limited resistance over time.

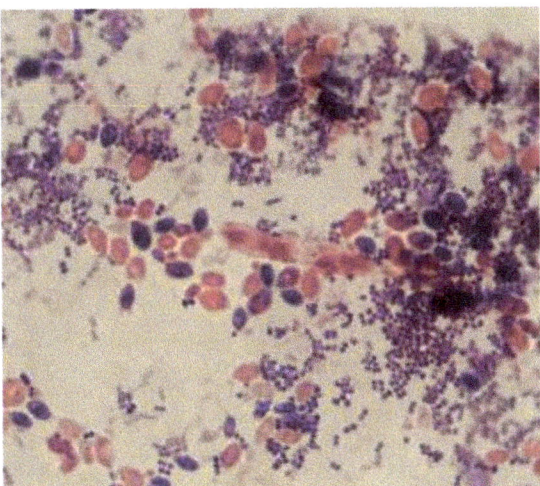

**Figure 6.** Microscopic images of Gram-stained smears performed directly from the biofilm developed on the surface of the voice prosthesis (Gram stain, ×1000).

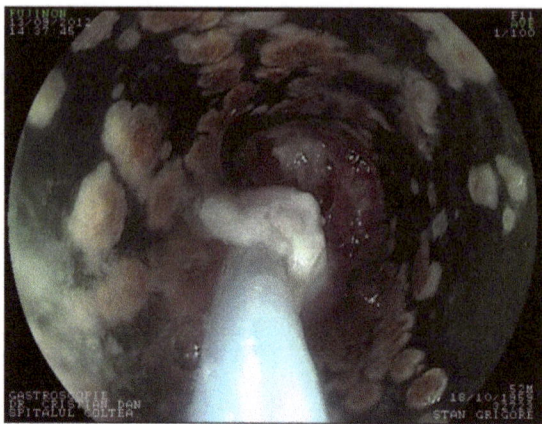

**Figure 7.** Biofilm, inlcuding *Candida* spp., *Staphilococcus aureus*, forming on the inner surface of the prosthesis.

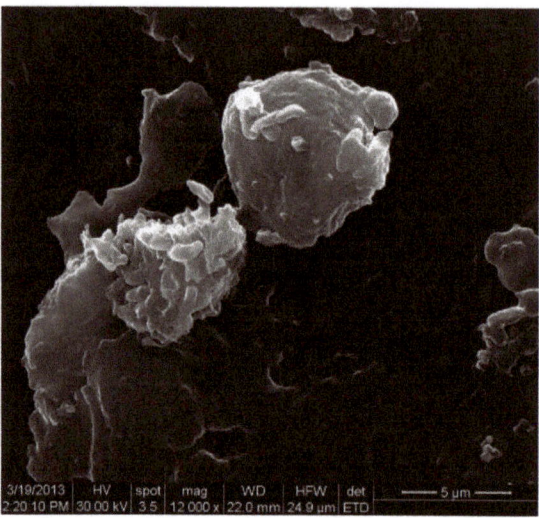

**Figure 8.** Electron-microscopy images of microbial biofilm developed on the surface of the voice prosthesis.

The follow-up period for the clinical part of the trial was 12 months for PDMS Ag nanoparticles prosthesis. Oncology status was followed-up for 24 months and was a secondary aspect of the clinical trial and with no relation to the aim of the study. However, the statistical analysis we performed in the ENT department of Colțea Clinical Hospital, related to the different forms of relapses of hypopharynx and cervical esophagus cancer concluded that only 34% of patients did not have a relapse of their cancer.

## 4. Discussion

The study describes the first prosthesis design using a combination of silicone elastomer and silver nanoparticles used for the reconstruction of the upper digestive tract. This project was based on the previously used Montgomery prosthesis which is a single silicone polymer device. Our main goal was to create an adequate polymer which can support the functions of the previous Montgomery prosthesis improved in terms of fungus colonization. Clinical outcome is dependent on the structural design of the prosthesis and on the capability of the biomaterial.

Along with the technique used to surgically implant the prosthesis a concurrent well-known problem appeared. Biofilm formation was observed in sample prosthesis. Infections resulting from microbial adhesion to medical surfaces have been observed on all prosthetic devices, regardless of the biomaterial nature, with severe economic and medical consequences. Biofilm-associated infections raise some clinical challenges, including disease, chronic inflammation, and rapidly acquired antibiotic resistance [37]. We compared clinical outcome in terms of biotolerance, functionality, and inner surface biofilm formation of PDMS Ag-nanoparticles implants with the original Montgomery tube.

Silicone based polymers have been used for reconstruction in the head and neck region but failed to address all the issues. Silver nanoparticles have proven their role in diminishing germ and fungus colonization of biomaterials. The blend that we used to develop the improved Montgomery prosthesis is similar to other blends that have already been used in biocompatible devices. Therefore, the method is already having its applications.

Raman spectrometry and mechanical testing provided us with basic and advanced data regarding the functional parameters of the prosthesis and these are consistent to other studies involving silicone/silver nanoparticles biomaterials [36]. By using this blending technique and receipts the polymer develops a network with cross-linkage on –Si–O– with low levels of cross-linking on –$CH_2$–$CH_2$– vinyl group which confers high levels of elasticity and, thus the possibility of high elastic energy accumulation.

Given the fact that the shear stress/shear strain curve has a quasilinear behavior up to 30 microns per millimeter reaching a plateau at shear strain ~100 microns we were able to say that this polymer is consistent with rubber-elastic materials. This behavior enables the polymer to return, after a deformation, to a quasi-reversible return to the initial state. All the data recovered from the shear stress/shear strain curve leads to the fact that this polymer has high flexibility which is mandatory for this type of prosthesis use.

Both samples, S1 and S2, interpreted in terms of toughness, show several features useful in biomechanical properties. In physical sense, toughness is really a measure of the energy absorbed before it breaks and estimated from the area underneath the stress-strain curve. Both samples show a transition from low toughness (high rubbery state with low energy absorbed) to high toughness where adsorbed energy is high and leads to breaking, losing the essential properties during the effort done for bolus transition.

In terms of quality of life, the reconstruction with synthetic prosthesis for most patients is well tolerated, considered satisfactory regarding silicone implant. In comparison to the original Montgomery tube, the PDMS with silver-nanoparticles has increased utility in terms of antibacterial and antifungal biofilm formation. The clinical results as shown on cohorts of patients after prosthesis implant and treated by a multidisciplinary approach, respective by monotherapy show a relatively good biocompatibility of the silicon rubber blended with silver nanoparticles [38–40].

To ensure that cytotoxicity due to silver impregnation is not posing any risks for our patients we determined the total silver levels in vitro which were below admitted levels (<1.1 µg $L^{-1}$). These data are consistent with results from a study made by Zhala Meran et al. who stated that prosthetic materials coated with silver nanoparticles are biocompatible with fibroblast cells [41]. According to SCHEER guidelines Montgomery prosthesis silicone elastomer mixed with silver nanoparticles meet the criteria for tolerable exposure (EN ISO 10993-17:2002) and for analytical contact conditions (EN ISO 10993-12) [42].

The limitation of the reconstructive method is derived from the inconsistency between mechanical properties of the Montgomery tube (given mechanical properties) and biomechanics of the esophagus for each patient. There is a wide variety of individual characteristics concerning anatomy landmarks and function preservation. The rehabilitation using this technique cannot overcome the prior functional status of each patient, hence the variation in function preservation. However, clinical outcome in terms of biocomplatibility, functionality, and biofilm formation prevention over repeated cycles of use for the Montgomery tube coated with silver nanoparticles showed that the rehabilitation method and the characteristics of the improved prosthesis are optimal for upper digestive tract reconstruction.

## 5. Conclusions

Silicon rubbers used in prosthesis for a specific surgery application (esophagus reconstruction) are the most appropriate solution in terms of morbidity, biocompatibility, functionality and bacterial and fungal biofilm formation.

The mechanical properties can be tailored by optimal recipes silicon oligomers/curing agent and curing temperatures, as shown previously. The fatigue strength, toughness, maximum shear strength are the key issues in designing Montgomery salivary silicone tube blended with silver nanoparticles with appropriate biomechanical behavior for each patient. Insertion of bacteriostatic agents, such as silver nanoparticles, decreases the fatigue strength, increases flexibility and offers optimal local protection solution against fungi development.

Furthermore, starting from the premises that including nanoparticles of different agents is a real possibility, we can state that this finding is useful in imagining a new concept to use bacteriostatic agents or other drugs for local therapy.

Prosthesis design needs to indulge both clinical outcome as well as design methods and research in the field of biomaterials. Transoral insertion of a prosthesis for esophagus reconstruction after cancer surgery has improved overall survival rates and the quality of life for these patients.

Further data and analysis will show eventual pitfalls of the technique.

## 6. Patents

Montgomery esophageal prosthesis are coded 878.3610 by Code of Federal regulations (21CFR 878). It is made of biocompatible silicon (recommended by Blue Book G95-1: ISO-10993 Biological Evaluation of Medical Devices Part1) tested for cytotoxicity, sensibility, implantation and sub-chronic and chronic toxicity. The reconstructive method is subject to Romanian patent for medical devices no. 130466 from 19.08.2014.

**Author Contributions:** Conceptualization: R.G., C.N., B.P., and Ş.V.G.B.; methodology: C.N., Ş.V.G.B., I.D.O., D.E. and G.S.M.; software: G.S.M.; validation: R.G., P.L.B., C.B.S.-A. and I.D.O.; formal analysis: R.G., C.N., and R.E.; investigation: C.N., P.L.B. and C.B.S.-A.; resources: R.E., C.N., A.N., P.L.B. and C.B.S.-A.; data curation: B.P., A.N., P.L.B. and C.B.S.-A. and I.D.O.; writing–original draft preparation: I.D.O., A.N., P.L.B. and C.B.S.-A.; writing–review & editing: D.E., G.S.M., A.N., P.L.B. and C.B.S.-A. and R.E.; visualization: B.P., G.S.M. and R.E.; supervision: Ş.V.G.B., R.G. and D.E.; project administration: B.P., I.D.O., A.N., D.E. and Ş.V.G.B.; funding acquisition: B.P., R.G., R.E., D.E. and Ş.V.G.B. All authors have read and agreed to the published version of the manuscript. All authors have equal contributions to this manuscript.

**Funding:** This research received no external funding.

**Institutional Review Board Statement:** The study was conducted according to the guidelines of the Declaration of Helsinki and approved by the Ethics Committee of COLTEA CLINICAL HOSPTAL and updated for this manuscript according to protocol code 20911 from 05.11.2021.

**Informed Consent Statement:** Informed consent was obtained from all subjects involved in the study.

**Data Availability Statement:** Data available on request due to privacy and ethical restrictions concerning patients' personal data. The data presented in this study are available on request from the corresponding author since main data is contained within the article.

**Acknowledgments:** The research performed by the interdisciplinary teams are supported by Coltea Clinical Hospital, University of Bucharest, Clinical Emergency Hospital and Romanian National Authority for Scientific Research, projects PCCDI-40/2018, PN II -PCCA No 210/2014. Data available on request due to privacy and ethical restrictions concerning patients' personal data. The data presented in this study are available on request from the corresponding author since main data is contained within the article. All authors have equal contribution to this research.

**Conflicts of Interest:** The authors declare no conflict of interest.

## References

1. Clark, G. *Cochlear Implants: Fundamentals and Applications*; Springer: Berlin, Germany, 2006.
2. Chugay, N.V.; Chugay, P.N.; Shiffman, M.A. *Body Sculpting with Silicone Implants*; Springer Science & Business Media: Berlin, Germany, 2014.
3. Montgomery, W.W.; Montgomery, S.K. Montgomery thyroplasty implant system. *Ann. Otol. Rhinol. Laryngol. Suppl.* **1997**, *170*, 1–16.
4. Cooper, J.D.; Todd, T.R.; Ilves, R.; Pearson, F.G. Use of the silicone tracheal T-tube for the management of complex tracheal injuries. *J. Thorac. Cardiovasc. Surg.* **1981**, *82*, 559–568. [CrossRef]
5. Liu, Q.; Shao, L.; Fan, H.; Long, Y.; Zhao, N.; Yang, S.; Xu, J. Characterization of maxillofacial silicone elastomer reinforced with different hollow microsphere. *J. Mater. Sci.* **2015**, *50*, 3976–3983. [CrossRef]
6. Sun, X.; Sun, H.; Li, H.; Peng, H. Developing Polymer Composite Materials: Carbon Nanotubes or Graphene? *Adv. Mater.* **2013**, *25*, 5153–5176. [CrossRef]
7. Smith, W.F.; Hashimi, J. *Foundation of Materials Science and Engineering*, 5th ed.; McGraw-Hill: New York, NY, USA, 2011.
8. Yua, L.; Deana, K.; Lib, L.; Yu, L. Polymer blends and composites from renewable resources. *Prog. Polym. Sci.* **2006**, *31*, 576–602. [CrossRef]
9. Mikitaev, A.K.; Ligidov, M.K.; Zaikov, G.E. *Polymer, Polymer Blends, Polymer Composites and Filled Poymers: Synthesis, Properties and Applications*; Nova Science Publishers, Inc.: New York, NY, USA, 2006.
10. Al-Qenaei, N. Nano Ceramic Fiber Reinforced Silicone Maxillofacial Prosthesis. Master's Thesis, Indiana University, Bloomington, IN, USA, 2010.
11. Zayed, S.M.; Alshimy, A.M.; Fahmy, A.E. Effect of Surface Treated Silicon Dioxide Nanoparticles on Some Mechanical Properties of Maxillofacial Silicone Elastomer. *Int. J. Biomater.* **2014**, *7*. [CrossRef] [PubMed]
12. Shakir, D.A.; Abdul-Ameer, F.M. Effect of nano-titanium oxide addition on some mechanical properties of silicone elastomers for maxillofacial prostheses. *J. Taibah Univ. Med Sci.* **2018**, *13*, 281–290. [CrossRef] [PubMed]
13. Luis, E.; Pan, H.M.; Sing, S.L.; Bajpai, R.; Song, J.; Yeong, W.Y. 3D Direct Printing of Silicone Meniscus Implant Using a Novel Heat-Cured Extrusion-Based Printer. *Polymers* **2020**, *12*, 1031. [CrossRef] [PubMed]
14. Lee, W.S.; Yeo, K.S.; Andriyana, A.; Shee, Y.G.; Mahamd Adikan, F.R. Effect of cyclic compression and curing agent concentration on the stabilization of mechanical properties of PDMS elastomer. *Mater. Des.* **2016**, *96*, 470–475. [CrossRef]
15. Williams, D.F. On the nature of biomaterials. *Biomaterials* **2009**, *30*, 5897–5909. [CrossRef] [PubMed]
16. Williams, D.F. There is no such thing as a biocompatible material. *Biomaterials* **2014**, *35*, 10009–10014. [CrossRef]
17. Williams, D.F. Regulatory biocompatibility requirements for biomaterials used in regenerative medicine. *J. Mater. Sci. Mater. Med.* **2015**, *26*, 89. [CrossRef]
18. Mir, M.; Ali, M.N.; Ansari, U.; Sami, J. Structure and motility of the esophagus from a mechanical perspective. *Esophagus* **2016**, *13*, 8–16. [CrossRef]
19. Sevilla García, M.A.; Suárez Fente, V.; Rodrigo Tapia, J.P.; Llorente Pendás, J.L. Insertion of Montgomery salivary bypass tube under local anesthesia in patients with pharyngocutaneous fistula following total laryngectomy. *Acta Otorrinolaringol. Esp.* **2004**, *55*, 244–246. [CrossRef]
20. Lörken, J.; Krampert, R.J.; Kau, W.A. Experiences with the Montgomery Salivary Bypass Tube (MSBT). *Dysphagia Spring* **1997**, *12*, 79–83. [CrossRef] [PubMed]
21. Holinger, P.H. Panel discussion: The historical development of laryngectomy. V. A century of progress of laryngectomies in the northern hemisphere. *Laryngoscope* **1975**, *85*, 322–332. [CrossRef] [PubMed]
22. Popescu, C.R. *Tratamentul Complex al Cancerului de Laringe*; Editura SAS: Bucuresti, Romania, 1994.
23. Lazar, V.; Chifiriuc, M.C. Architecture and physiology of microbial biofilms. *Roum. Arch. Microbiol. Immunol.* **2010**, *69*, 92–98.
24. Costerton, J.W.; Lappin-Scott, H.M. Behavior of bacteria in biofilms. *ASM News* **1989**, *55*, 650–654.
25. Carpentier, B. Les biofilms (2). *Bullentin Soc. Fr. Microbiol.* **1999**, *14*, 105–111.
26. Donlan, R.M.; Costerton, J.W. Biofilms: Survival mechanisms of clinically relevant microorganisms. *Clin. Microbiol. Rev.* **2002**, *15*, 167–193. [CrossRef]
27. Grumezescu, A.M. Essential oils and nanotechnology for combating microbial biofilms. *Curr. Org. Chem.* **2013**, *17*, 90–96. [CrossRef]
28. Ene, R.; Sinescu, R.D.; Ene, P.; Popescu, D.; Cirstoiu, M.M.; Cirstoiu, F.C. Proximal tibial osteosarcoma in young patients: Early diagnosis, modular reconstruction. *Rom. J. Morphol. Embriol.* **2015**, *56*, 413–417.
29. Popescu, D.; Ene, R.; Popescu, A.; Cirstoiu, M.; Sinescu, R.; Cirstoiu, C. Total hip joint replacement in young male patient with osteoporosis, secondary to hypogonadotropic hypogonadism. *Acta Endocrinol.* **2015**, *11*, 109–113. [CrossRef]
30. Harrison, L.B.; Sessions, R.B.; Hong, W.K. *Head and Neck Cancer: A Multidisciplinary Approach*, 3rd ed.; Lipppincott Williams & Wilkins: Philadelphia, PA, USA, 2009.

31. Bertesteanu, S.V.G.; Popescu, C.R.; Grigore, R.; Popescu, B. Pharyngoesophageal junction neoplasia-therapeutic management. *Chirurgia* **2012**, *1071*, 33–38.
32. Carlson, G.W.; Schusterman, M.A.; Guillamondegui, O.M. Total reconstruction of the hypopharynx and cervical esophagus: A 20-year experience. *Ann Plast Surg.* **1992**, *29*, 408–412. [CrossRef] [PubMed]
33. Agasti, N.; Kaushik, N.K. Synthesis of water soluble glycine capped silver nanoparticles and their surface selective interaction. *Mater. Res. Bull.* **2015**, *64*, 17–21. [CrossRef]
34. Cirstoiu, C.; Ene, R.; Panti, Z.; Ene, P.; Cirstoiu, M. Particularities of Shoulder Recovery After Arthroscopic Bankart Repair with Bioabsorbable and Metallic Suture Anchors. *Mater. Plast.* **2015**, *52*, 361–363.
35. Nica, M.; Cretu, B.; Ene, D.; Antoniac, I.; Gheorghita, D.; Ene, R. Failure Analysis of Retrieved Osteosynthesis Implants. *Materials* **2020**, *13*, 1201. [CrossRef]
36. Clarson, S.J.; Semlyen, J.A. *Siloxane Polymers*; Prentice Hall: Englewood Cliffs, NJ, USA, 1993.
37. Rodrigues, L.R. Inhibition of Bacterial Adhesion on Medical Devices. In *Bacterial Adhesion: Advances in Experimental Medicine and Biology*; Linke, D., Goldman, A., Eds.; Springer: Dordrecht, The Netherlands, 2011. [CrossRef]
38. Tran, Q.; Nguyen, N.; Le, A. Silver nanoparticles: Synthesis, properties, toxicology, applications and perspectives. *Adv. Nat. Sci. Nanosci. Nanotechnol.* **2013**, *4*, 1–20. [CrossRef]
39. Asghari, S.; Johari, S.; Lee, J.; Kim, Y.; Jeon, Y.; Choi, H.; Moon, M.; Yu, J. Toxicity of various silver nanoparticles compared to silver ions in Daphnia magna. *J. Nanobiotechnol.* **2012**, *10*, 1–11. [CrossRef]
40. Solano-Umaña, V.; Vega-Baudrit, J.R. *Silver Nanoparticles and PDMS Hybrid Nanostructure for Medical Applications*; IntechOpen: London, UK, 2018. [CrossRef]
41. Meran, Z.; Besinis, A.; De Peralta, T.; Handy, R.D. Antifungal properties and biocompatibility of silver nanoparticle coatings on silicone maxillofacial prostheses in vitro. *J. Biomed. Mater. Res. B Appl. Biomater.* **2018**, *106*, 1038–1051. [CrossRef] [PubMed]
42. European Comission. *Scheer Guidelines*; European Comission: Brussels, Belgium, 2019; pp. 16–17.

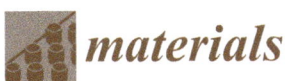

Article

# Does Printing Orientation Matter? In-Vitro Fracture Strength of Temporary Fixed Dental Prostheses after a 1-Year Simulation in the Artificial Mouth

Julian Nold *, Christian Wesemann, Laura Rieg, Lara Binder, Siegbert Witkowski, Benedikt Christopher Spies and Ralf Joachim Kohal

Medical Center–University of Freiburg, Center for Dental Medicine, Department of Prosthetic Dentistry, Faculty of Medicine, University of Freiburg, Hugstetter Str. 55, 79106 Freiburg, Germany; christian.wesemann@uniklinik-freiburg.de (C.W.); noemi.rieg@uniklinik-freiburg.de (L.R.); lara.binder@icloud.com (L.B.); siegbert.witkowski@uniklinik-freiburg.de (S.W.); benedikt.spies@uniklinik-freiburg.de (B.C.S.); ralf.kohal@uniklinik-freiburg.de (R.J.K.)
* Correspondence: julian.nold@uniklinik-freiburg.de; Tel.: +49-762-2704-9290

**Abstract:** Computer-aided design and computer-aided manufacturing (CAD–CAM) enable subtractive or additive fabrication of temporary fixed dental prostheses (FDPs). The present in-vitro study aimed to compare the fracture resistance of both milled and additive manufactured three-unit FDPs and bar-shaped, ISO-conform specimens. Polymethylmethacrylate was used for subtractive manufacturing and a light-curing resin for additive manufacturing. Three (bars) and four (FDPs) different printing orientations were evaluated. All bars (n = 32) were subjected to a three-point bending test after 24 h of water storage. Half of the 80 FDPs were dynamically loaded (250,000 cycles, 98 N) with simultaneous hydrothermal cycling. Non-aged (n = 40) and surviving FDPs (n = 11) were subjected to static loading until fracture. Regarding the bar-shaped specimens, the milled group showed the highest flexural strength (114 ± 10 MPa, $p = 0.001$), followed by the vertically printed group (97 ± 10 MPa, $p < 0.007$). Subtractive manufactured FDPs revealed the highest fracture strength (1060 ± 89 N) with all specimens surviving dynamic loading. During artificial aging, 29 of 32 printed specimens failed. The present findings indicate that both printing orientation and aging affect the strength of additive manufactured specimens. The used resin and settings cannot be recommended for additive manufacturing of long-term temporary three-unit FDPs.

**Keywords:** additive manufacturing; fracture strength; printing orientation; anisotropy; stereolithography (SLA); fixed dental prostheses

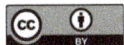

## 1. Introduction

The fabrication of fixed dental prostheses (FDPs) is rarely achieved in one session. Therefore, a temporary solution is needed to bridge the duration between preparation and cementation of the final FDP. A temporary restoration protects the prepared tooth from chemical, thermal, and physical irritations and restores chewing function, esthetics, and phonetics, as well as fixing the tooth position [1,2]. Long-term temporaries can also be used to test a new bite position [3]. While short-term temporaries can be manufactured chairside, long-term temporaries are fabricated in the dental laboratory based on conventional or digital impressions.

After conventional impression-taking, the tooth morphology can be restored using a wax-up to create a negative mold for subsequent fabrication of a temporary restoration made of chemically or light-curing resins. As an alternative, a digital workflow including computer-aided design (CAD) and computer-aided manufacturing (CAM) is feasible. This allows the manufacturing of the temporary and final FDP based on the identical data set [4].

In the case of CAD–CAM manufacturing, most of the material is discarded when the temporary restoration is milled, and reuse of the resulting waste is not possible at present [5]. In contrast, during additive manufacturing, only the volume of the temporary restoration and supporting structures are cured, making this procedure more resource-efficient.

The most widespread additive technology in dentistry is vat photopolymerization, whereby a liquid photopolymer in a vat is selectively cured by light-activated polymerization [6]. The two most established methods are stereolithography (SLA) and digital light processing (DLP). In the first case, the polymerization is performed by a directed UV-laser point; in the second case, a whole layer is simultaneously polymerized by a UV-light mask [7]. After printing, the parts have to be cleaned from excess monomer in isopropanol and then post-polymerized with UV-light.

The mechanical properties of additively manufactured parts are not only influenced by the material but also by the manufacturing process. The post-processing protocol is of crucial relevance. Post-curing time, the radiant power and wavelength of the UV-curing unit, as well as the temperature can influence the material properties [8,9]. Likewise, these are influenced by the printing orientation leading to an anisotropic behavior of the parts [10]. As reasons for this, the interlayer bond [11] and technology-based differences in the local polymerization process [12] are discussed. For geometric reference bodies, a vertical printing orientation when perpendicular loads are applied shows the highest load capacity [10]. However, little is known about to what extent this can be transferred to complex morphologies such as FDPs. In addition, the materials must withstand intraorally dynamic loads, a wet environment, and thermal stress.

Therefore, this study aimed to investigate first, the flexural strengths of subtractive manufactured versus additive manufactured reference bodies of different printing orientations according to ISO standards. The flexural strength is defined as the maximal stress reached during a three point flexural test, measured in MPa. Second, it compared the fracture strength of milled versus additive manufactured three-unit FDPs of different printing orientations by means of static loading. The fracture strength is defined as the exerted force at the moment of fracture during a static loading test, measured in N. Third, it investigated the impact of dynamical loading and thermal stress of a chewing simulator on fracture resistance. The null hypothesis assumed that neither the manufacturing method nor the printing orientation influenced the flexural and fracture strength.

## 2. Materials and Methods

### 2.1. Fabrication and Static Loading of Bar-Shaped Specimens

A bar-shaped specimen with the dimensions of $25 \times 2 \times 2$ mm was designed in a CAD software program (Tinkercad, Autodesk, San Rafael, CA, USA) and exported as a standard tessellation language (STL) file. Acting as our control group, eight bar specimens were subtractive manufactured out of the commonly used polymethylmethacrylate (PMMA) blanks for provisional restorations (inCoris, Dentsply Sirona, Charlotte, NC, USA). This was achieved using a five-axis milling machine (MC X5, Dentsply Sirona) quipped with the recommended PMMA bur set (0.5, 1.0, and 2.5 mm bur, Sirona) and the highest quality setting (inLab Software, Sirona). For additive manufacturing of 24 bar specimens, the design was digitally orientated in a vertical, diagonal, and horizontal position on the print platform (PreForm Software, Formlabs, Boston, MA, USA). Eight specimens of each orientation were printed using an acrylic resin (Denture Teeth, Formlabs) and an SLA printer (Form2, Formlabs) using a layer height of 50 µm (Figure 1).

Postprocessing of the printed samples included a 10 min wash in 99% isopropanol (Form Wash, Formlabs) followed by UV-curing for 60 min at 60 °C (Form Cure, Formlabs). After removing the supports, this post-curing process was repeated twice with the samples being submerged in vaseline. This was done to prevent an oxygen inhibition layer and, therefore, a layer of uncured resin that would negatively affect biocompatibility when used in the patient's mouth. The objects were rotated by 180° in-between the latter two post-curing steps.

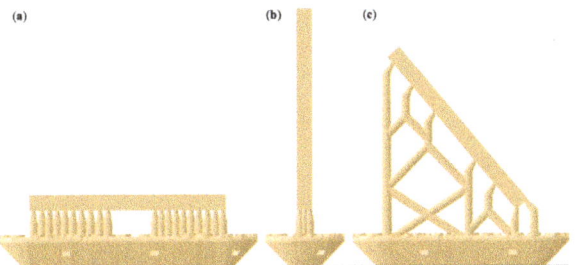

**Figure 1.** Illustration of the bar-shaped specimens in an (**a**) horizontal, (**b**) vertical, and (**c**) diagonal printing orientation including support structures and rafts.

After finishing, they were placed in distilled water for 24 h at 37 °C and measured in height and width with a digital caliper (accuracy of 0.01 µm; DealMux, Guangzhou, China). The flexural strength of both materials and the influence of the printing orientation were determined in a three-point bending test in accordance with ISO 4049 [13] as well as ISO 10477 [14]. The three-point bending test until fracture was performed using a universal testing machine (Z010/TN2S, ZwickRoell, Ulm, Germany) with a loading span of 20 mm and a crosshead speed of 1 mm/min. The maximum flexural strength, $\sigma$, in megapascal (MPa) was calculated with the following Equation (1):

$$\sigma = \frac{3FL}{2bd^2} \tag{1}$$

$F$ is the maximum load in Newton, $l$ is the distance between the supports in millimeters (20 mm), $w$ is the width in millimeters (2 mm), and $h$ is the height in millimeters (2 mm).

## 2.2. Fabrication and Static and Dynamic Loading of FDPs

### 2.2.1. Preparation of Specimens

For the standardized fabrication of three-unit FDPs, the upper right first molar (tooth 16, according to the FDI scheme) was removed from a phantom model (KaVo Dental, Biberach, Germany), and the upper right second premolar (15) and second molar (17) were prepared with a circular chamfer of 0.8 mm and an occlusal reduction of 1.5 mm. This situation was digitized with a model scanner (inEos X5, inLab software, Dentsply Sirona), and a three-unit FDP was designed following the recommended settings of the inLab software for the fabrication of long-term temporaries out of inCoris PMMA blanks. This resulted in connector sizes of 15.05 mm² mesial and 14.07 mm² distal of the pontic 16 (Figure 2).

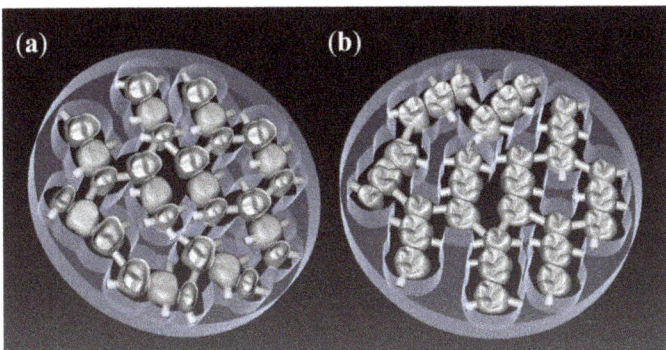

**Figure 2.** Ten fixed dental prostheses (FDPs) nested into one olymethylmethacrylate(PMMA) blank (inCoris, Dentsply Sirona): (**a**) bottom view, (**b**) top view.

As our control group for both aged and non-aged specimens, 16 milled FPDs (M1 n = 8, M2 n = 8) were manufactured, similar to the bar-shaped specimens, out of PMMA blanks (inCoris, MC X5 milling machine, Dentsply Sirona) (Figure 3).

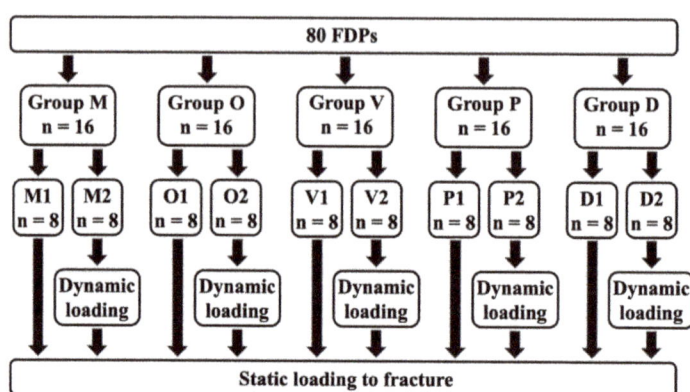

**Figure 3.** Groups: (M) milled, (O) occlusal, (V) vertical, (P) palatal, (D) diagonal, (1) non-aged, (2) aged.

For additive manufacturing of the FDPs (n = 64), four printing orientations were used (Figure 4). Group occlusal (O): Occlusal surface pointing down towards the print platform. Group vertical (V): The distal side of the FDP is facing the print platform. Group palatal (P): The palatal side of the FDP is facing the print platform. Group diagonal (D): Positioning at a 45° angle with the mesial side facing the print platform.

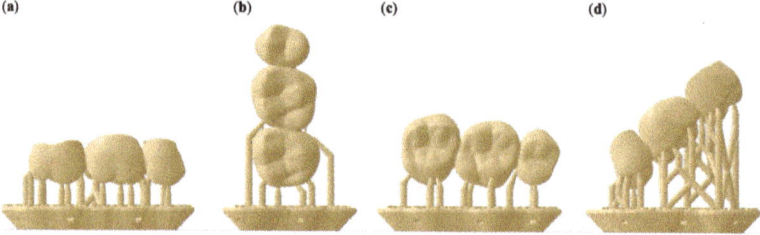

**Figure 4.** Illustration of the FDP specimens in an (**a**) occlusal, (**b**) vertical, (**c**) palatal, and (**d**) diagonal printing orientation including support structures and rafts.

The supports were only placed on the outside of the FDP; no internal supports were used. All FDPs of groups O, V, P, and D were printed and post-processed similar to the bar-shaped specimens.

A total of 80 FDPs were produced, consisting of five groups of 16 specimens each.

#### 2.2.2. Preparation of Object Holders

For designing a standardized object holder, the scan of the dental model was reduced to the area from stump 15 to 17 and exported. A cylindric bottom part with a diameter of 4 cm and a height of 1.5 cm was generated using a CAD software program (Tinkercad, Autodesk) and merged with the reduced dental model into a single STL file (MeshMixer, Autodesk) (Figure 5).

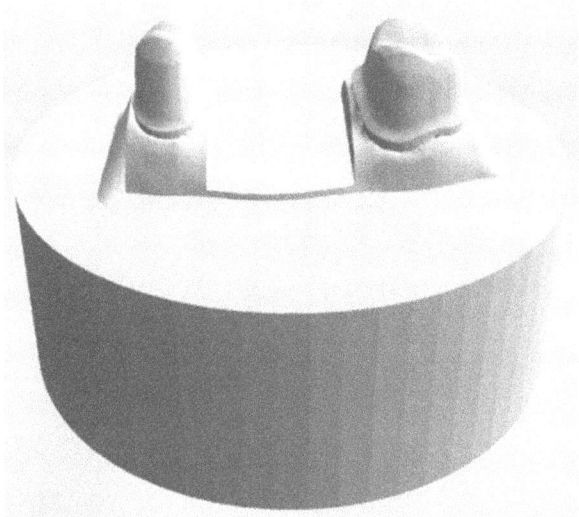

**Figure 5.** Design of the object holder with two prepared teeth.

Based on this design, 80 object holders were printed in acrylic resin (Rigid, Formlabs) on the SLA printer (Form2, Formlabs) using a layer height of 50 µm. After the print was completed the object holders were cleaned for 15 min using 99% isopropanol (Form Wash, Formlabs) and UV-cured for 30 min at 60 °C (Form Cure, Formlabs).

All FDPs were cemented to their object holders with zinc oxide-based cement for temporary cementation (TempBond NE, Kerr, Bioggio, Switzerland) following the recommendations of the manufacturers at a controlled pressure of 80 N.

*2.3. Dynamic Loading with Simultaneous Hydrothermal Cycling*

The 16 samples of all five groups were subdivided into (1) eight specimens remaining as manufactured and (2) eight that were artificially loaded and aged in a computer-controlled dual-axis chewing simulator (CS4.8, Willytec, Munich, Germany) by means of dynamic loading and hydrothermal cycling.

Dynamic loading consisted of a vertical load of 98 N applied at the center of the occlusal surface by means of a three-point support (mesio buccal, mesio palatal, and distobuccal cusp) of 16 with a subsequent lateral side shift of 0.5 mm under load. To simulate one year of clinical loading, 250,000 cycles were chosen [15]. Hydrothermal cycling included an exposure to water set at 5 °C for 30 s, a drain time of 10 s, followed by an exposure of 30 s to water set at 55 °C. The status of the FDPs was visually controlled twice per day.

*2.4. Static Loading*

All bridges, the non-loaded as well as those that survived the dynamic loading procedure in the artificial chewing simulator, were loaded until fracture at the previously described three-point contact of 16 at a speed of 10 mm/min using the universal testing machine (Z010/TN2S, ZwickRoell). The maximum load (Fmax) was recorded.

*2.5. Statistical Analysis*

Normal distribution (Kolmogorov–Smirnov test) and variance homogeneity (Levene-test) of the data were verified. Afterward, the flexural strength (MPa) of the bar-shaped specimens and the maximum load (Fmax) of the FDPs were analyzed by one-way ANOVA with post-hoc Bonferroni pairwise comparisons. The analysis was performed with a statistical software program (SPSS Statistics, v22.0, IBM, Armonk, NY, USA). The significance level was set at α < 0.05.

## 3. Results

### 3.1. Static Loading of Bar-Shaped Specimens

The group of milled bars showed the highest mean fracture strength with 113.6 ± 9.8 MPa (Table 1). All printed groups showed significantly lower values ($p$ = 0.001), with the vertically printed bars showing significantly higher flexural strength compared to the diagonally and horizontally printed groups ($p$ < 0.007).

**Table 1.** Mean and standard deviation (SD) of the flexural strength of the subtractive and additive manufactured bars in megapascals (MPa).

| Technology | Group | N | Mean | SD |
|---|---|---|---|---|
| subtractive | milled | 8 | 113.6 * MPa | 9.8 MPa |
| additive | horizontal | 8 | 82.8 ** MPa | 4.2 MPa |
| additive | vertical | 8 | 96.9 *** MPa | 9.9 MPa |
| additive | diagonal | 8 | 83.4 * MPa | 3.6 MPa |

Groups with the same asterisks count did not differ significantly from each other.

### 3.2. Dynamic Loading with Simultaneous Hydrothermal Cycling of FDPs

While all milled specimens sustained the artificial loading (group M2), the additive manufactured specimens failed more often. In group P2 and O2, all specimens fractured. In group D2 only one and in group V2 two out of eight specimens survived the aging procedure (Figure 6).

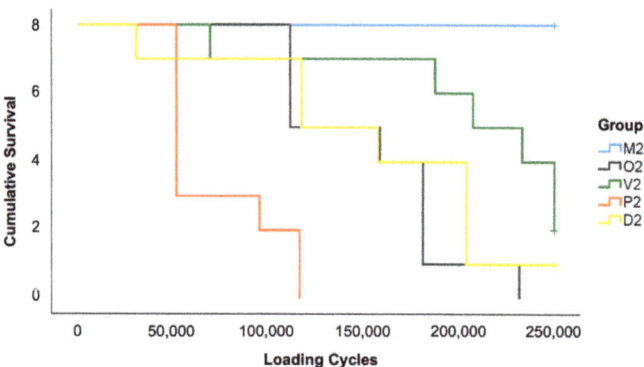

**Figure 6.** Kaplan–Meier survival rates of the FDPs during thermodynamic loading.

### 3.3. Static Loading of FDPs

One-way ANOVA of the untreated samples revealed significant differences between the groups ($p$ = 0.001). The mean fracture load of group M1 (1060.1 ± 88.9 N) showed significantly higher values compared with all additive manufactured specimens, except group D1 ($p$ = 0.311). Among the printed specimens, D1 showed the highest load capacity (931.7 ± 151.3 N) and P1 the lowest (727.6 ± 107.3 N, $p$ > 0.011).

When comparing M1 with M2 (1064.3 ± 61.3 N), no significant difference was found ($p$ = 0.931). The two surviving FDPs from group V2 showed a fracture strength of 983.5 N and 674.3 N, whereas the surviving specimen of group D2 fractured at an applied load of 1075.2 N (Figure 7).

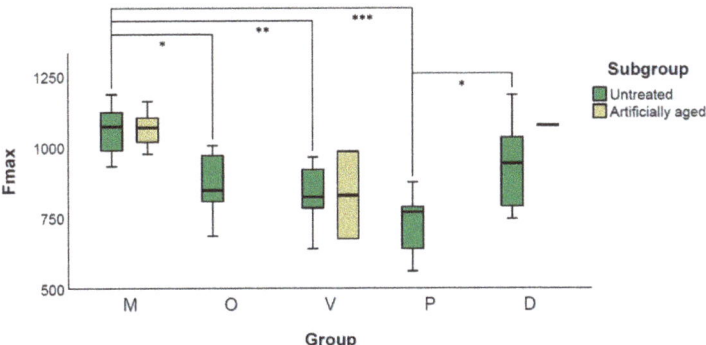

**Figure 7.** Grouped Boxplot of Fmax (N) of untreated and artificial loaded FDPs. Additive manufactured specimens revealed a total failure during artificial aging in group O and P, one survivor in D and two in V represented by the upper and lower limits of the box. * indicates $p < 0.05$; ** indicates $p < 0.01$, *** indicates $p < 0.001$.

*3.4. Fracture Analysis*

All 16 subtractive manufactured FDPs fractured into two parts when statically loaded (Figure 8). Nine samples fractured between crown 15 and its connector (Table 2); the other seven showed a fracture affecting 15, the connector, and 16. During artificial aging, 29 out of 32 additive manufactured FDPs fractured. Of those, 93% fractured into two pieces. The prevalent failure patterns were a fractured connector of 15 (83%), a fractured pontic (76%), and a fractured premolar crown (72%). All statically loaded specimens fractured into multiple pieces.

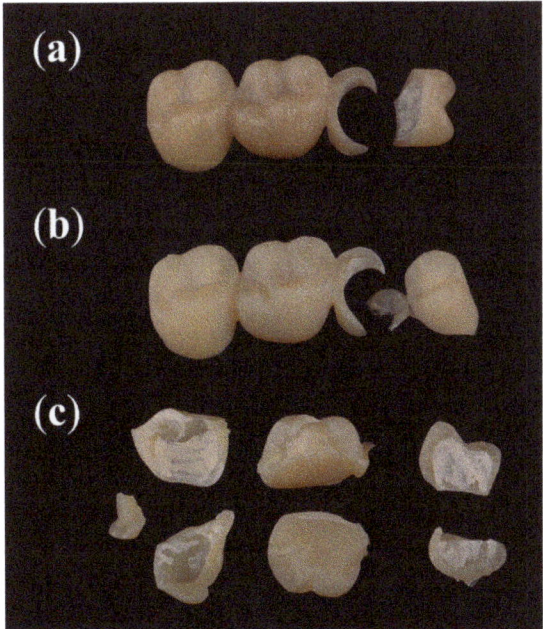

**Figure 8.** Most common fracture patterns: (**a**) statically loaded subtractive manufactured FDPs and (**b**) dynamically loaded additive manufactured FDPs fractured into two pieces, while (**c**) statically loaded additive manufactured FDPs fractured into multiple pieces.

Table 2. Areas of failures during dynamic and static loading of FDPs.

| Technology | Loading | N | Crown 15 | Connector 1 | Pontic 16 | Connector 2 | Crown 17 |
|---|---|---|---|---|---|---|---|
| subtractive | dynamic | 0 | 0 | 0 | 0 | 0 | 0 |
|  | static | 16 | 16 | 16 | 7 | 0 | 0 |
| additive | dynamic | 32 | 21 | 24 | 22 | 8 | 7 |
|  | static | 35 | 34 | 35 | 34 | 34 | 31 |

## 4. Discussion

In this in vitro study, the effect of printing orientation of additive manufactured temporary FDPs on fracture strength was compared to subtractive manufactured samples. The fracture strength was statically determined according to available ISO standards using bar-shaped specimens as well as statically and dynamically by means of artificial loaded FDPs. As a result, the fracture resistance was significantly affected by the manufacturing technique, the printing orientation, and in the case of the additive manufactured FPDs, the applied loading procedure. Therefore, the null hypothesis had to be rejected. Subtractive manufactured specimens showed the highest loading capacity. A vertical printing orientation revealed the highest values for bar-shaped specimens, whereas a diagonal printing orientation showed the highest values for FDPs. Dynamic loading with simultaneous hydrothermal cycling did not affect the fracture strength of the subtractive manufactured FDPs, while most of the additive manufactured specimens failed during this procedure.

The combined testing of bar-shaped specimens and FDPs was intended to evaluate whether the results of standardized ISO-conform specimens can be transferred to complex organic morphologies. Since the materials are exposed to complex loads and temperature fluctuations in the oral cavity, the FDPs were additionally dynamically loaded and hydrothermally cycled in the chewing simulator. A vertical load of 98 N representing applied forces during mastication was applied [16]. This is consistent with comparable studies [17]. Additionally, each loading cycle included a lateral movement by means of a 0.5 mm side shift with the applied load of the antagonist. This simulates complex masticatory motions and represents higher stress compared to solely vertically applied forces [18]. Furthermore, since some materials are known to be less fatigue-resistant when exposed to an aqueous environment [19,20], hydrothermal cycling in water changing the temperature from 5 to 55 °C every 30 s was included during dynamic loading. In previous studies, it was discussed that rigid sample holders led to a reduction in the fracture load and may not reflect the biological conditions [8,21]. For this reason, customized sample holders were made of resin instead of prefabricated steel mounts to mimic the dampening effect of the periodontal fiber apparatus between the alveolar bone and teeth.

The choice of cementation material can affect the fracture strength of crowns [22]. In this study, eugenol-free temporary cement was used for cementation. Nakamura et al. [23] showed that their adhesively cemented zirconia crowns achieved higher fracture loads compared to those cemented conventionally. In addition, Stawarczyk et al. [22] showed that leucite reinforced glass-ceramic crowns achieved significantly higher fracture loads using an adhesive cement acting as a stress breaker, but no such effect was found for resin-based crowns. Whether adhesive cementation would have resulted in higher fracture loading capacities in this study remains unknown. However, adhesive cementation of temporary FDPs is currently not to be considered a clinical standard procedure.

All bar specimens achieved significantly higher flexural strength than the 50 MPa required by the ISO 10477:2020 standard [14], but only the subtractive manufactured bar specimens achieved more than the required 100 MPa of the ISO 14049:2019 standard [13]. The vertical printing orientation showed the highest mean flexural strength of all printed bar specimens (96.9 MPa) with an increase of 16% compared to the other additive manufactured bars. This is in accordance with Unkovskiy et al. [10] who showed that the specimens with layer orientation parallel to the axial load achieved superior flexural strength. The horizontal and diagonal printing orientation showed similar results. Meanwhile, new materials containing ceramic fillers are available on the market which may reveal improved strength.

Regarding the FDPs, a high failure rate of the additive manufactured groups under dynamic loading with simultaneous thermocycling occurred. Therefore, the additive manufactured groups with and without artificial aging could not be compared to each other due to the resulting low sample size. For the subtractive manufactured FDPs, artificial aging did not end in a statistically significant difference regarding fracture strength. Static loading of the FDPs revealed that the subtractive manufactured group showed a significantly higher fracture strength compared to all additive manufactured specimen, except those printed in a diagonal orientation. In accordance with Park et al. [11], the group with the palatal printing orientation of the FDPs exhibited the lowest fracture strength. The diagonally printed FDPs showed the highest load capacity, but the differences to the vertical and occlusal printing orientations are minor and might not be of clinical relevance.

The data obtained in the present investigation for FDPs are not directly comparable to other studies. Many factors such as the span length and design of the FDPs influence the load capacity. Reymus et al. compared different parameters that affect the fracture strength of CAD–CAM fabricated temporary FDPs [8]. The load capacities in their investigation ranged from 777 to 1050 N, depending on the used resin. Milled samples showed comparable results to the printed ones (881 N), but the control group using chairside autopolymerizing bis-acryl methacrylate exhibited significantly lower fracture strengths (552 N). This is in agreement with the values of Park et al., who showed comparable fracture strength values for FDPs after milling, SLA, and DLP printing, but reduced results for chairside autopolymerizing [11].

The fracture analysis revealed that the milled FDPs fractured under static load into two pieces, while the additive manufactured ones fractured into multiple pieces. The pontic was prone to fracture longitudinally under static loading. It could be explained by the force exerted through the round shape of the indenter resulting in a transversal force and spreading the buccal and palatal cusps apart. This effect is to be expected to be less pronounced during the dynamic loading with a force of only 98 N, explaining the different fracture behaviors.

The anisotropy of additive materials caused by the printing orientation is known [24]. The demonstrated increased load capacity of the vertically printed bar-shaped specimens is in line with previous investigations [10,24]. For the two most common technologies, SLA and DLP, this can be explained by two different phenomena. In the case of SLA, the laser speed is slower in the marginal areas and leads to a higher degree of polymerization than in central areas [12]. When vertically printed, the ratio is improved in favor of the marginal areas [25]. Using DLP, the UV-light is projected over an assembly of micro-mirrors, resulting in a simultaneously polymerized layer consisting of a multitude of voxels. In the vertical direction, the voxels are polymerized without gaps forming columns layer by layer. In the lateral direction, however, the voxels are separated from each other by thin interstitial areas showing a reduced degree of polymerization. These areas correspond to the boundaries of each micro-mirror, which may represent a potential weakness [12]. When vertically oriented, long columns are present, whereas flat orientation results in many short columns with correspondingly numerous interstitial areas. If the anisotropy of the parts is not explained by the interlayer bonding, but by varying laser speed between marginal and central regions, it is comprehensible that complex morphologies such as FDPs can show a different optimal printing orientation compared to bar-shaped specimens. In this study, a diagonal printing orientation showed the best results for FDPs. This is consistent with the results of Park et al., who showed increased loading capacity when FDPs were diagonally printed [11]. However, the effect of printing orientation for SLA and DLP is overlaid by other factors. Layer height [24], post-processing parameters such as wavelength [8], and radiant power [9], as well as water absorption [26], have a greater influence on the mechanical properties.

The described weakening effect through water absorption is in line with our results of the artificially aged groups. The non-aged specimens withstood at least 559 N and up to 1183 N during static loading. However, almost all failed during dynamic loading with 98 N and simultaneous thermocycling. Väyrynen et al. used geometric reference bodies to investigate the influence of printing orientation and water storage on fracture strength [26]. Printing orientation showed a minor influence with slightly better values for vertical and diagonal orientation. In contrast, water storage of 14 days reduced the load capacity of the specimens by about 50%. Berli et al. demonstrated that two out of three investigated additively manufactured resins absorbed significantly more water than milled polymers [27]. For both materials, the fracture strength after water storage was reduced by about one-third. This is in accordance with our results of the additive manufactured and artificially aged FDPs that showed a comparable fracture strength to the non-aged groups after being no longer subjected to an aqueous environment. The third printable resin in their study, which showed only low water uptake, exhibited almost the same strength in the water-saturated as in the dry state. The water uptake is reversible [27], which explains why the surviving FDPs after dynamic loading and drying showed comparable loading capacity to the initial state.

The resin used in this study has no ceramic fillers. Newer resins that incorporate ceramic particles might show improved mechanical properties. Artificial saliva would have allowed for a closer representation of the intraoral situation, but because of the risk of mineral depositions, only the use of distilled water is allowed in the chewing simulator.

In summary, the printing orientation affected the flexural strength of standardized bars and the fracture strength of the FDPs. Assuming varying laser speeds as the reason for those results, the morphology of the printed object is of decisive importance. General recommendations for the printing orientation can, therefore, not be given. The effect of water storage and artificial aging of the additive manufactured specimens has to be regarded as detrimental. This fatiguing resulted in failure significantly below the initial load capacity of the additive manufactured specimens. Accordingly, when using materials for restorations in patients, not only ISO conform flexural tests are required, but also the validation of fatigue after simulated long-term loading and water immersion under clinically realistic conditions is highly important.

## 5. Conclusions

The subtractive manufactured bars and FDPs showed the highest strength in all experiments. The strength of the additive manufactured specimens was affected by the printing orientation. While vertical printing was superior for the bar-shaped specimens in terms of flexural strength, diagonal printing orientation showed the highest fracture strength for the FDPs. According to our results, the palatal printing orientation should be avoided. Additive manufacturing of the utilized material for the FDPs showed acceptable fracture strength in the dry state, but dynamic loading with simultaneous hydrothermal cycling decreased the strength in a clinically relevant way.

**Author Contributions:** Conceptualization, J.N. and R.J.K.; methodology, J.N.; validation B.C.S.; investigation, J.N., S.W., L.R. and L.B.; formal analysis, C.W. and B.C.S.; supervision, R.J.K.;writing—original draft preparation, J.N. and C.W; writing—review and editing, R.J.K. and B.C.S. All authors have read and agreed to the published version of the manuscript.

**Funding:** This research received no external funding.

**Institutional Review Board Statement:** Not applicable.

**Informed Consent Statement:** Not applicable.

**Data Availability Statement:** Data is contained within the article.

**Acknowledgments:** All materials used were provided by the manufacturing companies (Dentsply Sirona, Formlabs). The article processing charge was funded by the Baden-Wuerttemberg Ministry of

Science, Research and Art and the University of Freiburg in the funding programme Open Access Publishing.

**Conflicts of Interest:** The authors declare no conflict of interest.

## References

1. Burns, D.R.; Beck, D.A.; Nelson, S.K. A review of selected dental literature on contemporary provisional fixed prosthodontic treatment: Report of the Committee on Research in Fixed Prosthodontics of the Academy of Fixed Prosthodontics. *J. Prosthet. Dent.* **2003**, *90*, 474–497. [CrossRef]
2. Burke, F.J.T.; Murray, M.C.; Shortall, A.C.C. Trends in indirect dentistry: 6. Provisional restorations, more than just a temporary. *Dent. Update* **2005**, *32*, 443–444. [CrossRef] [PubMed]
3. Fox, C.W.; Abrams, B.L.; Doukoudakis, A. Provisional restorations for altered occlusions. *J. Prosthet. Dent.* **1984**, *52*, 567–572. [CrossRef]
4. Davidowitz, G.; Kotick, P.G. The use of CAD/CAM in dentistry. *Dent. Clin. N. Am.* **2011**, *55*, 559–570. [CrossRef] [PubMed]
5. Wemken, G.; Spies, B.C.; Pieralli, S.; Adali, U.; Beuer, F.; Wesemann, C. Do hydrothermal aging and microwave sterilization affect the trueness of milled, additive manufactured and injection molded denture bases? *J. Mech. Behav. Biomed. Mater.* **2020**, *111*, 103975. [CrossRef] [PubMed]
6. ASTM. *ASTM Standard Terminology for Additive Manufacturing—General Principles—Terminology*; ASTM: West Conshohocken, PA, USA, 2015.
7. Groth, C.; Kravitz, N.D.; Jones, P.E.; Graham, J.W.; Redmond, W.R. Three-dimensional printing technology. *J. Clin. Orthod.* **2014**, *48*, 475–485. [PubMed]
8. Reymus, M.; Fabritius, R.; Keßler, A.; Hickel, R.; Edelhoff, D.; Stawarczyk, B. Fracture load of 3D-printed fixed dental prostheses compared with milled and conventionally fabricated ones: The impact of resin material, build direction, post-curing, and artificial aging—an in vitro study. *Clin. Oral Investig.* **2019**, *24*, 701–710. [CrossRef] [PubMed]
9. Zguris, Z. *How Mechanical Properties of Stereolithography 3D Prints Are Affected by UV Curing*; Formlabs Inc.: Somerville, MA, USA, 2016.
10. Unkovskiy, A.; Bui, P.H.-B.; Schille, C.; Geis-Gerstörfer, J.; Huettig, F.; Spintzyk, S. Objects build orientation, positioning, and curing influence dimensional accuracy and flexural properties of stereolithographically printed resin. *Dent. Mater.* **2018**, *34*, e324–e333. [CrossRef]
11. Park, S.-M.; Park, J.-M.; Kim, S.-K.; Heo, S.-J.; Koak, J.-Y. Comparison of flexural strength of three-dimensional printed three-unit provisional fixed dental prostheses according to build directions. *J. Korean Dent. Sci.* **2019**, *12*, 13–19. [CrossRef]
12. Monzón, M.; Ortega, Z.; Hernández, A.; Paz, R.; Ortega, F. Anisotropy of photopolymer parts made by digital light processing. *Materials* **2017**, *10*, 64. [CrossRef]
13. International Organization for Standardization. *ISO 4049:2019—Dentistry—Polymer-Based Restorative Materials*; ISO: Geneva, Switzerland, 2019.
14. International Organization for Standardization. *ISO 10477:2020—Dentistry—Polymer-Based Crown and Veneering Materials*; ISO: Geneva, Switzerland, 2020.
15. DeLong, R.; Sakaguchi, R.L.; Douglas, W.H.; Pintado, M.R. The wear of dental amalgam in an artificial mouth: A clinical correlation. *Dent. Mater.* **1985**, *1*, 238–242. [CrossRef]
16. Schindler, H.J.; Stengel, E.; Spiess, W.E.L. Feedback control during mastication of solid food textures—A clinical-experimental study. *J. Prosthet. Dent.* **1998**, *80*, 330–336. [CrossRef]
17. Reeponmaha, T.; Angwaravong, O.; Angwarawong, T. Comparison of fracture strength after thermo-mechanical aging between provisional crowns made with CAD/CAM and conventional method. *J. Adv. Prosthodont.* **2020**, *12*, 218–224. [CrossRef] [PubMed]
18. Wimmer, T.; Huffmann, A.M.S.; Eichberger, M.; Schmidlin, P.R.; Stawarczyk, B. Two-body wear rate of PEEK, CAD/CAM resin composite and PMMA: Effect of specimen geometries, antagonist materials and test set-up configuration. *Dent. Mater.* **2016**, *32*, e127–e136. [CrossRef] [PubMed]
19. Lang, R.; Rosentritt, M.; Behr, M.; Handel, G. Fracture resistance of PMMA and resin matrix composite-based interim FPD materials. *Int. J. Prosthodont.* **2003**, *16*, 381–384. [PubMed]
20. Stawarczyk, B.; Ender, A.; Trottmann, A.; Özcan, M.; Fischer, J.; Hämmerle, C.H.F. Load-bearing capacity of CAD/CAM milled polymeric three-unit fixed dental prostheses: Effect of aging regimens. *Clin. Oral Investig.* **2012**, *16*, 1669–1677. [CrossRef]
21. Mahmood, D.J.H.; Linderoth, E.H.; Vult Von Steyern, P. The influence of support properties and complexity on fracture strength and fracture mode of all-ceramic fixed dental prostheses. *Acta Odontol. Scand* **2011**, *69*, 229–237. [CrossRef]
22. Stawarczyk, B.; Beuer, F.; Ender, A.; Roos, M.; Edelhoff, D.; Wimmer, T. Influence of cementation and cement type on the fracture load testing methodology of anterior crowns made of different materials. *Dent. Mater. J.* **2013**, *32*, 888–895. [CrossRef]
23. Nakamura, K.; Mouhat, M.; Nergård, J.M.; Lægreid, S.J.; Kanno, T.; Milleding, P.; Örtengren, U. Effect of cements on fracture resistance of monolithic zirconia crowns. *Acta Biomater. Odontol. Scan.* **2016**, *2*, 12–19. [CrossRef]
24. Dizon, J.R.C.; Espera, A.H.; Chen, Q.; Advincula, R.C. Mechanical characterization of 3D-printed polymers. *Addit. Manuf.* **2018**, *20*, 44–67. [CrossRef]

25. Puebla, K.; Arcaute, K.; Quintana, R.; Wicker, R.B. Effects of environmental conditions, aging, and build orientations on the mechanical properties of ASTM type I specimens manufactured via stereolithography. *Rapid Prototyp.* **2012**, *18*, 374–388. [CrossRef]
26. Väyrynen, V.O.E.; Tanner, J.; Vallittu, P.K. The anisotropicity of the flexural properties of an occlusal device material processed by stereolithography. *J. Prosthet. Dent.* **2016**, *116*, 811–817. [CrossRef] [PubMed]
27. Berli, C.; Thieringer, F.M.; Sharma, N.; Müller, J.A.; Dedem, P.; Fischer, J.; Rohr, N. Comparing the mechanical properties of pressed, milled, and 3D-printed resins for occlusal devices. *J. Prosthet. Dent.* **2020**, *124*, 780–786. [CrossRef] [PubMed]

# PICN Nanocomposite as Dental CAD/CAM Block Comparable to Human Tooth in Terms of Hardness and Flexural Modulus

Yohei Kawajiri [1,2], Hiroshi Ikeda [2,*], Yuki Nagamatsu [2], Chihiro Masaki [1], Ryuji Hosokawa [1] and Hiroshi Shimizu [2]

1. Division of Oral Reconstruction and Rehabilitation, Department of Oral Functions, Kyushu Dental University, Fukuoka 803-8580, Japan; r16kawajiri@fa.kyu-dent.ac.jp (Y.K.); masaki@kyu-dent.ac.jp (C.M.); hosokawa@kyu-dent.ac.jp (R.H.)
2. Division of Biomaterials, Department of Oral Functions, Kyushu Dental University, Fukuoka 803-8580, Japan; yuki-naga@kyu-dent.ac.jp (Y.N.); r14shimizu@fa.kyu-dent.ac.jp (H.S.)
* Correspondence: r16ikeda@fa.kyu-dent.ac.jp; Tel.: +81-93-582-1131

**Abstract:** Polymer infiltrated ceramic network (PICN) composites are an increasingly popular dental restorative material that offer mechanical biocompatibility with human enamel. This study aimed to develop a novel PICN composite as a computer-aided design and computer-aided manufacturing (CAD/CAM) block for dental applications. Several PICN composites were prepared under varying conditions via the sintering of a green body prepared from a silica-containing precursor solution, followed by resin infiltration. The flexural strength of the PICN composite block (107.8–153.7 MPa) was similar to a commercial resin-based composite, while the Vickers hardness (204.8–299.2) and flexural modulus (13.0–22.2 GPa) were similar to human enamel and dentin, respectively. The shear bond strength and surface free energy of the composite were higher than those of the commercial resin composites. Scanning electron microscopy and energy dispersive X-ray spectroscopic analysis revealed that the microstructure of the composite consisted of a nanosized silica skeleton and infiltrated resin. The PICN nanocomposite block was successfully used to fabricate a dental crown and core via the CAD/CAM milling process.

**Keywords:** CAD/CAM; polymer infiltrated ceramic network; nanocomposite; silica; restorative material; dental material; biomimetics; dental core; dental crown; mechanical properties

## 1. Introduction

The fabrication of dental prostheses has shifted from conventional craftsmanship to digital techniques based on computer-aided design and computer-aided manufacturing (CAD/CAM) [1–3]. Specifically, recent advances in CAD/CAM technologies have allowed for the production of dental crowns, inlays, bridges and cores using block materials and the CAD/CAM milling process. In materials science, contemporary CAD/CAM blocks are categorized into three groups, namely metal-based (e.g., titanium alloy [4] and Co-Cr alloy [5]), ceramic-based (e.g., feldspathic porcelain [6], lithium disilicate glass [7] and zirconia [8]), or resin-based (e.g., acrylic resin [9] and resin composite (hereafter composite) [10]). An investigation of new composites already in use (e.g., poly(ether-ether-ketone) (PEEK) [11]) and some interesting research on new materials with hierarchized geometry [12] and biomechanical problems [13–15] (i.e., bruxism) have also been conducted thus far.

CAD/CAM blocks that offer excellent biocompatibility and mechanical properties in the oral environment have been practically implemented, but their mechanical properties differ from those of human tooth [16]. To overcome this issue, dental material development should consider biomimetics [17,18]. Biomimetic materials imitate a biological function and tissue morphology, where such dental materials have been previously investigated and reported [16,19–21]. Biomimetic dental restorative materials for prostheses should imitate the properties of natural tooth and its components, such as enamel and dentin [22]. Previous reports on the development of restorative materials that mimic tooth morphology and function [23,24] have demonstrated that highly biocompatible materials show promise as next-generation dental CAD/CAM blocks.

The realization of long-term tooth restoration using a dental material without fatal failure of the tooth or the restorative material is important. External stress tends to be concentrated at the interface of dissimilar materials with different mechanical properties [25]. The differences in the mechanical properties of a natural tooth, such as the hardness and elastic modulus, between the enamel and dentin are drastic. Further, the dentin–enamel junction, which is the gradient structure for connecting the enamel and dentin, moderates the stress concentration at the interface, thereby avoiding fatal failure of the natural tooth [26]. With regard to biomimetics, the mechanical properties of the restoration material and natural teeth should be the same. However, the Vickers hardness ($H_V$) and the elastic modulus (E) of the recent CAD/CAM materials, such as zirconia ($H_V$ = ca. 1300–1641, E = ca. 146–210 GPa [27]), lithium disilicate glass ($H_V$ = ca. 580–676, E = ca. 95–96 GPa [27]), and resin-composites ($H_V$ = ca. 65–98, E = ca. 9–15 GPa [10]), differ from those of dentin ($H_V$ = ca. 20–90 [28], E = 16–25 GPa [29–31]) and enamel ($H_V$ = ca. 270–420 [28], E = 48–105 GPa [32,33]).

The CAD/CAM material that offers mechanical properties that most closely mimic human enamel, thereby ensuring mechanical biocompatibility, is polymer infiltrated ceramic network (PICN) composite [34–40]. PICN composites have a dual network microstructure comprising a ceramic skeleton with infiltrated resin. This structure differs from conventional dispersed-filler (DF) composites, which comprise filler dispersed in a resin matrix [41]. PICN composite CAD/CAM blocks have been applied to indirect tooth restoration [42,43], where several basic and clinical studies have used a commercially available PICN composite named VITA ENAMIC, which comprises a silicate glass ceramic skeleton with infiltrated acrylic resin [34]. The previous studies have demonstrated that the PICN composites suitably mimic human enamel, specifically in terms of mechanical properties [16,44]. However, differences between the mechanical properties of PICN composites and teeth remain, thus there is room for further improvement.

This study aimed to develop a novel PICN composite CAD/CAM block material to mimic the mechanical properties of enamel and dentin. The PICN composite block was produced using a novel process.

## 2. Materials and Methods

The composition of the precursor solution was optimized to obtain a monolithic block without fatal cracks, and six PICN composites were prepared under different preparation conditions (sintering time, type of infiltration resin monomer, and polymerization schedule) (see Appendix A). The mechanical properties (flexural strength, flexural modulus, and Vickers hardness) of the PICN composite blocks were evaluated, and the bonding properties to resin cement were assessed based on shear bond strength (SBS) and surface free energy (SFE). Further, the microstructure of the PICN composite was determined using scanning electron microscopy (SEM). The resultant PICN composite block was used to produce a dental crown and core via CAD/CAM milling.

### 2.1. Materials

The regents used to produce the PICN composite are listed in Table 1. The resulting PICN composites were compared to the commercial composites (i.e., control samples) listed in Table 2.

Table 1. Reagents used for preparation of PICN composites.

| Acronym | Material Type | Manufacturer | Product Name | Purity (%) |
| --- | --- | --- | --- | --- |
| Silica | Nanoparticles | NiPPON AEROSIL, Tokyo, Japan | OX50 | 99.8 |
| HEMA | Monomer | FujiFilm Wako Chemical, Osaka, Japan | 2-hydroxyethy methacrylate | 95.0 |
| TEGDMA | Monomer | FujiFilm Wako Chemical, Osaka, Japan | Triethylene glycol dimethacrylate | 90.0 |
| POE | Solvent | FujiFilm Wako Chemical, Osaka, Japan | 2-phenoxyethanol | 99.0 |
| PrOH | Solvent | FujiFilm Wako Chemical, Osaka, Japan | 1-propanol | 99.5 |
| BAPO | Light-initiator | FujiFilm Wako Chemical, Osaka, Japan | Phenylbis (2, 4, 6-trimethyl-benzoyl) phosphine oxide | 97.0 |
| γ-MPTS | Silane coupling agent | Shin-Etsu Chemical, Tokyo, Japan | 3-methacryl oxypropyl trimethoxysilane | 99.9 |
| UDMA | Monomer | Sigma-Aldrich, St. Louis, MO, USA | Urethane dimethacrylate | 97.0 |
| BPO | Heat-initiator | Alfa Aesar, Lancashire, UK | Benzoyl peroxide | 97.0 |

Table 2. Commercial resin composite control samples.

| Acronym | Material Type | Product | Manufacturer | Monomer Composition | Filler Composition |
| --- | --- | --- | --- | --- | --- |
| DC* | Direct resin composite | Clear fill DC core Auto Mix ONE | Kuraray Noritake Dentall, Tokyo, Japan | Bis-GMA, methacrylic monomer, TEGDMA, other | Silica, Alumina, Silica-based glass |
| AV | Indirect resin composite (CAD/CAM block) | KATANA AVENCIA Block | Kuraray Noritake Dentall, Tokyo, Japan | UDMA, methacrylic monomer, other | Silica, Aulmina |

* The specimen was formed via a light-curing by following manufacture's instructions and used for the experiment.

### 2.2. Preparation of PICN Composite

The PICN composites were produced using a novel process, as illustrated in Figure 1. This process included seven steps, as follows: (I) preparation of light-curable precursor solution, (II) molding of precursor, (III) light-curing of precursor to form a green body, (IV) sintering of green body to form a porous body, (V) infiltration of resin monomer into sintered porous body, (VI) heat-polymerization of the infiltrated body, and (VII) cutting the PICN composite to give CAD/CAM blocks. Six different PICN composites were produced by varying the preparation conditions, namely the sintering duration at 1150 °C, type of infiltrated resin monomer, and polymerization schedule for the infiltrated resin monomer.

The precursor solution (PS-1, see Appendix A and Table A1) were prepared with varying proportions of monomers (2-hydroxyethy methacrylate (HEMA) and triethylene glycol di-methacrylate (TEGDMA)) and solvents (2-phenoxyethanol (POE) and 1-propanol (PrOH)) with a fixed content of $SiO_2$ nanoparticles and light initiator (phenylbis (2, 4, 6-trimethyl-benzoyl) phosphine oxide (BAPO). The reagents were mixed using a planetary centrifugal mixer (ARE-310, THINKY Corp., Tokyo, Japan) at 2000 rpm for 6 min, and defoamed for 1 min using the defoam mode of the mixer to remove microbubbles from the solution. The precursor solution was poured into transparent silicone mold (height = 20 mm; diameter = 18 mm) and light-cured using a light-irradiator (α-LIGHT II N, J. Morita Corp., Suita, Japan) for 10 min. The samples were dried in an oven at 80 °C for 1 week to fabricate a green body. The green bodies were sintered in a furnace according to the following heating schedule: heating from room temperature to 220 °C at 50 °C/h; isothermal hold at 220 °C for 6 h; heating to 600 °C at 100 °C/h; isothermal hold for 3 h; heating to 1150 °C at 100 °C/h; isothermal hold for 1, 2, or 3 h (Table 3); and cooling to room temperature inside the furnace. The sintered body was a porous silica block, which was immersed in a silane solution of γ-MPTS (0.5 g), ethanol (8.5 g), distilled water (1.0 g), and 1M $HNO_3$ (100 μL) at room temperature for 3 h and dried in an oven (DY300, Yamato Scientific Co., Ltd., Tokyo, Japan) at 80 °C for 3 h. The silanized porous silica block was immersed in a resin monomer containing 0.5 wt% BPO at room temperature for 3 days.

The monomer infiltrated silica block was heat-polymerized using the appropriate schedule for the monomer composition (Table 3) to give the PICN composite. The PICN composite was cut into blocks (12 × 15 × 10 mm³) to obtain CAD/CAM blocks.

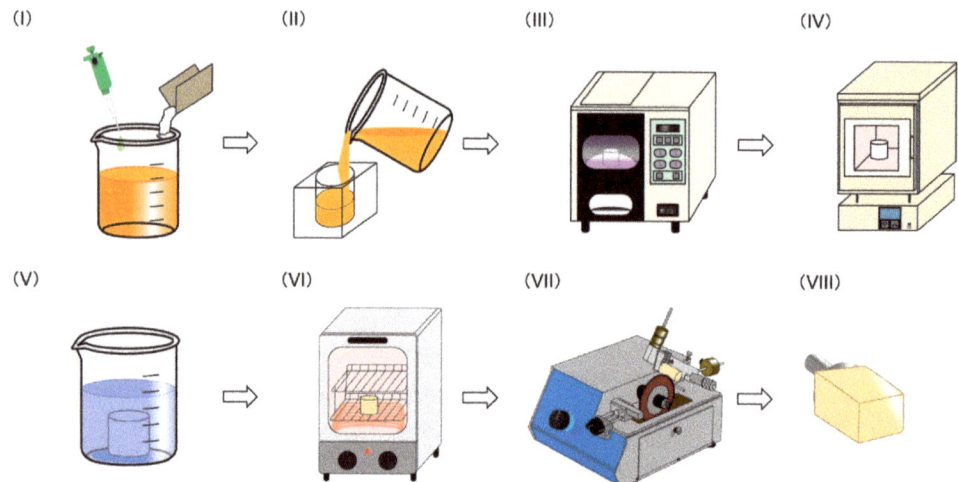

**Figure 1.** Fabrication of the polymer infiltrated ceramic network (PICN) composite to produce computer-aided design and computer-aided manufacturing (CAD/CAM) blocks: (I) preparation of light-curable precursor solution, (II) molding of precursor, (III) light-curing of precursor to form a green body, (IV) sintering of green body to form a porous body, (V) infiltration of resin monomer into the sintered porous body, (VI) heat-polymerization of the infiltrated body, and (VII) cutting of the PICN composite into (VIII) CAD/CAM blocks.

**Table 3.** Preparation conditions for the PICN composites (sintering time at 1150 °C, infiltrated resin monomer, and polymerization schedule).

| Sample Name | Sintering Time | Monomer | Polymerization Schedule |
|---|---|---|---|
| 2h-T-100 | 2 h | TEGDMA * | 100 °C 1d *** |
| 2h-T-60 | 2 h | TEGDMA * | 60 °C 5d → 80 °C 1d **** |
| 2h-U-100 | 2 h | UDMA+TEGDMA ** | 100 °C 1d *** |
| 1h-U-60 | 1 h | UDMA+TEGDMA ** | 60 °C 5d → 80 °C 1d **** |
| 2h-U-60 | 2 h | UDMA+TEGDMA ** | 60 °C 5d → 80 °C 1d **** |
| 3h-U-60 | 3 h | UDMA+TEGDMA ** | 60 °C 5d → 80 °C 1d **** |

* Infiltrated resin monomer is TEGDMA only. ** Infiltrated resin monomer is a mixture of UDMA and TEGDMA (4:1 weight ratio). *** Infiltrated resin was heat-polymerized at 100 °C for 1 day. **** Infiltrated resin was heat-polymerized at 60 °C for 5 days and at 80 °C for 1 day.

### 2.3. Three-Point Bending Test

Each sample was cut and polished using emery papers up to #2000 to produce bar-shaped samples (width = 4 mm; length = 14 mm; thickness = 1.2 mm) (n = 10). The flexural strength and modulus of the samples were determined via three-point bending testing according to the standard procedure given in ISO 6872: 2008 [45]. A universal testing machine (AGS-H, Shimadzu Corp., Kyoto, Japan) with a support span of 12 mm and crosshead speed of 1 mm/min was used [10].

### 2.4. Vickers Hardness

After the three-point bending test, the fractured samples were used for the measurement of Vickers hardness according to the standard procedure given in ISO 6872: 2008 [45]. A hardness tester (HMV-G21ST, Shimadzu Corp., Kyoto, Japan) with a load of 200 g and dwell time of 15 s was used (n = 10) [39].

## 2.5. Inorganic Content

After hardness testing, the samples were weighed using an electric balance and calcined at 600 °C for 3 h in air to remove all organic matter. According to the literature [46], the organic matter in the sample, such as poly-UDMA and poly-TEGDMA, would be completely combusted at that temperature. The residue after calcination was weighed, and the inorganic content of the sample was calculated as the difference between the specimen weight before and after calcination (n = 10).

## 2.6. Shear Bond Strength

The SBS between the samples and a commercial resin cement was measured using a conventional procedure [47]. Disk-shaped samples (diameter = 10 mm, thickness = 1.5 mm) (n = 20) were polished using emery papers up to #1000. Silane primer (Porcelain primer, SHOFU Inc., Kyoto, Japan) was applied on the sample surface, and the resin cement (Resicem, SHOFU Inc., Kyoto, Japan) was loaded on the sample surface and cured using the light irradiator for 5 min. The cement-cured sample was held under ambient conditions for 60 min, and stored in distilled water at 37 °C for 24 h. The samples were divided into two groups to establish the properties before and after thermocycling, denoted as the 0-thermocycle and 20,000-thermocycle groups, respectively. Thermocycling was conducted by alternately immersing the samples in water baths at 5 and 55 °C for 20,000 cycles of 60 s in each bath. SBS testing of the 0-thermocycle and 20,000-thermocycle group samples was performed using the universal testing machine (n = 10). After SBS testing, the cement-debonded surface was observed using an optical microscope to classify the failure modes as one of three types, namely adhesive failure at the cement–sample interface, cohesive failure within the sample, or mixed adhesive and cohesive failure.

## 2.7. Surface Free Energy

The SFE of the samples (n = 10) was determined based on the contact angles between the sample surface and two liquids, namely distilled water and diiodomethane (Kanto Chemical Co., Inc. Tokyo, Japan). A contact angle meter (DMe-211, Kyowa Interface Science Co., Ltd., Saitama, Japan) was used under ambient conditions at 20 ± 3 °C (n = 10). The SFE was calculated using the Owens–Wendt theory [48] as follows:

$$\sqrt{\gamma_{L1}^d \gamma_S^d} + \sqrt{\gamma_{L1}^p + \gamma_s^p} = \frac{\gamma_{L1}^{total}(1 + \cos\theta_{L1})}{2}, \quad (1)$$

$$\sqrt{\gamma_{L2}^d \gamma_S^d} + \sqrt{\gamma_{L2}^p + \gamma_s^p} = \frac{\gamma_{L2}^{total}(1 + \cos\theta_{L2})}{2}, \quad (2)$$

$$\sqrt{\gamma^{total}} = \gamma^d + \gamma^p \quad (3)$$

where $\theta$ denotes the contact angle for the liquids, the subscript indices L1 and L2 indicate water and diiodomethane, respectively, and $\gamma^{total}$, $\gamma^p$, and $\gamma^d$ are the total SFE, polar (hydrogen) SFE component, and dispersive SFE component of the sample, respectively. The SFE values for water and diiodomethane were based on previously reported values [48].

## 2.8. Microstructural Analysis

SEM and elemental mapping images of the samples were acquired using SEM (JCM-6000Plus NeoScope, JEOL Ltd., Tokyo, Japan) equipped with an energy dispersive X-ray spectroscopy (EDX) spectrometer.

## 2.9. CAD/CAM Milling of PICN Composite Block

The PICN composite block was milled to form a dental crown (maxillary right first premolar) (n = 1) and dental core (maxillary right first premolar) (n = 1) using a commercial CAD/CAM system (inLab MC X5, Dentsply Sirona Inc., Charlotte, NC, USA).

## 2.10. Statistical Analysis

Statistical analysis was performed using EZR software (Saitama Medical Center, Jichi Medical University, Saitama, Japan). Analysis of the flexural strength, flexural modulus, Vickers hardness, SBS and SFE was conducted using one-way analysis of variance (ANOVA) for multiple comparisons in the groups. Tukey's post hoc test was performed for the statistically significant groups. A significance level ($p$) of 0.05 was used for all analyses.

## 3. Results

### 3.1. Mechanical Properties

The mechanical properties and inorganic contents of the PICN composites and commercial composites are given in Table 4. The flexural strength of the PICN composites was influenced by the preparation conditions, namely sintering time, infiltrated resin monomer, and polymerization schedule, where the highest flexural strength (153.7 MPa) was achieved in sample 2h-U-60. Further, the flexural modulus and Vickers hardness of the PICN composites increased with sintering time. The inorganic content of the PICN composites increased with increasing the sintering time from 71.2 wt% to 89.6 wt%. The 2h-U-60 composite was chosen as the representative PICN composite for the subsequent steps, including SBS analysis, SFE analysis, SEM-EDX analysis, and CAD/CAM milling fabrication.

**Table 4.** Mechanical properties and inorganic content of the PICN composites and commercial composites (DC and AV) given as mean values (with standard deviation). Different letters indicate a significant difference between the groups ($p < 0.05$, Tukey test, n = 10).

| Sample Name | Flexural Strength (MPa) | Flexural Modulus (GPa) | Vickers Hardness | Inorganic Content (wt%) |
|---|---|---|---|---|
| 2h-T-100 | 107.8 (8.0) a | 13.4 (1.3) a | 204.8 (12.8) a | 71.8 (3.1) a |
| 2h-T-60 | 117.6 (6.5) a | 13.0 (1.1) a | 200.8 (13.0) a | 71.2 (3.3) a |
| 2h-U-100 | 119.0 (13.6) a | 13.5 (1.6) a | 210.3 (10.1) a | 73.0 (3.4) a |
| 1h-U-60 | 130.8 (19.2) ab | 14.3 (1.9) a | 213.6 (13.7) a | 73.2 (2.9) a |
| 2h-U-60 | 153.7 (9.6) b | 16.9 (2.0) ab | 218.3 (16.9) a | 75.6 (3.3) a |
| 3h-U-60 | 129.9 (25.2) ab | 22.2 (3.6) c | 299.2 (30.1) b | 89.6 (5.6) b |
| DC | 143.4 (11.5) b | 8.3 (0.9) d | 82.7 (7.02) c | 69.4 (0.9) a |
| AV | 208.0 (24.8) c | 11.8 (2.2) a | 72.5 (7.16) c | 60.6 (1.5) c |

### 3.2. Shear Bond Strength

The SBS test results of the PICN composite (2h-U-60) and commercial composites (DC and AV) before and after 20,000 thermocycles are given in Figure 2. Before thermocycling groups, there was difference between the PICN composite and AV. After thermocycling, the SBS of the PICN composite was significantly higher than those of DC and AV. Further, there was no significant change in the SBS value of the PICN composite between before and after thermocycling, while the SBSs of DC and AV significantly decreased.

AV exhibited the fewest cohesive failures before thermocycling, followed by the PICN composite and then DC (Figure 3). After thermocycling, AV exhibited the fewest, followed by DC and PICN composite. There was no difference in the incidence of cohesive failure of the PICN composite before and after thermocycling.

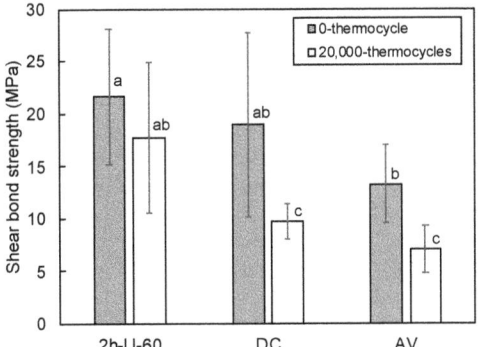

**Figure 2.** Shear bond strength of the PICN composite (2h-U-60) and commercial composites (DC and AV) at 0 and 20,000 thermocycles. Different letters indicate a significant difference between the groups ($p < 0.05$, Tukey test, n = 10), and the vertical bars denote standard deviation.

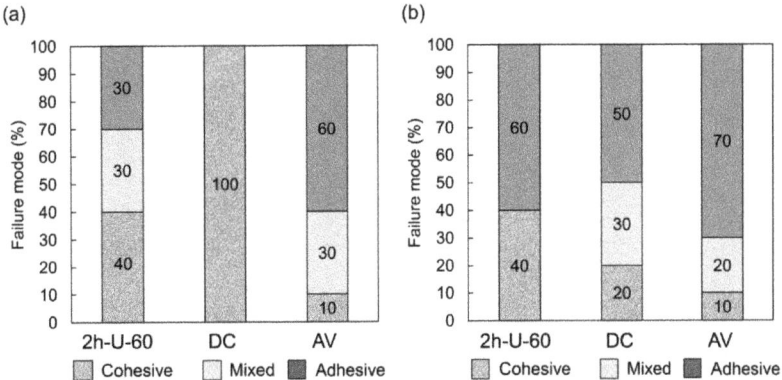

**Figure 3.** Failure modes of the PICN composite (2h-U-60) and commercial composites (DC and AV) after shear bond strength testing at (**a**) 0 and (**b**) 20,000 thermocycles (n = 10).

### 3.3. Surface Free Energy

The PICN composite (2h-U-60) exhibited a higher total SFE (Figure 4a) and polar SFE component (Figure 4b) than the commercial composites (DC and AV), as well as the lowest dispersive SFE component (Figure 4c).

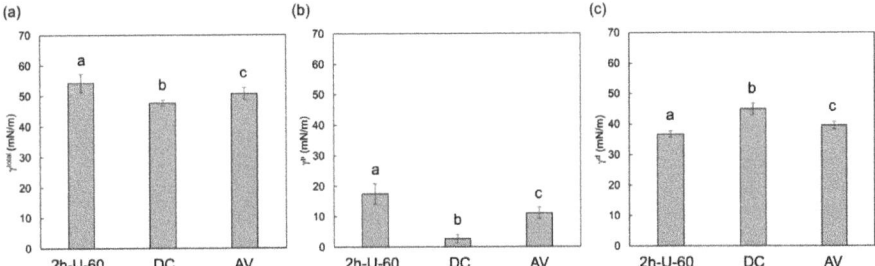

**Figure 4.** SFE of the PICN composite (2h-U-60) and commercial composites (DC and AV) given as (**a**) total SFE ($\gamma^{total}$); (**b**) polar component of SFE ($\gamma^p$); (**c**) dispersive component of SFE ($\gamma^d$). Different letters indicate a significant difference between the groups ($p < 0.05$, Tukey test, n = 10), and the vertical bars denote standard deviation.

## 3.4. Microstructure

The EDX spectra of the PICN composite (2h-U-60) was compared to those of the commercial composites (DC and AV) (Figure 5). The PICN composite exhibited peaks attributed to silicon and oxygen, which corresponded to the silica skeleton, as well as a carbon peak due to the infiltrated resin. AV exhibited silicon and oxygen peaks related to its silica fillers, and carbon peaks due to the resin matrix, while DC exhibited peaks attributed to silicon, oxygen and carbon, as well as aluminum, barium, zirconium due to the barium glass and zirconia fillers.

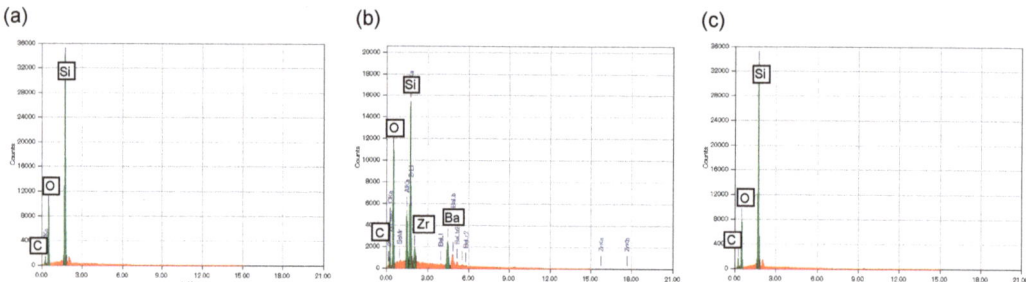

**Figure 5.** Energy dispersive X-ray spectroscopy (EDX) spectra of (**a**) PICN composite (2h-U-60); (**b**) DC commercial composite; and (**c**) AV commercial composite.

SEM and EDX elemental mapping images were acquired to evaluate the silica ($SiO_2$) inorganic component (oxygen and silicon) and the resin component (carbon) (Figure 6). The PICN composite exhibited a uniform PICN nanostructure, while DC and AV comprised nano- and in microsized dispersed-filler structures, respectively.

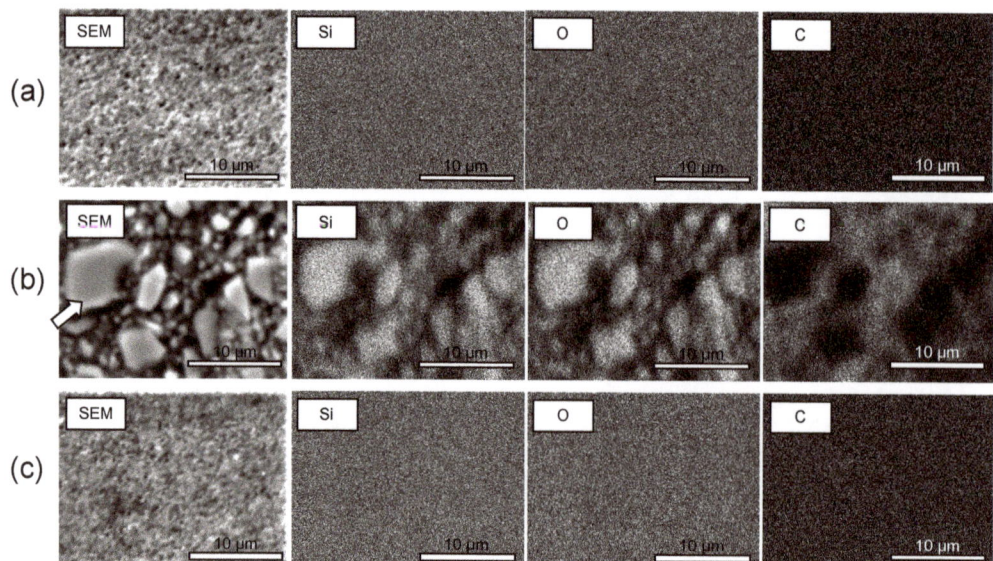

**Figure 6.** SEM images and EDX elemental mapping images of silicon (Si), oxygen (O), and carbon (C) of (**a**) PICN composite (2h-U-60); (**b**) DC commercial composite; and (**c**) AV commercial composite. The white arrow in (Figure c) indicates the filler. The silica skeleton (Figure **a**) and the silica nanoparticles (Figure **c**) were homogeneous in nanoscale.

## 3.5. CAD/CAM Milling

The PICN composite was used to produce a CAD/CAM block, which was milled to give a dental crown and dental core (Figure 7). The prepared PICN composite monolith block did not exhibit any cracks, while the milled crown and core exhibited no fatal damage such as edge chipping.

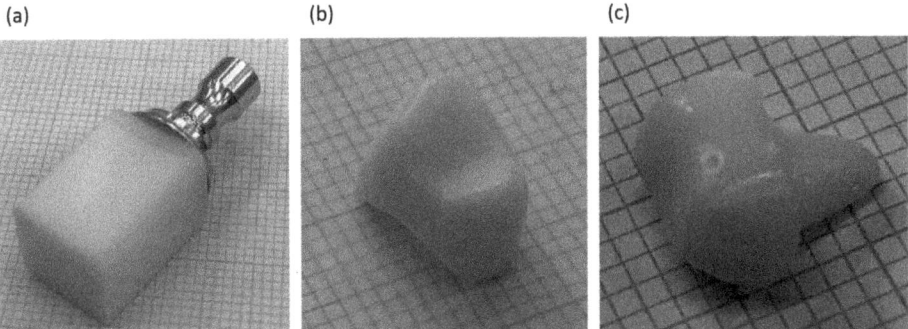

**Figure 7.** Digital photographs of the PICN composite (2h-U-60) (**a**) CAD/CAM block; (**b**) dental crown (maxillary right first premolar); and (**c**) dental core (maxillary right first premolar).

## 4. Discussion

The effect of the PICN composite preparation conditions on the mechanical properties was evaluated (Table 4). The infiltrated resin monomer affected the flexural strength, where the addition of UDMA (2h-U-60; 153.7 MPa) significantly enhanced the flexural strength compared to the composite prepared with only TEGDMA (2h-T-60; 117.7 MPa). TEGDMA has a lower strength than UDMA, and is usually used to dilute UDMA [49,50], which led to the superior flexural strength of the UDMA-infiltrated samples compared to the TEGDMA-infiltrated samples. The flexural strength was also affected by polymerization schedule, and was significantly higher in the sample polymerized at 60 °C for 5 days followed by 80 °C for 1 day (2h-U-60; 153.7 MPa) compared that polymerized at 100 °C for 1 day (2h-U-100; 119.0 MPa). Polymerization led to volume shrinkage, which typically generates internal stress within the sample [51]. Slower polymerization moderated internal stress in the sample [52], thus the internal stress during polymerization of the infiltrated monomer resin in the 2h-U-60 sample was less than that of the 2h-U-100 sample. Sintering time affected both the Vickers hardness and flexural modulus of the PICN composite, which increased with increasing sintering time in 1h-U-60, 2h-U-60, and 3h-U-60. Sintering of the silica particles progressed over time, which led to a stronger silica skeleton after a longer sintering time. This phenomenon was supported by the increase in inorganic (silica) content of the sample from 73.2 wt% for 1 h sintering (1h-U-60) to 89.6 wt% for 3 h (3h-U-60).

Vickers hardness and flexural modulus are import mechanical properties in dental restorative materials, where the Vickers hardness of the PICN composites (200.8–299.2) was significantly higher than those of the commercial composites (82.7 for DC and 72.5 for AV). This hardness is closer to that of enamel (270–420 [28]) rather than dentin (20–90 [28]), where the 3h-U-60 sample exhibited a particularly compatible hardness with enamel. The flexural modulus of the PICN composites (13.0–22.2 GPa) was also higher than those of the commercial composites (8.3 for DC and 11.8 for AV). These values were more similar to those of dentin (16–25 GPa [29–31]) compared to enamel (48–105 GPa [32,33]). Overall, the PICN composite was mechanically biocompatible with the hardness of enamel and flexural (elastic) modulus of dentin. The mechanical properties of the proposed PICN composite emulates the Vickers hardness and elastic modulus of enamel more closely than dentin, unlike previously reported PICN composites [34,38,53].

The superior SBS of the PICN composite with the resin cement compared to the commercial composites (DC and AV) led to the PICN composite undergoing cohesive failure after thermocycling more often than the other composites. This was attributed to the preferable bond durability between the PICN composite and resin cement, which was related to its surface properties. The SFE analysis revealed that the polar SFE component and total SFE of the PICN composite were significantly higher than those of commercial composites. A previous study [54] demonstrated that the large polar SFE component of this type of composite is indicative of a large number of surface silanol groups, where the active site of the silane coupling agent allowed for higher bond strength to the resin cement. This facilitated effective bonding between the resin cement (with silane primer) and the PICN composite.

The microstructure of the PICN was too fine for observation using SEM-EDX analysis (Figure 6). This demonstrated that the structure of the proposed PICN composite comprised a nanoscale silica skeleton with infiltrated resin. Thus, the proposed nanocomposite had a finer ceramic skeleton than previously reported microscale PICN composites [34,36,37].

To demonstrate the possible fabrication of a dental crown or core using the prepared PICN nanocomposite block, we attempted to mill the PICN nanocomposite block using the commercial CAD/CAM milling system. The PICN composite CAD/CAM block was successfully milled to form a dental crown and core without fatal damages (Figure 7).

Within the limitation of this study, the Vickers hardness and elastic modulus of the PICN nanocomposite block are comparable to those of enamel and dentin. These findings suggest the application potential of the proposed PICN nanocomposite as a biomimetic dental restorative material. The presented PICN nanocomposite clearly exhibited comparable Vickers hardness and lower elastic modulus than those of the alkali-aluminosilicate-glass skeleton (e.g., VITA ENAMIC; $H_V$ = ca. 177–190, E = ca. 29–38 GPa [10,34] or zirconia skeleton ($H_V$ = ca. 300, E = ca. 44 GPa [55]). Thus, the elastic modulus of the presented PICN nanocomposite is relatively similar to that of dentin. This can be ascribed to the microstructure of the presented PICN nanocomposite because the ceramic skeleton is consistent with the nanosized silica. The restorative material (e.g., a crown) developed using the presented PICN nanocomposite may overcome the problems caused by the difference in hardness between the opposite tooth and restorative material and by the difference in elastic modulus between the abutment tooth and restorative material. In the future, the wear and fatigue behaviors of the PICN nanocomposite are expected to be studied. In addition, in vivo studies will be conducted to compare the mechanical behaviors of such materials with those of conventional restorative materials.

## 5. Conclusions

A monolithic PICN nanocomposite block comprising a silica skeleton and infiltrated UDMA-based resin was prepared by optimizing the processing conditions. The PICN nanocomposite exhibited a similar Vickers hardness to enamel and flexural modulus to dentin, as well as excellent bond properties with resin cement. The PICN nanocomposite block was used to form a biomimetic dental crown and core via CAD/CAM milling. The proposed PICN nanocomposite shows great promise as a mechanically biocompatible restorative material.

**Author Contributions:** Conceptualization, H.I. and H.S.; methodology, Y.K. and H.I.; software, Y.K. and Y.N.; validation, Y.K. and H.I.; formal analysis, Y.K. and C.M.; investigation, Y.K., Y.N., and H.I.; resources, Y.K., C.M., and H.I.; data curation, Y.K. and H.I.; writing—original draft preparation, Y.K. and H.I.; writing—review and editing, Y.N., C.M., R.H., and H.S.; visualization, R.H.; supervision, H.I., R.H., and H.S.; project administration, H.I. and H.S.; funding acquisition, H.I. and H.S. All authors have read and agreed to the published version of the manuscript.

**Funding:** This work was supported by JSPS KAKENHI Grant Numbers 20K21685 and by Japanese Association for Dental Science.

**Data Availability Statement:** The date presented in this study are available on request from the corresponding author.

**Conflicts of Interest:** The authors declare no conflict of interest.

## Appendix A

*Optimization of Precursor Solution*

Six precursor solutions, referred to as PS-1 to PS-6, were prepared with varying proportions of monomers (HEMA and TEGDMA) and solvents (POE and PrOH) with a fixed content of $SiO_2$ nanoparticles and light initiator (BAPO) (supplemental Table). The reagents were mixed using the planetary centrifugal mixer. Monolithic porous silica blocks with a cylindrical shape (height = 20 mm; diameter = 18 mm) were formed using the precursor solutions via sintering. The green bodies were sintered in a furnace according to the following heating schedule: heating from room temperature to 220 °C at 50 °C/h; isothermal hold at 220 °C for 6 h; heating to 600 °C at 100 °C/h; isothermal hold for 3 h; heating to 1150 °C at 100 °C/h; isothermal hold for 2 h; and cooling to room temperature inside the furnace.

The monolithic porous silica blocks produced using precursor solutions PS-2, PS-3, PS-4, PS-5 and PS-6 formed fatal cracks during the sintering due to shrinkage stress. However, the monolithic porous silica block formed using PS-1 exhibited no cracks despite shrinking during the sintering process. Thus, PS-1 was used further in the present study, and the resulting monolithic porous silica blocks were successfully used to fabricate monolithic PICN composite blocks via the subsequent infiltration and polymerization processing steps.

Crack generation is a complicated phenomenon, and the mechanism through which cracking was suppressed in the PS-1 PICN composite has not yet been clarified. However, it is speculated that the appropriate ratio of resin monomers (HEMA and TEGDMA) and solvents (POE and PrOH) provided sufficient mechanical strength within the green body during light curing, which allowed for the structure to overcome the shrinkage stress generated during the subsequent sintering step. A PICN composite CAD/CAM block material must be capable of forming a monolithic block without fatal cracks. However, typical PICN composites tend to crack due to shrinkage during the sintering process. Therefore, determination of the optimal precursor solution composition was a critical step to ensure that monolithic blocks without fatal cracks were produced.

**Table A1.** Composition (g) of the precursor solutions.

| Precursor Solution | Monomer | | Solvent | | Nanoparticles | Initiator |
|---|---|---|---|---|---|---|
| | HEMA | TEGDMA | POE | PrOH | Silica | BAPO |
| PS-1 | 8.0 | 0.8 | 1.8 | 7.0 | 22.0 | 0.4 |
| PS-2 | 16.0 | 1.6 | 0 | 0 | 22.0 | 0.4 |
| PS-3 | 8.8 | 0 | 1.8 | 7.0 | 22.0 | 0.4 |
| PS-4 | 0 | 8.8 | 1.8 | 7.0 | 22.0 | 0.4 |
| PS-5 | 8.0 | 0.8 | 8.8 | 0 | 22.0 | 0.4 |
| PS-6 | 8.0 | 0.8 | 0 | 8.8 | 22.0 | 0.4 |

## References

1. Alghazzawi, T.F. Advancements in CAD/CAM technology: Options for practical implementation. *J. Prosthodont. Res.* **2016**, *60*, 72–84. [CrossRef] [PubMed]
2. Spitznagel, F.A.; Boldt, J.; Gierthmuehlen, P.C. CAD/CAM ceramic restorative materials for natural teeth. *J. Dent. Res.* **2018**, *97*, 1082–1091. [CrossRef] [PubMed]
3. Yamaguchi, S.; Lee, C.; Karaer, O.; Ban, S.; Mine, A.; Imazato, S. Predicting the debonding of CAD/CAM composite resin crowns with AI. *J. Dent. Res.* **2019**, *98*, 1234–1238. [CrossRef] [PubMed]
4. Yilmaz, B.; Alshahrani, F.A.; Kale, E.; Johnston, W.M. Effect of feldspathic porcelain layering on the marginal fit of zirconia and titanium complete-arch fixed implant-supported frameworks. *J. Prosthet. Dent.* **2018**, *120*, 71–78. [CrossRef] [PubMed]

5. Kim, H.R.; Jang, S.H.; Kim, Y.K.; Son, J.S.; Min, B.K.; Kim, K.H.; Kwon, T.Y. Microstructures and mechanical properties of Co-Cr dental alloys fabricated by three CAD/CAM-based processing techniques. *Materials* **2016**, *9*, 596. [CrossRef] [PubMed]
6. Blackburn, C.; Rask, H.; Awada, A. Mechanical properties of resin-ceramic CAD-CAM materials after accelerated aging. *J. Prosthet. Dent.* **2018**, *119*, 954–958. [CrossRef] [PubMed]
7. Lawson, N.C.; Bansal, R.; Burgess, J.O. Wear, strength, modulus and hardness of CAD/CAM restorative materials. *Dent. Mater.* **2016**, *32*, e275–e283. [CrossRef] [PubMed]
8. Ban, S. Chemical durability of high translucent dental zirconia. *Dent. Mater. J.* **2020**, *39*, 12–23. [CrossRef]
9. McLaughlin, J.B.; Ramos, V.J.; Dickinson, D.P. Comparison of fit of dentures fabricated by traditional techniques versus CAD/CAM technology. *J. Prosthodont.* **2019**, *28*, 428–435. [CrossRef] [PubMed]
10. Lauvahutanon, S.; Takahashi, H.; Shiozawa, M.; Iwasaki, N.; Asakawa, Y.; Oki, M.; Finger, W.J.; Arksornnukit, M. Mechanical properties of composite resin blocks for CAD/CAM. *Dent. Mater. J.* **2014**, *33*, 705–710. [CrossRef] [PubMed]
11. Souza, J.C.M.; Correia, M.S.T.; Oliveira, M.N.; Silva, F.S.; Henriques, B.; Novaes de Oliveira, A.P.; Gomes, J.R. PEEK-matrix composites containing different content of natural silica fibers or particulate lithium-zirconium silicate glass fillers: Coefficient of friction and wear volume measurements. *Biotribology* **2020**, *24*, 100147. [CrossRef]
12. Nakonieczny, D.S.; Antonowicz, M.; Paszenda, Z.K. Cenospheres and their application advantages in biomedical engineering—A systematic review. *Rev. Adv. Mater. Sci.* **2020**, *59*, 115–130. [CrossRef]
13. Faus-Matoses, V.; Ruiz-Bell, E.; Faus-Matoses, I.; Ozcan, M.; Salvatore, S.; Faus-Llacer, V.J. An 8-year prospective clinical investigation on the survival rate of feldspathic veneers: Influence of occlusal splint in patients with bruxism. *J. Dent.* **2020**, *99*, 103352. [CrossRef]
14. Nakonieczny, D.S.; Marcin, B.; Sambok, A.; Antonowicz, M.; Paszenda, Z.K.; Ziębowicz, A.; Krawczyk, C.; Ziębowicz, B.; Lemcke, H.; Kałużyński, P. Ageing of zirconia dedicated to dental prostheses for bruxers part 1: Influence of accelerating ageing for surface topography and mechanical properties. *Rev. Adv. Mater. Sci.* **2019**, *58*, 189–194. [CrossRef]
15. D'Addazio, G.; Santilli, M.; Rollo, M.L.; Cardelli, P.; Rexhepi, I.; Murmura, G.; Al-Haj Husain, N.; Sinjari, B.; Traini, T.; Ozcan, M.; et al. Fracture resistance of zirconia-reinforced lithium silicate ceramic crowns cemented with conventional or adhesive systems: An in vitro study. *Materials* **2020**, *13*, 2012. [CrossRef] [PubMed]
16. Eldafrawy, M.; Nguyen, J.F.; Mainjot, A.K.; Sadoun, M.J. A functionally graded PICN material for biomimetic CAD-CAM blocks. *J. Dent. Res.* **2018**, *97*, 1324–1330. [CrossRef]
17. Ritchie, R.O. The conflicts between strength and toughness. *Nat. Mater.* **2011**, *10*, 817–822. [CrossRef]
18. Wilmers, J.; Bargmann, S. Nature's design solutions in dental enamel: Uniting high strength and extreme damage resistance. *Acta Biomater.* **2020**, *107*, 1–24. [CrossRef] [PubMed]
19. Du, J.; Niu, X.; Rahbar, N.; Soboyejo, W. Bio-inspired dental multilayers: Effects of layer architecture on the contact-induced deformation. *Acta Biomater.* **2013**, *9*, 5273–5279. [CrossRef] [PubMed]
20. Madfa, A.A.; Yue, X.G. Dental prostheses mimic the natural enamel behavior under functional loading: A review article. *Jpn. Dent. Sci. Rev.* **2016**, *52*, 2–13. [CrossRef]
21. Al-Jawoosh, S.; Ireland, A.; Su, B. Fabrication and characterisation of a novel biomimetic anisotropic ceramic/polymer-infiltrated composite material. *Dent. Mater.* **2018**, *34*, 994–1002. [CrossRef]
22. Zafar, M.S.; Amin, F.; Fareed, M.A.; Ghabbani, H.; Riaz, S.; Khurshid, Z.; Kumar, N. Biomimetic aspects of restorative dentistry biomaterials. *Biomimetics* **2020**, *5*, 34. [CrossRef] [PubMed]
23. Petrini, M.; Ferrante, M.; Su, B. Fabrication and characterization of biomimetic ceramic/polymer composite materials for dental restoration. *Dent. Mater.* **2013**, *29*, 375–381. [CrossRef] [PubMed]
24. Oshima, M.; Inoue, K.; Nakajima, K.; Tachikawa, T.; Yamazaki, H.; Isobe, T.; Sugawara, A.; Ogawa, M.; Tanaka, C.; Saito, M.; et al. Functional tooth restoration by next-generation bio-hybrid implant as a bio-hybrid artificial organ replacement therapy. *Sci. Rep.* **2014**, *4*, 6044. [CrossRef] [PubMed]
25. Kim, J.W.; Bhowmick, S.; Chai, H.; Lawn, B.R. Role of substrate material in failure of crown-like layer structures. *J. Biomed. Mater. Res. Part B* **2007**, *81*, 305–311. [CrossRef] [PubMed]
26. Imbeni, V.; Kruzic, J.; Marshall, G.; Marshall, S.; Ritchie, R. The dentin–enamel junction and the fracture of human teeth. *Nat. Mater.* **2005**, *4*, 229–232. [CrossRef] [PubMed]
27. Homaei, E.; Farhangdoost, K.; Tsoi, J.K.H.; Matinlinna, J.P.; Pow, E.H.N. Static and fatigue mechanical behavior of three dental CAD/CAM ceramics. *J. Mech. Behav. Biomed. Mater.* **2016**, *59*, 304–313. [CrossRef] [PubMed]
28. Warkentin, M.; Freyse, C.; Specht, O.; Behrend, D.; Maletz, R.; Janda, R.; Ottl, P. Correlation of ultrasound microscopy and Vickers hardness measurements of human dentin and enamel—A pilot study. *Dent. Mater.* **2018**, *34*, 1036–1040. [CrossRef] [PubMed]
29. Xu, H.H.; Smith, D.T.; Jahanmir, S.; Romberg, E.; Kelly, J.R.; Thompson, V.P.; Rekow, E.D. Indentation damage and mechanical properties of human enamel and dentin. *J. Dent. Res.* **1998**, *77*, 472–480. [CrossRef]
30. Kinney, J.H.; Balooch, M.; Marshall, G.W.; Marshall, S.J. A micromechanics model of the elastic properties of human dentine. *Arch. Oral. Biol.* **1999**, *44*, 813–822. [CrossRef]
31. Fong, H.; Sarikaya, M.; White, S.; Snead, M. Nano-mechanical properties profiles across dentin–enamel junction of human incisor teeth. *Mater. Sci. Eng. C* **1999**, *7*, 119–128. [CrossRef]
32. Ausiello, P.; Rengo, S.; Davidson, C.L.; Watts, D.C. Stress distributions in adhesively cemented ceramic and resin-composite Class II inlay restorations: A 3D-FEA study. *Dent. Mater.* **2004**, *20*, 862–872. [CrossRef] [PubMed]

33. He, L.H.; Swain, M.V. Nanoindentation derived stress-strain properties of dental materials. *Dent. Mater.* **2007**, *23*, 814–821. [CrossRef] [PubMed]
34. Della Bona, A.; Corazza, P.H.; Zhang, Y. Characterization of a polymer-infiltrated ceramic-network material. *Dent. Mater.* **2014**, *30*, 564–569. [CrossRef] [PubMed]
35. Nguyen, J.F.; Ruse, D.; Phan, A.C.; Sadoun, M.J. High-temperature-pressure polymerized resin-infiltrated ceramic networks. *J. Dent. Res.* **2014**, *93*, 62–67. [CrossRef] [PubMed]
36. El Zhawi, H.; Kaizer, M.R.; Chughtai, A.; Moraes, R.R.; Zhang, Y. Polymer infiltrated ceramic network structures for resistance to fatigue fracture and wear. *Dent. Mater.* **2016**, *32*, 1352–1361. [CrossRef]
37. He, L.H.; Swain, M. A novel polymer infiltrated ceramic dental material. *Dent. Mater.* **2011**, *27*, 527–534. [CrossRef] [PubMed]
38. Li, J.; Cui, B.C.; Lin, Y.H.; Deng, X.L.; Li, M.; Nan, C.W. High strength and toughness in chromatic polymer-infiltrated zirconia ceramics. *Dent. Mater.* **2016**, *32*, 1555–1563. [CrossRef] [PubMed]
39. Ikeda, H.; Nagamatsu, Y.; Shimizu, H. Preparation of silica-poly (methyl methacrylate) composite with a nanoscale dual-network structure and hardness comparable to human enamel. *Dent. Mater.* **2019**, *35*, 893–899. [CrossRef]
40. Facenda, J.C.; Borba, M.; Corazza, P.H. A literature review on the new polymer-infiltrated ceramic-network material (PICN). *J. Esthet. Restor. Dent.* **2018**, *30*, 281–286. [CrossRef] [PubMed]
41. Mainjot, A.K.; Dupont, N.M.; Oudkerk, J.C.; Dewael, T.Y.; Sadoun, M.J. From artisanal to CAD-CAM blocks: State of the art of indirect composites. *J. Dent. Res.* **2016**, *95*, 487–495. [CrossRef] [PubMed]
42. Goujat, A.; Abouelleil, H.; Colon, P.; Jeannin, C.; Pradelle, N.; Seux, D.; Grosgogeat, B. Mechanical properties and internal fit of 4 CAD-CAM block materials. *J. Prosthet. Dent.* **2018**, *119*, 384–389. [CrossRef] [PubMed]
43. Conejo, J.; Ozer, F.; Mante, F.; Atria, P.J.; Blatz, M.B. Effect of surface treatment and cleaning on the bond strength to polymer-infiltrated ceramic network CAD-CAM material. *J. Prosthet. Dent.* **2020**. [CrossRef] [PubMed]
44. Ludovichetti, F.S.; Trindade, F.Z.; Werner, A.; Kleverlaan, C.J.; Fonseca, R.G. Wear resistance and abrasiveness of CAD-CAM monolithic materials. *J. Prosthet. Dent.* **2018**, *120*, 318. [CrossRef]
45. ISO. *ISO 6872. Dentistry—Ceramic Materials*, 3rd ed.; International Organization for Standardization: Geneva, Switzerland, 2008.
46. Alarcon, R.T.; Gaglieri, C.; Bannach, G. Dimethacrylate polymers with different glycerol content. *J. Therm. Anal. Calorim.* **2018**, *132*, 1579–1591. [CrossRef]
47. Yano, H.T.; Ikeda, H.; Nagamatsu, Y.; Masaki, C.; Hosokawa, R.; Shimizu, H. Effects of alumina airborne-particle abrasion on the surface properties of CAD/CAM composites and bond strength to resin cement. *Dent. Mater. J.* **2020**. [CrossRef] [PubMed]
48. Owens, D.K.; Wendt, D.T. Estimation of the surface free energy of polymers. *J. Appl. Polym. Sci.* **1969**, *13*, 1741–1747. [CrossRef]
49. Floyd, C.J.; Dickens, S.H. Network structure of Bis-GMA-and UDMA-based resin systems. *Dent. Mater.* **2006**, *22*, 1143–1149. [CrossRef]
50. Lin, C.H.; Lin, Y.M.; Lai, Y.L.; Lee, S.Y. Mechanical properties, accuracy, and cytotoxicity of UV-polymerized 3D printing resins composed of Bis-EMA, UDMA, and TEGDMA. *J. Prosthet. Dent.* **2020**, *123*, 349–354. [CrossRef]
51. Ferracane, J.L. Developing a more complete understanding of stresses produced in dental composites during polymerization. *Dent. Mater.* **2005**, *21*, 36–42. [CrossRef] [PubMed]
52. Gad, M.M.; Fouda, S.M.; ArRejaie, A.S.; Al-Thobity, A.M. Comparative effect of different polymerization techniques on the flexural and surface properties of acrylic denture bases. *J. Prosthodont.* **2019**, *28*, 458–465. [CrossRef] [PubMed]
53. Kang, L.; Zhou, Y.; Lan, J.; Yu, Y.; Cai, Q.; Yang, X. Effect of resin composition on performance of polymer-infiltrated feldspar-network composites for dental restoration. *Dent. Mater. J.* **2020**, *39*, 900–908. [CrossRef] [PubMed]
54. Yano, H.T.; Ikeda, H.; Nagamatsu, Y.; Masaki, C.; Hosokawa, R.; Shimizu, H. Correlation between microstructure of CAD/CAM composites and the silanization effect on adhesive bonding. *J. Mech. Behav. Biomed. Mater.* **2020**, *101*, 103441. [CrossRef] [PubMed]
55. Li, K.; Kou, H.; Rao, J.; Liu, C.; Ning, C. Fabrication of enamel-like structure on polymer-infiltrated zirconia ceramics. *Dent. Mater.* **2021**. [CrossRef] [PubMed]

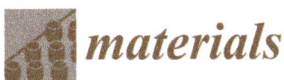 

*Article*

# Effect of Cement Layer Thickness on the Immediate and Long-Term Bond Strength and Residual Stress between Lithium Disilicate Glass-Ceramic and Human Dentin

João Paulo Mendes Tribst [1,*], Alison Flavio Campos dos Santos [1], Giuliane da Cruz Santos [1], Larissa Sandy da Silva Leite [1], Julio Chávez Lozada [2], Laís Regiane Silva-Concílio [1], Kusai Baroudi [1] and Marina Amaral [1]

[1] Department of Dentistry, University of Taubaté (UNITAU), Taubaté 12020-340, Brazil; flaviosantosdr@outlook.com (A.F.C.d.S.); giucs90@gmail.com (G.d.C.S.); larissasandy.ls@gmail.com (L.S.d.S.L.); regiane1@yahoo.com (L.R.S.-C.); d_kusai@yahoo.co.uk (K.B.); marinamaral_85@yahoo.com.br (M.A.)
[2] Department of Operative Dentistry, FO-National University of Córdoba, Córdoba 5016, Argentina; juliochavezlozada@gmail.com
\* Correspondence: joao.tribst@gmail.com

**Abstract:** This study tested whether three different cement layer thicknesses (60, 120 and 180 μm) would provide the same bonding capacity between adhesively luted lithium disilicate and human dentin. Ceramic blocks were cut to 20 blocks with a low-speed diamond saw under cooling water and were then cemented to human flat dentin with an adhesive protocol. The assembly was sectioned into 1 mm$^2$ cross-section beams composed of ceramic/cement/dentin. Cement layer thickness was measured, and three groups were formed. Half of the samples were immediately tested to evaluate the short-term bond strength and the other half were submitted to an aging simulation. The microtensile test was performed in a universal testing machine, and the bond strength (MPa) was calculated. The fractured specimens were examined under stereomicroscopy. Applying the finite element method, the residual stress of polymerization shrinkage according to cement layer thickness was also calculated using first principal stress as analysis criteria. Kruskal–Wallis tests showed that the "cement layer thickness" factor significantly influenced the bond strength results for the aged samples ($p = 0.028$); however, no statistically significant difference was found between the immediately tested groups ($p = 0.569$). The higher the cement layer thickness, the higher the residual stress generated at the adhesive interface due to cement polymerization shrinkage. In conclusion, the cement layer thickness does not affect the immediate bond strength in lithium disilicate restorations; however, thinner cement layers are most stable in the short term, showing constant bond strength and lower residual stress.

**Keywords:** dental bonding; polymerization; finite element analysis; dental materials

## 1. Introduction

When performing a ceramic restoration, the most recommended protocol is the use of resin-based cements combined to adhesive protocols during the cementation procedure [1,2]. This recommendation aims to achieve a clinical long-lasting bond between ceramic/resin cement and between resin cement/dental tissues [3,4]. In addition, the resin cements are easily handled, have an adequate setting time, and have the potential for both mechanical and chemical bonding [2,5].

However, the vertical misfit, or cement thickness, between the restoration and tooth preparation is an important factor which affects the success and survival of ceramic restorations [6]. The literature recommends a cement layer thickness around 50–100 μm for resin cements in ceramic crowns [7]. Furthermore, the bonding properties have been shown to be significantly reduced for cement thickness of 450–500 μm due to the residual stress of polymerization shrinkage [7,8]. May et al. [7] demonstrated a significant effect of the cement thickness on the failure loads of feldspathic ceramic crowns, showing that the cement layer thickness can be directly associated with the gap formation, increasing the tensile stresses on the crown's intaglio surface and decreasing failure loads.

For that reason, several clinical reports have aimed to control the luting procedure and reduce the thickness of the cement layer by applying some kind of pressure during the restoration placement [9–12]. However, sometimes the beneficial effect of a thinner cement layer is not evidenced in these reports [9–11] and not always associated as an important factor in the clinical failures involving indirect dental restorations [13,14].

According to the literature, the cement space of ceramic crowns may vary for computer-aided design/computer-aided manufacturing (CAD/CAM) materials; additionally, there is no consensus on the best treatment option to improve the mechanical performance and bond durability. Previous clinical studies showed the mean internal adaptation of milled ceramic crowns ranged from 220 to 295 µm [15]. The mean discrepancies ranged from 137 to 175 µm for the same crown in different regions and from 148 to 203 µm for fixed dental prostheses [16,17]. A previous in vitro study evaluated the influence of occlusal resin cement space (50, 100, and 300 µm) on the fatigue performance of anatomical ceramic crowns bonded to a dentin analogue preparation [18]. According to the authors, the variation in the cement space did not affect the fatigue performance of CAD/CAM crowns [18]. Therefore, it is noticeable that previous studies have demonstrated the inverse relationship between the thickness of cement layer and bond strength, but this is not a consensus due to the wide variety of cement thicknesses considered in these previous reports. In addition, the evaluation of variation of cement thicknesses as an arithmetical progression could be useful to demonstrate how the linear increase in the thickness of cement layer could affect the bond strength values.

However, in addition to the residual stress, the exposed cement layer could expand by water sorption during the aging process [19] and therefore can present failures such as slow crack growth [20,21], which reduces the survival of composites and ceramics [14–16]. This phenomenon is responsible for the failure of the majority of dental biomaterials that are placed in the oral environment. Water sorption is also responsible for degradation of resin-based cements [22], and a thick marginal cement layer would be more exposed to the oral environment. In this sense, aging simulations in in vitro studies should be performed to elucidate the long-term bond strength achieved by dental materials and dental tissues [20–23]. Finite element analysis (FEA) is a numerical method that can be applied to elucidate the effect of polymerization shrinkage on stress; however, it was not performed in association with in vitro measurements of immediate and short-term bond strength. The association of this information could be useful to assist the comprehension of adhesive interface stability in restorative dentistry.

The aim of the present study was to evaluate the effect of different cement layer thicknesses on immediate and aged microtensile bond strength between lithium disilicate and dentin and to evaluate the residual stress of polymerization shrinkage according to the cement layer thickness using first principal stress analysis. The null hypothesis was that the cement layer thickness would not affect bond strength or residual stresses in the ceramic-dentin interface.

## 2. Materials and Methods

### 2.1. Sample Preparation

After approval of the university institutional ethical review board (Process n° 4.075.061), 24 first human molars donated from the university's human teeth bank were embedded by root portions into chemically cured acrylic resin (JET, Classico, Cotia, Brazil) and had their occlusal surface flattened under constant cooling water using sandpaper #600 until dentin exposure was achieved. In sequence, the teeth were cleaned in ultrasonic bath with water for 10 min and stored until the luting procedure.

Lithium disilicate glass-ceramic blocks (IPS e.max CAD, IvoclarVivadent, Schaan, Liechtenstein) were sectioned with a low-speed diamond saw under constant cooling water (Isomet 1000, Buehler, Lake Bluff, IL, USA) to 24 blocks (6 × 6 × 7 mm$^3$). The ceramic surfaces were ground flat with grit SIC papers (600, 800, and 1200 grit) using a polishing machine (EcoMet/AutoMet 250, Buehler, Lake Bluff, IL, USA) under cooling water. Then, the ceramic blocks were crystallized following the manufacturer's instructions (850 °C/10 min). The blocks were randomly divided into three groups according to cementation weight (500 g, 1000 g or 3000 g) to obtain different cement layer thicknesses. For surface treatment, the ceramic blocks were etched with 10% hydrofluoric acid (Condacporcelana, FGM, Joinville, Brazil) for 20 s, rinsed with water, and dried with an oil-free air jet. Silane coupling agent (Monobond Plus, IvoclarVivadent, Schaan, Liechtenstein) was then applied on the surface with 60 s of volatilization time.

The flattened dentin adhesive area was etched with 37% phosphoric acid for 15 s (Condac37, FGM, Joinville, Brazil), followed by a rinse of water for 20 s. The surface was dried with absorbent paper, and then the dental adhesive (Excite F DSC, IvoclarVivadent, Schaan, Liechtenstein) was applied and light cured for 15 s using the LED light curing device (BluePhase, IvoclarVivadent, Schaan, Liechtenstein). The luting procedure was performed with a dual cure resin cement (Variolink II, IvoclarVivadent, Schaan, Liechtenstein) following the manufacturer's instructions. After positioning the ceramic blocks with resin cement on flat dentin, different loads (500, 1000 or 3000 g weight) were applied to the ceramic blocks to obtain different cement layer thicknesses. The excess cement was removed with a brush, and then light curing was performed for 40 s (BluePhase, IvoclarVivadent, Schaan, Liechtenstein), starting at the proximal margins on each side of the tooth.

After 24 h of storage into distilled water, 1 mm$^2$ cross-section beams composed of ceramic/cement/dentin were obtained by means of a precision cutting machine (Isomet 1000, Buehler, Lake Bluff, IL, USA) under constant cooling water. The external beams of each block were delimited and removed.

### 2.2. Cement Thickness Measurement

Before testing the specimens, the cement layer thickness was examined by stereomicroscopy (Stereo Discovery V20, Zeiss, Gottingen, Germany), and three linear measurements in each sample were performed by a single calibrated operator. As standardization, each sample cement thickness average value was assumed as representative and considered a simplified homogeneous cement layer. Then, the samples (beams) were divided according to the cement layer in three different groups ($n$ = 20) of thicknesses (60 μm [59.74 ± 8.41 μm], 120 μm [119.89 ± 21.85 μm] and 180 μm [182.66 ± 98.66]).

### 2.3. Microtensile Bond Strength (μTBS)

Half of the samples were considered baseline and were immediately tested, while the other half of the beams were subjected to storage in distilled water at 37 °C for 140 days for a posterior bond strength test. The final dimensions of each specimen were measured with a digital caliper and recorded.

To perform the μTBS, the specimens were glued to the testing device (OG01, Odeme, Lucerne, Brazil) with cyanoacrylate (Superbonder, Loctite, Dusseldorf, Germany). The setup was carried out in a universal testing machine (MBio, BioPDI, São Carlos, Brazil; 0.5 mm/min), and the bond strength (MPa) was calculated using the ratio between load at failure (N) and the adhesive area (mm$^2$).

### 2.4. Assessment of Residual Polymerization Shrinkage Stress

To assess the stress magnitude generated between the different cement layer thicknesses, the finite element method was applied. A three-dimensional (3D) model of an in vitro sample was modeled containing 8 mm of length with 1 mm$^2$ of adhesive area. This model was replicated, and three different cement layer thicknesses were simulated in different models as well as the in vitro setup. The resultant Figure 1 summarizes the models considered in the present study. The geometries were imported into analysis software (ANSYS 19.2, ANSYS Inc., Houston, TX, USA) in STEP format (Standard for the Exchange of Product Model Data) and a mesh was generated using tet-10 element type. To reduce meshing error, a convergence test was performed to determine the appropriate mesh density (number of elements and nodes) with a threshold level set at 10% [24]. The material properties were assumed to be homogeneous, linear and with elastic behavior. The elastic modulus and Poisson ratio assigned for each material were derived from the literature (Table 1).

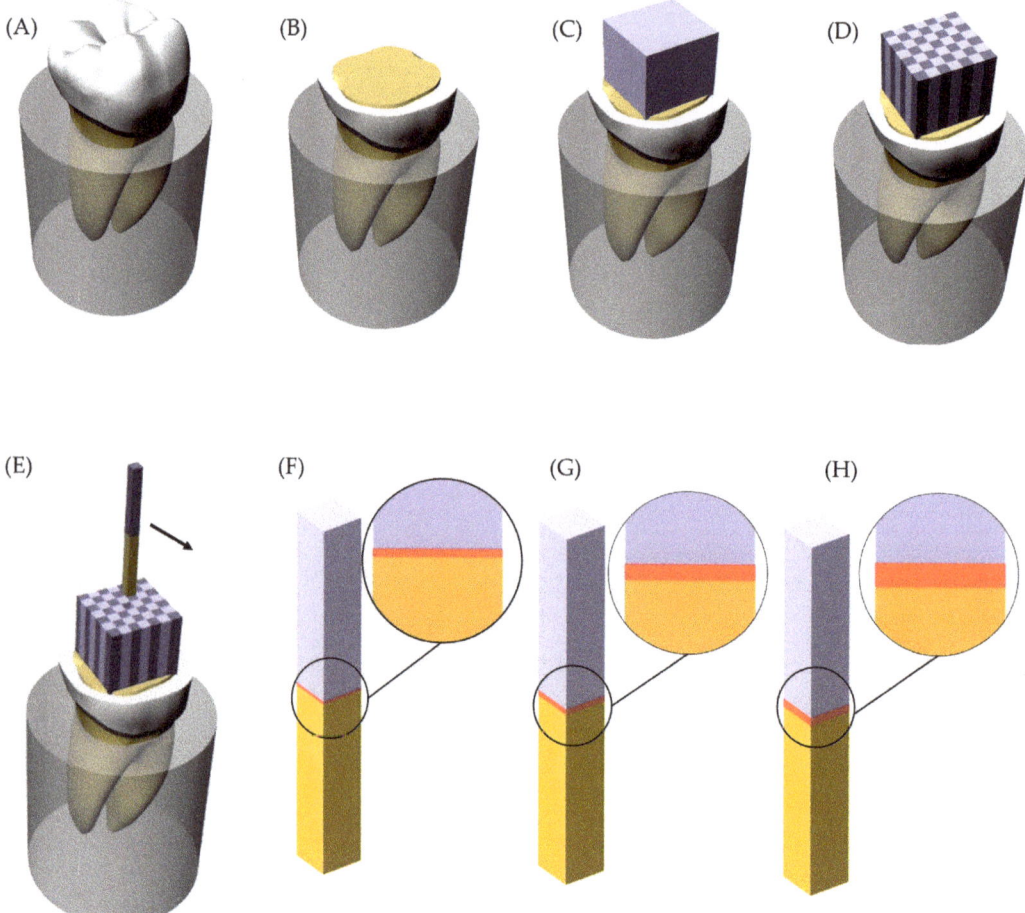

**Figure 1.** Sample preparation scheme and groups. (**A**) Sound tooth embedded into acrylic resin; (**B**) Flattened tooth with exposed dentin tissue; (**C**) Lithium disilicate glass-ceramic block cemented; (**D**) Sectioned sample with the beams separated; (**E**) Beam removed from the position; (**F**) Groups with 60 μm of cement layer thickness; (**G**) Groups with 120 μm of cement layer thickness and (**H**) Groups with 180 μm of cement layer thickness.

The external bases of the beam were fixed on the Z-axis (based in three-dimensional Cartesian coordinates oriented vertically). The adhesive interfaces were considered bonded. The polymerization shrinkage was simulated by thermal analogy, similar to previous reported FEA simulations involving polymeric dental materials [24,25]. The linear thermal expansion coefficient calculated was 0.005766. This information was inserted in the analysis software and temperature was reduced by 1 °C. A linear static structural analysis was performed to calculate stress magnitude in the dentin adhesive surface, cement layer, and lithium disilicate adhesive surface. The stress maps and peaks were recorded and tabled for the comparison between the models.

Table 1. Material properties considered to calculate the residual stress.

| Material | Elastic Modulus (GPa) | Poisson Ratio | Volumetric Shrinkage (%) | References |
|---|---|---|---|---|
| Enamel | 18 | 0.30 | - | [25] |
| Lithium Disilicate glass-ceramic | 95.0 | 0.30 | - | [24] |
| Resin cement | 7.0 | 0.24 | 1.74 | [25] |

## 2.5. Data Analysis

The bond strength (MPa) data were calculated, and the normality was rejected (Figure 2).

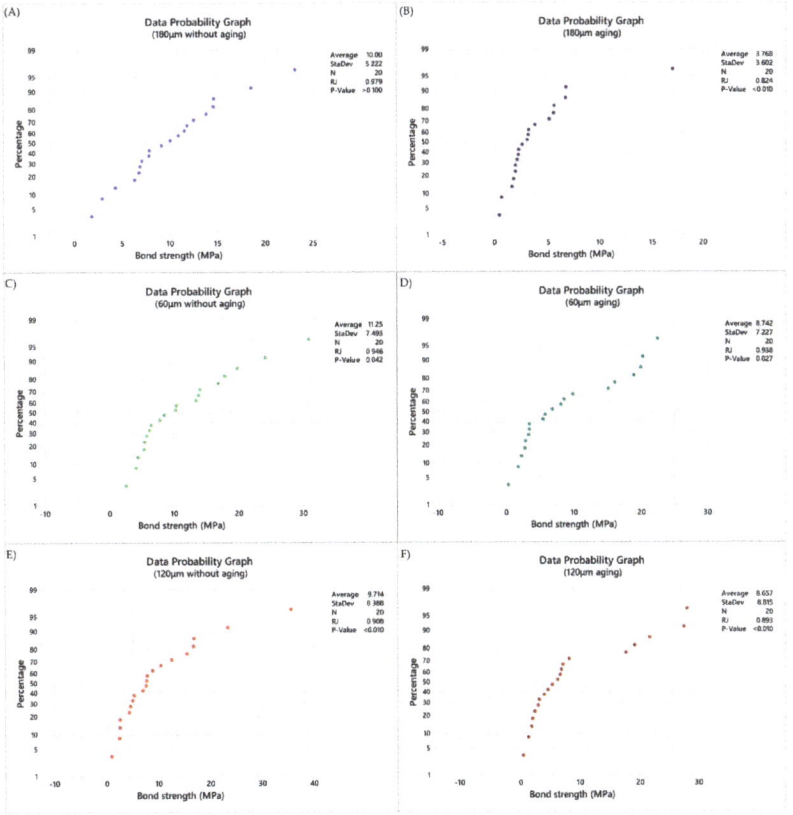

Figure 2. Normality data plot (Ryan–Joiner) applied in the present study. (A) Data probability graph in immediate tested samples with 180 μm of cement layer thickness, (B) Data probability graph in aged samples with 180 μm of cement layer thickness, (C) Data probability graph in immediate tested samples with 120 μm of cement layer thickness, (D) Data probability graph in aged samples with 120 μm of cement layer thickness, (E) Data probability graph in immediate tested samples with 60 μm of cement layer thickness, (F) Data probability graph in aged samples with 60 μm of cement layer thickness.

The µTBS results were statistically analyzed by Kruskal–Wallis and MINITAB Macro Dunn's tests ($\alpha$ = 0.05) for both groups of samples: immediately tested and tested after aging simulation. This macro performs multiple comparisons in a nonparametric setting. For that, the output was performed considering the number of comparisons ($k$), $k = \frac{k(k-1)}{2}$, the family alpha ($\alpha$), the Bonferroni individual alpha ($\beta$), $B = \frac{\alpha}{k}$ and the 2-sided critical z-value.

The stress data (MPa) was qualitatively analyzed using the colorimetric stress maps and the stress peaks were used for the quantitative comparison assuming that values recorded from the same region with more than 10% of difference between the models are significant.

## 3. Results

The mean values of µTBS ranged between 11.24 and 3.76 MPa (Table 2). Kruskal–Wallis tests showed that there were no significant group differences (adjusted for ties) considering the immediate bond strength ($p$ = 0.569).

**Table 2.** Means (in MPa) and standard deviations (±value) of the µTBS Test.

| Cement Thickness (µm) | Immediate | After Aging |
|---|---|---|
| 60 | 11.2 ± 7.4 | 8.7 ± 7.2 |
| 120 | 9.7 ± 8.3 | 8.6 ± 8.8 |
| 180 | 10.0 ± 5.2 | 3.7 ± 3.6 |

However, the statistical test showed that the "cement layer thickness" factor significantly influenced the bond strength results for the aged samples ($p$ = 0.028). Detailed statistical characteristic are summarized in Table 3. After post-hoc pairwise comparison, the aged groups showed significant differences between 60 and 180 µm cement thicknesses ($p$ = 0.0125) and between 120 and 180 µm cement thicknesses ($p$ = 0.0390).

**Table 3.** Descriptive statistics from Kruskal–Wallis tests (MPa versus Cement layer).

| | Immediate | | | | After Aging | | |
|---|---|---|---|---|---|---|---|
| Cement (µm) | Median | Mean Rank | Z-Value | Cement (µm) | Median | Mean Rank | Z-Value |
| 60 | 9.19 | 32.5 | 0.61 | 60 | 6.08 | 35.9 | 1.69 |
| 120 | 7.52 | 27.1 | −1.06 | 120 | 5.54 | 33.5 | 0.94 |
| 180 | 9.45 | 31.9 | 0.45 | 180 | 2.69 | 22.1 | −2.63 |
| Overall | | 30.5 | | Overall | | 30.5 | |

The median and standard deviation of each value are summarized in Figure 3 for immediate tested groups and Figure 4 for aged groups. The bond strength data distribution considering sign confidence intervals and pair wise comparison can be observed in Figure 3 for the samples tested immediately after the cementation procedure and in Figure 4 for the aged samples. The achieved confidence calculated during the multiple comparisons statistic is summarized in Table 4 for immediate tested groups and Table 5 for aged groups.

Mixed failures (association of adhesive and cohesive failures) were predominant in all groups. The failure analysis is summarized in Figure 5.

After the numerical calculation process, the stress results (MPa) can be observed in the ceramic adhesive surface, cement layer and dentin adhesive layer which compose the adhesive interface (Figures 6 and 7). In the cement layer (Figure 6), there is a visibly higher amount of stress with a higher volume of resin material concentrated in the bonded surfaces and with a lower magnitude at the center of the material. In the adhesive surface for dentin tissue and ceramic material (Figure 7), there is a similar stress pattern between surfaces from the same model; however, the higher the cement layer thickness, the higher the calculated stress magnitude (Table 6).

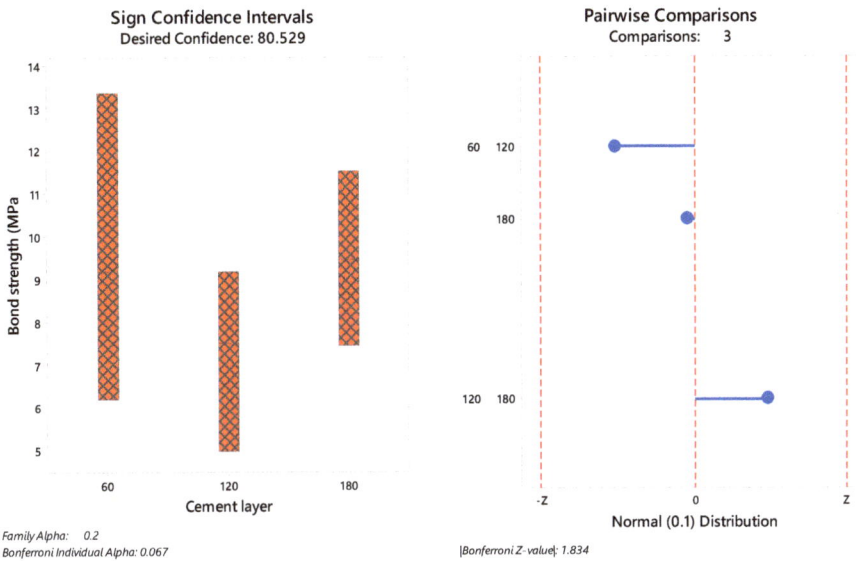

**Figure 3.** Multiple comparison chart for immediate tested groups (60, 120 and 180 µm). The sign of confidence was calculated considering family alpha = 0.2 and Bonferroni individual alpha = 0.067. The pairwise comparison demonstrated 1.83 as the Bonferroni Z-value without a visible difference between the evaluated cement layers.

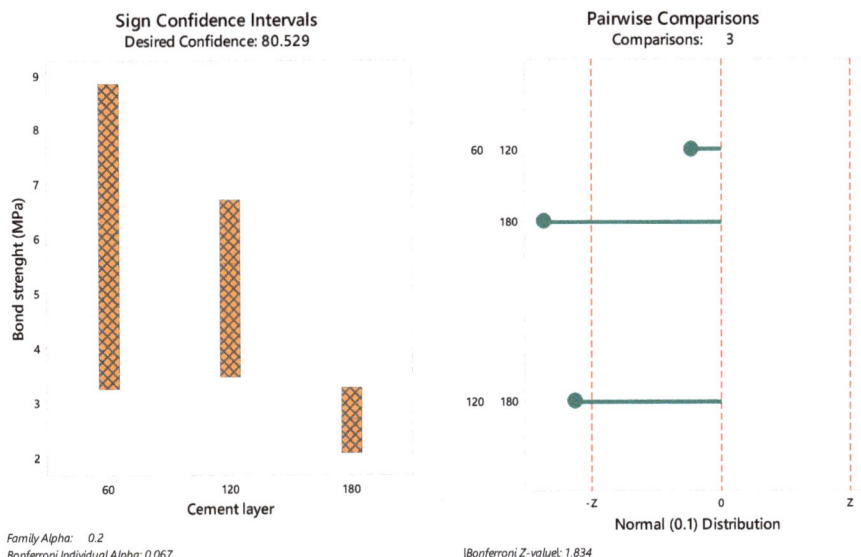

**Figure 4.** Multiple comparison chart for aged groups (60, 120 and 180 µm). The sign of confidence was calculated considering family alpha = 0.2 and Bonferroni individual alpha = 0.067. The pairwise comparison demonstrated 1.83 as the Bonferroni Z-value with visible differences between the evaluated cement layers.

**Table 4.** Confidence intervals, achieved confidence and data position according to the cement layer thickness for the immediate tested groups.

| Cement Thickness (μm) | CI for η | Achieved Confidence | Position |
|---|---|---|---|
| 60 | (6.27; 13.21) | 73.68% | (8; 13) |
|  | (6.20; 13.37) | 80.53% | Interpolation |
|  | (6.04; 13.70) | 88.47% | (7; 14) |
| 120 | (5.09; 8.65) | 73.68% | (8; 13) |
|  | (4.98; 9.18) | 80.53% | Interpolation |
|  | (4.75; 10.31) | 88.47% | (7; 14) |
| 180 | (7.68; 11.43) | 73.68% | (8; 13) |
|  | (7.44; 11.52) | 80.53% | Interpolation |
|  | (6.92; 11.71) | 88.47% | (7; 14) |

**Table 5.** Confidence intervals, achieved confidence and data position according to the cement layer thickness for aged groups.

| Cement Thickness (μm) | CI for η | Achieved Confidence | Position |
|---|---|---|---|
| 60 | (3.24; 8.42) | 73.68% | (8; 13) |
|  | (3.23; 8.84) | 80.53% | Interpolation |
|  | (3.23; 9.72) | 88.47% | (7; 14) |
| 120 | (3.71; 6.64) | 73.68% | (8; 13) |
|  | (3.45; 6.71) | 80.53% | Interpolation |
|  | (2.90; 6.86) | 88.47% | (7; 14) |
| 180 | (2.10; 3.10) | 73.68% | (8; 13) |
|  | (2.06; 3.27) | 80.53% | Interpolation |
|  | (1.99; 3.64) | 88.47% | (7; 14) |

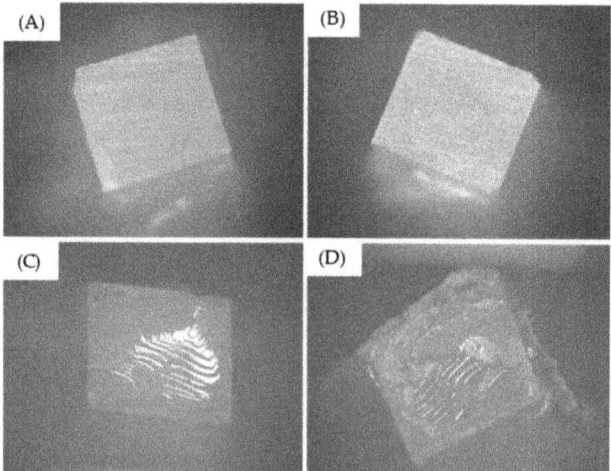

**Figure 5.** Predominant failure type observed after the testing. (**A**,**B**) Purely adhesive failures and (**C**,**D**) mixed failures.

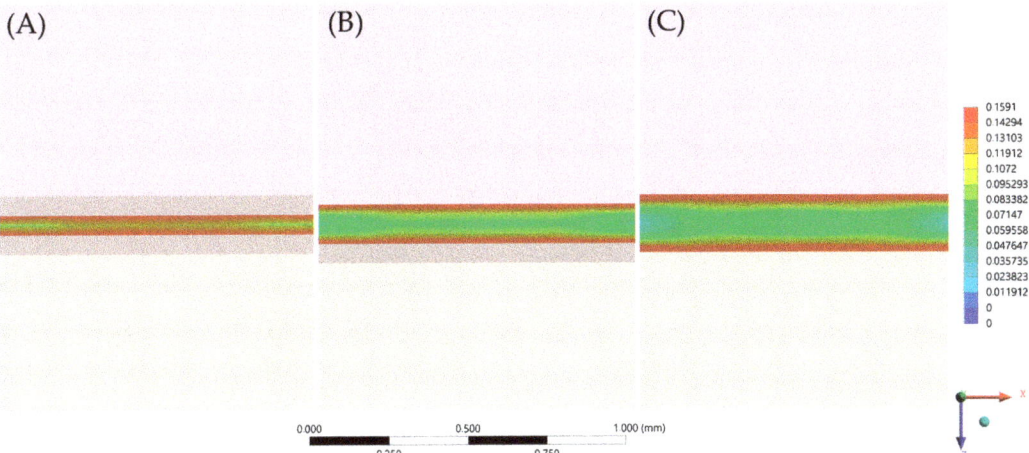

**Figure 6.** First principal stress (tensile) distribution in the cement layer for each evaluated group. (**A**) Models with 60 μm of cement layer thickness; (**B**) Models with 120 μm of cement layer thickness and (**C**) Models with 180 μm of cement layer thickness.

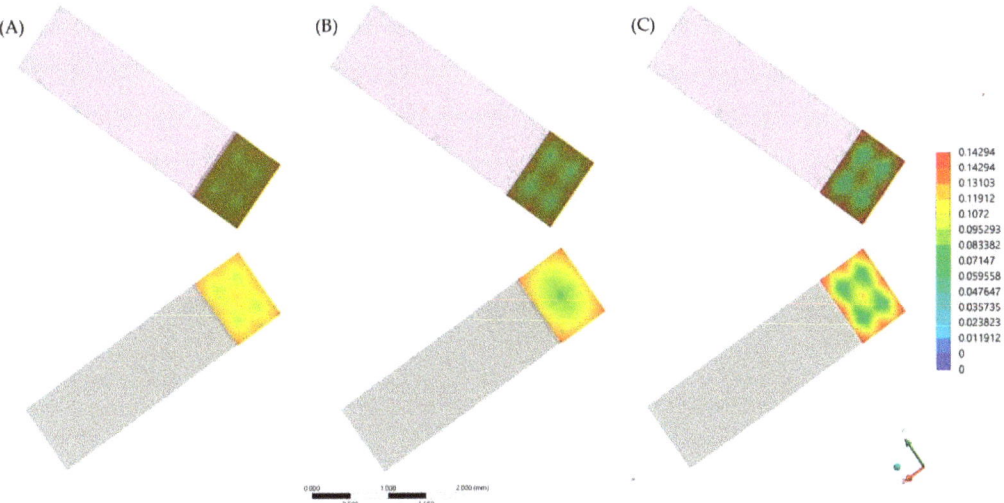

**Figure 7.** First principal stress (tensile) distribution in the ceramic (upper row) and dentin tissue (lower row) for each evaluated group. (**A**) Models with 60 μm of cement layer thickness; (**B**) Models with 120 μm of cement layer thickness and (**C**) Models with 180 μm of cement layer thickness.

**Table 6.** Stress peaks (in MPa) calculated * for each adhesive interface component.

| Cement Thickness (μm) | Cement | Ceramic Adhesive Surface | Dentin Adhesive Surface |
|---|---|---|---|
| 60 | 0.14 | 0.13 | 0.13 |
| 120 | 0.15 | 0.13 | 0.13 |
| 180 | 0.17 | 0.15 | 0.15 |

* Values obtained using the maximum probe software tool.

## 4. Discussion

The present study aimed to evaluate the effect of different cement layer thicknesses on immediate and aged microtensile bond strength between lithium disilicate and crown dentin, beside the residual stress of polymerization shrinkage. The results from both in vitro and in silico methods showed that the cement layer thickness can affect the bond strength and adhesive interface behavior. Therefore, the null hypothesis was rejected.

An adequate cementation procedure is a critical step to the success and longevity of ceramic restorations, since these biomaterials rely on adhesion not only for retention but also for resistance [12]. Unfortunately, the adhesive resin luting cement is a challenging procedure and involves multiple technique-sensitive steps [9–12]. Therefore, the present study demonstrates that the effect of a neglected cementation step will affect not the immediate but the long-term bond strength, probably compromising the restoration prognosis.

In addition to the bond strength, the fracture resistance of adhesively cemented ceramic restorations has been associated with the cement film thickness [26]. However, different parameters may affect the thickness of resin cement, and because of this, it is possible to observe reports showing average cement film thickness of 106.74 μm for the heat-pressing lithium disilicate ceramic and 340.35 μm for the milled CAD/CAM restorations. Despite the fact that the acceptable cement thickness of the International Standard Organization (ISO) is no more than 50 μm [26], there is a noticeable variation in the clinically achieved cement layer thickness.

In the present study, during the sample manufacturing process, the average cement thickness was in the range of 60 to 180 μm (Figure 1). It is possible to observe an indirect proportion between cement layer thickness and bond strength in literature [27]. In addition, a significant association between lower ceramic fracture load and thicker cement layer was already reported, indicating that a thin cement layer is more favorable for improved restoration mechanical response [27].

The stress maps calculated with the finite element method showed that the region of highest tensile stress magnitude was at the periphery of the cement layer; this formed in a centripetal behavior during the volumetric shrinkage. These results are in agreement with a previous study that found critical flaws at the margin of samples for μTBS [28] and also with a previous study that evaluated different resinous cement materials with a similar setup [28].

According to the literature, during the cementation procedure, the resinous cement should completely fill the space between the restoration and the tooth with no marginal discrepancy [29]. However, the cement film thickness can be strongly influenced by the type of luting cement and the seating force applied [29]. The present study applied different seating forces to obtain different values of cement thicknesses; however, it was necessary to verify each of the samples in the microscopy and to calculate the cement layer thickness with the analysis software before affirming the average cement layer per group.

Another reason that can justify the reduced bond strength in thicker cement layer group is the presence of porosity in the materials that could be relatively prominent in thicker layers of resin cement [27]. In addition, some authors proposed that a combination of surface preparation and the luting cement could act to move the fracture origin from the porcelain/cement interface to the cement surface [18,24,27].

The literature has reported that the lowest shrinkage stress (photoelastic analysis) was observed for the thinnest layer (25 μm) and proportionally increased with higher thicknesses (100 μm, 200 μm, and 400 μm) [30]. However, after the aging simulation, the authors reported that the use of thicker cement layers might have a positive clinical effect, resulting in the creation of expansion stress that could potentially influence the sealing of the marginal gap and enhance restoration-tooth retention [30]. This assumption was based on the expansion stresses found in the thinner cement layer group. The present study showed that there is a difference in the bond strength after the aging simulation regardless of the cement layer thickness, suggesting that the aging effect will be deleterious also for higher cement layer thicknesses and not only in the thinnest groups.

Thicker resin cement layers (verified by 3-dimensional microcomputed tomography) were also reported to promote higher polymerization shrinkage on stresses in ceramic [31]. At the same time, a thicker cement layer exposes more polymeric material to the oral environment, increasing its susceptibility to aging degradation. This suggested degradation susceptibility in larger areas of exposed cement could have contributed to the worst behavior found when 180 μm was considered, which in addition to the higher amount of residual stress, culminated in a significantly lower value of bond strength after aging in comparison with 120 μm and 60 μm layer thicknesses. The difference in stress peak in dentin tissue was approximately 13% between 120 to 180, while this same difference was approximately 1.5% between 120 μm to 60 μm. Therefore, it is possible to hypothesize that the stress state generated in the polymerization shrinkage is not a perfect linear regression as a function of the cement thickness.

The space planned for the resin cement layer in the digital workflow did not affect the fracture resistance of lithium disilicate veneers [32], simulating 120.4 μm, 174.9 μm (near the cement thickness simulated in the present study) and 337.2 μm of cement thicknesses. Therefore, the present study suggests that the use of thinner cement layers should be indicated to guarantee bond strength and adhesive interface integrity instead of improvements in the load-to-fracture values. The thickness of resin cement is considered a critical factor for the prognosis of indirect restorations. A greater thickness of cement increases the stress at the walls of the tooth cavity because of the polymerization shrinkage [33]. Therefore, not only could the bond strength be benefited with a thin cement layer, the cusp deflection could also be reduced in partial restorations. Thus, cement layer thickness has an important role in the mechanical behavior of adhesively cemented ceramic restorations. Further studies should be developed considering the bond strength with different ageing times, including lap shear, tensile and peel stresses evaluations.

## 5. Conclusions

During the restoration cementation procedure, a thicker cement layer thickness will not negatively affect the immediate bond strength. However, due to the higher volume of material, a higher magnitude of residual stress will be present and, during aging, the bond strength will be dampened. Therefore, to improve bond durability, thinner (60–120 μm) cement layer should be recommended.

**Author Contributions:** Conceptualization, J.P.M.T.; L.R.S.-C.; K.B. and M.A.; methodology, J.P.M.T.; A.F.C.d.S.; G.d.C.S.; L.S.d.S.L.; L.R.S.-C. and M.A.; software, J.P.M.T. and M.A.; validation, J.P.M.T.; J.C.L.; L.R.S.-C.; K.B. and M.A.; formal analysis, J.P.M.T.; A.F.C.d.S.; G.d.C.S.; L.S.d.S.L. and M.A.; investigation, J.P.M.T.; A.F.C.d.S.; G.d.C.S.; L.S.d.S.L.; J.C.L. and M.A.; resources, J.P.M.T.; L.R.S.-C.; K.B. and M.A.; data curation, J.P.M.T. and M.A.; writing—original draft preparation, J.P.M.T.; A.F.C.d.S.; G.d.C.S.; L.S.d.S.L.; J.C.L.; L.R.S.-C.; K.B. and M.A.; writing—review and editing, J.P.M.T.; L.R.S.-C.; K.B. and M.A.; visualization, J.P.M.T. and M.A.; supervision, M.A.; project administration, M.A.; funding acquisition, J.P.M.T.; A.F.C.d.S.; G.d.C.S.; L.S.d.S.L.; J.C.L.; L.R.S.-C.; K.B. and M.A. All authors have read and agreed to the published version of the manuscript.

**Funding:** This research was funded by Fundação de Amparo à Pesquisa do Estado de São Paulo grant number FAPESP 2019/20801-4 and Universidade de Taubaté with studentship PRPPG ODO_296_2019.

**Institutional Review Board Statement:** Not applicable.

**Informed Consent Statement:** Not applicable.

**Data Availability Statement:** Data available on request.

**Acknowledgments:** The authors would like to thank São Paulo Research Foundation (FAPESP) with the grant 2019/20801-4 and Universidade de Taubaté with studentship PRPPG ODO_296_2019.

**Conflicts of Interest:** The authors declare no conflict of interest.

## References

1. Lohbauer, U.; Scherrer, S.S.; Della Bona, A.; Tholey, M.; van Noort, R.; Vichi, A.; Kelly, J.R.; Cesar, P.F. ADM guidance-Ceramics: All-ceramic multilayer interfaces in dentistry. *Dent. Mater.* **2017**, *33*, 585–598. [CrossRef] [PubMed]
2. Mante, F.K.; Ozer, F.; Walter, R.; Atlas, A.M.; Saleh, N.; Dietschi, D.; Blatz, M.B. The current state of adhesive dentistry: A guide for clinical practice. *Compend. Contin. Educ. Dent.* **2013**, *34*, 2–8.
3. Tribst, J.; Anami, L.C.; Özcan, M.; Bottino, M.A.; Melo, R.M.; Saavedra, G. Self-etching primers vs acid conditioning: Impact on bond strength between ceramics and resin cement. *Oper. Dent.* **2018**, *43*, 372–379. [CrossRef] [PubMed]
4. Rangel, J.H.R.; Faria, M.S.; D'Ajuda, T.C.S.; Monteiro, A.F.; Weitzel, I.S.S.L.; Silva-Concílio, L.R.; Amaral, M. Failure load and shear bond strength of indirect materials bonded to enamel after aging. *Gen. Dent.* **2021**, *69*, 24–29. [PubMed]
5. Blatz, M.B.; Sadan, A.; Kern, M. Resin-ceramic bonding: A review of the literature. *J. Prosthet. Dent.* **2003**, *89*, 268–274. [CrossRef]
6. Tribst, J.P.M.; Dal Piva, A.M.d.O.; Penteado, M.M.; Borges, A.L.S.; Bottino, M.A. Influence of ceramic material, thickness of restoration and cement layer on stress distribution of occlusal veneers. *Braz. Oral Res.* **2018**, *32*, e118. [CrossRef]
7. May, L.G.; Kelly, J.R.; Bottino, M.A.; Hill, T. Effects of cement thickness and bonding on the failure loads of CAD/CAM ceramic crowns: Multi-physics FEA modeling and monotonic testing. *Dent. Mater.* **2012**, *28*, e99–e109. [CrossRef]
8. Aker Sagen, M.; Dahl, J.E.; Matinlinna, J.P.; Tibballs, J.E.; Rønold, H.J. The influence of the resin-based cement layer on ceramic-dentin bond strength. *Eur. J. Oral Sci.* **2021**, *129*, e12791. [CrossRef]
9. Al Hamad, K.Q.; Al Quran, F.A.; AlJalam, S.A.; Baba, N.Z. Comparison of the accuracy of fit of metal, Zirconia, and lithium disilicate crowns made from different manufacturing techniques. *J. Prosthodont.* **2019**, *28*, 497–503. [CrossRef]
10. Al Hamad, K.Q.; Al Rashdan, B.A.; Al Omari, W.M.; Baba, N.Z. Comparison of the fit of lithium disilicate crowns made from conventional, digital, or conventional/digital techniques: Fit of lithium disilicate crowns. *J. Prosthodont.* **2019**, *28*, e580–e586. [CrossRef] [PubMed]
11. Adolfi, D.; Tribst, J.P.M.; Adolfi, M.; Dal Piva, A.M.d.O.; Saavedra, G.d.S.F.A.; Bottino, M.A. Lithium disilicate crown, Zirconia hybrid abutment and platform switching to improve the esthetics in anterior region: A case report. *Clin. Cosmet. Investig. Dent.* **2020**, *12*, 31–40. [CrossRef]
12. Bhandari, S.; Rajagopal, P.; Bakshi, S. An interdisciplinary approach to reconstruct a fractured tooth under an intact all ceramic crown: Case report with four years follow up. *Indian J. Dent. Res.* **2011**, *22*, 587–590. [CrossRef] [PubMed]
13. Farah, R.I.; Aldhafeeri, A.F.; Alogaili, R.S. A technique to facilitate ceramic veneer cementation. *J. Prosthet. Dent.* **2018**, *120*, 194–197. [CrossRef]
14. Soares-Rusu, I.; Villavicencio-Espinoza, C.A.; de Oliveira, N.A.; Wang, L.; Honório, H.M.; Rubo, J.H.; Francisconi, P.; Borges, A. Clinical evaluation of lithium disilicate veneers manufactured by CAD/CAM compared with heat-pressed methods: Randomized controlled clinical trial. *Oper. Dent.* **2021**, *46*, 4–14. [PubMed]
15. Passos Rocha, E.; Bruniera Anchieta, R.; Alexandre da Cunha Melo, R.; Henrique Dos Santos, P.; Gonçalves Assunção, W.; Isquierdo de Souza, F.; Paula Martini, A. Clinical outcomes of minimally invasive ceramic restorations executed by dentists with different levels of experience. Blind and prospective clinical study. *J. Prosthodont. Res.* **2021**, *65*, 191–197. [CrossRef] [PubMed]
16. Haddadi, Y.; Bahrami, G.; Isidor, F. Accuracy of crowns based on digital intraoral scanning compared to conventional impression-a split-mouth randomised clinical study. *Clin. Oral Investig.* **2019**, *23*, 4043–4050. [CrossRef] [PubMed]
17. Benic, G.I.; Sailer, I.; Zeltner, M.; Gütermann, J.N.; Özcan, M.; Mühlemann, S. Randomized controlled clinical trial of digital and conventional workflows for the fabrication of zirconia-ceramic fixed partial dentures. Part III: Marginal and internal fit. *J. Prosthet. Dent.* **2019**, *121*, 426–431. [CrossRef]
18. Venturini, A.B.; Wandscher, V.F.; Marchionatti, A.M.E.; Evangelisti, E.; Ramos, G.F.; Melo, R.M.; May, L.G.; Baldissara, P.; Valandro, L.F. Effect of resin cement space on the fatigue behavior of bonded CAD/CAM leucite ceramic crowns. *J. Mech. Behav. Biomed. Mater.* **2020**, *110*, 103893. [CrossRef] [PubMed]
19. Feilzer, A.J.; de Gee, A.J.; Davidson, C.L. Relaxation of polymerization contraction shear stress by hygroscopic expansion. *J. Dent. Res.* **1990**, *69*, 36–39. [CrossRef]
20. Melo, R.M.; Pereira, C.; Ramos, N.C.; Feitosa, F.A.; Dal Piva, A.M.d.O.; Tribst, J.P.M.; Özcan, M.; Jorge, A.O.C. Effect of pH variation on the subcritical crack growth parameters of glassy matrix ceramics. *Int. J. Appl. Ceram. Technol.* **2019**, *16*, 2449–2456. [CrossRef]
21. Amaral, M.; Weitzel, I.S.S.L.; Silvestri, T.; Guilardi, L.F.; Pereira, G.K.R.; Valandro, L.F. Effect of grinding and aging on subcritical crack growth of a Y-TZP ceramic. *Braz. Oral Res.* **2018**, *32*, e32. [CrossRef] [PubMed]
22. Yiu, C.K.Y.; King, N.M.; Carrilho, M.R.O.; Sauro, S.; Rueggeberg, F.A.; Prati, C.; Carvalho, R.M.; Pashley, D.H.; Tay, F.R. Effect of resin hydrophilicity and temperature on water sorption of dental adhesive resins. *Biomaterials* **2006**, *27*, 1695–1703. [CrossRef] [PubMed]
23. Wendler, M.; Stenger, A.; Ripper, J.; Priewich, E.; Belli, R.; Lohbauer, U. Mechanical degradation of contemporary CAD/CAM resin composite materials after water ageing. *Dent. Mater.* **2021**, *37*, 1156–1167. [CrossRef] [PubMed]
24. De Andrade, G.S.; Pinto, A.B.A.; Tribst, J.P.M.; Chun, E.P.; Borges, A.L.S.; de Siqueira Ferreira Anzaloni Saavedra, G. Does overlay preparation design affect polymerization shrinkage stress distribution? A 3D FEA study. *Comput. Methods Biomech. Biomed. Engin.* **2021**, *24*, 1026–1034. [CrossRef]

25. Ausiello, P.; Dal Piva, A.M.d.O.; Borges, A.L.S.; Lanzotti, A.; Zamparini, F.; Epifania, E.; Mendes Tribst, J.P. Effect of shrinking and no shrinking dentine and enamel replacing materials in posterior restoration: A 3D-FEA study. *Appl. Sci.* **2021**, *11*, 2215. [CrossRef]
26. Mn, E.W.A.; Mh, G. Internal adaptation, marginal accuracy and microleakage of a pressable versus a machinable ceramic laminate veneers. *J. Dent.* **2012**, *40*, 670–677.
27. Rojpaibool, T.; Leevailoj, C. Fracture resistance of lithium disilicate ceramics bonded to enamel or dentin using different resin cement types and film thicknesses. *J. Prosthodont.* **2017**, *26*, 141–149. [CrossRef]
28. Barbon, F.J.; Moraes, R.R.; Isolan, C.P.; Spazzin, A.O.; Boscato, N. Influence of inorganic filler content of resin luting agents and use of adhesive on the performance of bonded ceramic. *J. Prosthet. Dent.* **2019**, *122*, 566.e1–566.e11. [CrossRef] [PubMed]
29. Ozer, F.; Pak-Tunc, E.; EsenDagli, N.; Ramachandran, D.; Sen, D.; Blatz, M.B. Shear bond strength of luting cements to fixed superstructure metal surfaces under various seating forces. *J. Adv. Prosthodont.* **2018**, *10*, 340–346. [CrossRef]
30. Sokolowski, G.; Krasowski, M.; Szczesio-Wlodarczyk, A.; Konieczny, B.; Sokolowski, J.; Bociong, K. The Influence of Cement Layer Thickness on the Stress State of Metal Inlay Restorations—Photoelastic Analysis. *Materials* **2021**, *14*, 599. [CrossRef]
31. Sampaio, C.S.; Barbosa, J.M.; Cáceres, E.; Rigo, L.C.; Coelho, P.G.; Bonfante, E.A.; Hirata, R. Volumetric shrinkage and film thickness of cementation materials for veneers: An in vitro 3D microcomputed tomography analysis. *J. Prosthet. Dent.* **2017**, *117*, 784–791. [CrossRef] [PubMed]
32. Farag, S.M.; Ghoneim, M.M.; Afifi, R.R. Effect of Die Spacer Thickness on the Fracture Resistance of CAD/CAM Lithium Disilicate Veneers on Maxillary First Premolars. *Clin. Cosmet. Investig. Dent.* **2021**, *13*, 223–230. [CrossRef] [PubMed]
33. Campaner, L.M.; Alves Pinto, A.B.; Demachkia, A.M.; Paes-Junior, T.J.d.A.; Pagani, C.; Borges, A.L.S. Influence of Cement Thickness on the Polymerization Shrinkage Stress of Adhesively Cemented Composite Inlays: Photoelastic and Finite Element Analysis. *Oral* **2021**, *1*, 17. [CrossRef]

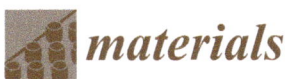 

*Article*

# Masking Ability of Monolithic and Layered Zirconia Crowns on Discolored Substrates

Cristina Gasparik [1], Manuela Maria Manziuc [1,*], Alexandru Victor Burde [1], Javier Ruiz-López [2], Smaranda Buduru [1] and Diana Dudea [1]

1. Department of Prosthetic Dentistry and Dental Materials, Iuliu Hatieganu University of Medicine and Pharmacy, 32 Clinicilor Street, 400006 Cluj-Napoca, Romania; gasparik.cristina@umfcluj.ro (C.G.); abv.alex@yahoo.com (A.V.B.); smarandabuduru@yahoo.com (S.B.); ddudea@umfcluj.ro (D.D.)
2. Department of Optics, Faculty of Science, Edificio Mecenas, Campus Fuente Nueva S/N, University of Granada, 18071 Granada, Spain; jruizlo@ugr.es
* Correspondence: manuelamanziuc@yahoo.com; Tel.: +40-7-4222-9113

**Abstract:** There is scarce information on the colorimetric behavior of monolithic and layered zirconia crowns in combination with various abutment colors. This study evaluated the masking ability on discolored substrates of monolithic and layered zirconia crowns. Anterior crowns were fabricated using 3Y-TZP zirconia and layering ceramic and divided into three groups: monolithic (ML), bi-layer (BL), and tri-layer (TL). The crowns were placed over eleven substrates (ND1-ND9, zirconia, metal), and CIE $L^*$, $a^*$, $b^*$, $C^*$, and $h°$ color coordinates were measured in the cervical, middle, and incisal areas with a spectrophotometer. Masking ability was calculated using the color difference formula, and values were interpreted according to the perceptibility and acceptability thresholds. Data were analyzed statistically ($\alpha = 0.001$). The $L^*$ coordinate was not significantly different between BL and TL crowns, regardless of the measurement area or substrate ($p \geq 0.001$). In the middle area, the $L^*$ coordinate of the ML group was statistically different from the BL and TL groups only for zirconia and metal substrates, while in the incisal area, only for ND7 and metal substrates. The $a^*$ coordinate was significantly different between the ML and layered crowns for all measurement areas and substrates (except zirconia). The $b^*$ and $C^*$ coordinates differed significantly between the groups only in the cervical area ($p < 0.001$). The ML crown had better masking ability than the BL and TL crowns. However, the color differences for ML crowns were below the acceptability threshold for ND2, ND3, and ND7 substrates in the cervical and middle areas and below perceptibility threshold only for the incisal area. The lowest masking ability of the crowns was found for ND9 and metal substrates in all measurement areas.

**Keywords:** zirconia; crown; color; masking ability

## 1. Introduction

Tooth discoloration is a common clinical condition encountered in daily dental practice. It affects one or multiple teeth, and several factors may be involved in the etiology: caries and tertiary dentin formation, hemorrhage into the pulp chamber, endodontic procedures, and materials, as well as metabolic or idiopathic causes [1,2]. The esthetic improvement of tooth discoloration can be achieved by bleaching with oxidizing agents or prosthetic treatments when it is aimed to restoring the tooth with either a veneer or a full crown. Nevertheless, the procedure's success is highly dependent on the skills and intuition of the dentist and dental technician since masking a discolored substrate is rarely a predictable process.

Today, there is an immense variety of dental materials available for the fabrication of indirect restorations. However, dental zirconia stands out because of its versatility, combining high strength with acceptable esthetics, allowing an entirely digitized fabrica-

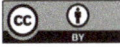

tion process, and permitting additional individualization through conventional ceramic layering methods.

The second generation of 3 mol% yttria-stabilized tetragonal zirconia polycrystal (3Y-TZP) zirconia has a reduced amount of aluminum oxide in its composition, compared to the first generation [3]. This material is sintered at higher temperatures, increasing grain size and reducing porosities, consequently improving the translucency. 3Y-TZP zirconia is indicated for monolithic or veneered restorations [4]. Traditional layering, over-pressing, file-splitting (CAD-on), and the cut-back technique are some veneering methods that can be combined with zirconia crowns [5].

Several factors influence the color appearance of zirconia restorations. Besides chemical composition and structure [3,6], other factors such as material thickness [5,7,8], processing parameters [9,10], shading technique and veneering material [11], substrate type and color [12–16], and luting agent [14,17–19] contribute to the overall color of the restoration.

According to the International Commission on Illumination (Commission Internationale de L'Éclairage—CIE), currently, the CIEDE2000 total color difference formula ($\Delta E_{00}$) [20], associated with the CIE L* a* b* color space, is widely implemented in clinical dentistry and dental research due to its better correlation with visual perception [21] and is recommended for total color difference computation by the International Standard Organization [22]. However, the use of the $\Delta E_{00}$ color difference formula alone is irrelevant unless the respective well-known visual 50:50% perceptibility and acceptability thresholds, determined in [23] and recommended in the latest guidance on color measurements for dentistry [22], are used for judging the significance of color differences [24].

In the past, the masking ability of a restorative material was evaluated using the color difference formulas ($\Delta E_{ab}$ or $\Delta E_{00}$), the translucency parameter (TP), or the contrast ratio (CR); notwithstanding, a recent systematic review concluded that the most appropriate method to assess the masking ability is using the color difference formula associated with the perceptibility (PT) and acceptability thresholds (AT) [25].

Several recent studies evaluated the masking ability and shade reproduction of dental materials [26–30]. The studies investigated the properties of monolithic samples when placed over discolored substrates. However, only a limited number and color of substrates were evaluated, while in clinical practice, the appearance of dental discoloration is highly variable.

Although extensive research has been recently conducted on the masking ability of restorative materials [12–19,31–38], there is still missing information on how color differences might impact visual perception when translucent restorations are evaluated over different discolored substrates. Furthermore, there is little information about the colorimetric behavior of monolithic and layered zirconia crowns in combination with various abutment colors. Most studies evaluated the masking ability using rectangular or disc samples [12,13,15–17,19,31–38], which do not reproduce the clinical conditions met in the oral cavity.

Therefore, this study aimed to evaluate the masking ability of monolithic and layered zirconia crowns in each of the three areas (cervical, middle incisal) on eleven different discolored substrates. The null hypotheses were: (1) there were no significant differences in CIE L*, a*, b*, C*, and h° color coordinates between the monolithic and the layered zirconia crowns on the different discolored substrates; (2) the masking ability of monolithic and layered zirconia crowns on discolored substrates was acceptable.

## 2. Materials and Methods

This study used 3Y-TZP zirconia (Katana HT10, Kuraray Noritake Dental Inc., Tokyo, Japan) to fabricate anterior full coverage monolithic and layered crowns.

### 2.1. Crowns Fabrication

A phantom head's upper right central incisor (DSE Expert, KaVo, Biberach, Germany) was prepared with a 1 mm circumferential chamfer finish line, 6° axial taper, 1 mm axial, and 1.5 mm incisal reductions. The prepared tooth was digitized using a laboratory scanner (InEos X5, Dentsply Sirona, Bensheim, Germany).

Three-dimensional designs of the crowns were made with Exocad Dental CAD 2.4 (v.2.4, Exocad GmbH, Darmstadt, Germany) software. The following two designs were considered: a full-contour crown design with 1 mm labial thickness (monolithic group) and a partial veneer crown design (layered group) with 0.4 mm thickness of the framework on the labial surface and 0.6 mm space for the veneering ceramic (Figure 1).

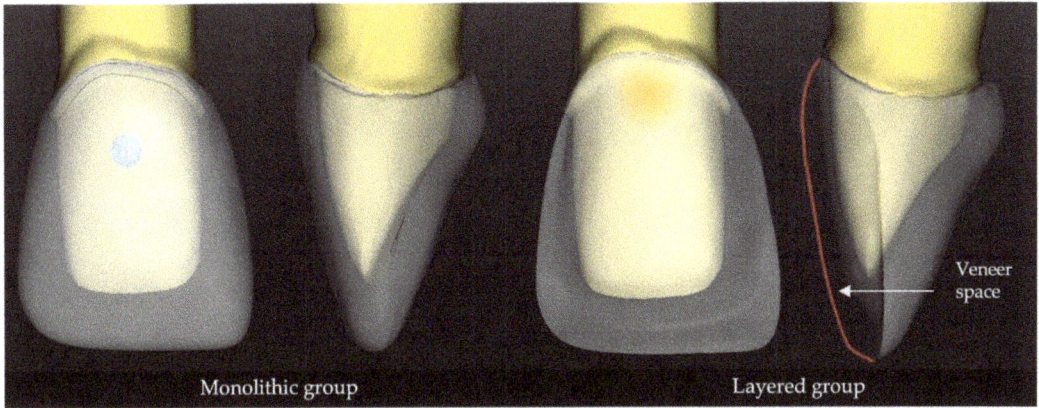

**Figure 1.** The 3D design of the monolithic and layered restorations in the CAD software.

The restorations were dry-milled under continuous vacuuming (Imes iCore 250i, Imes iCore GmbH, Eiterfeld, Germany) using a 3Y-TZP zirconia blank and then sintered at 1500 °C for 2 h (Mihm Vogt HT2, GmbH, Stutensee, Germany). The finishing of the sintered crowns was done using silicone discs (Meister SC51, Kuraray Noritake Dental Inc., Tokyo, Japan). The labial surface of the layered group was sandblasted using aluminum oxide (50 microns, 2 bars), and impurities were removed from the crown surfaces by immersing the restorations in an ultrasonic cleaner with distilled water for 10 min (Figure 2).

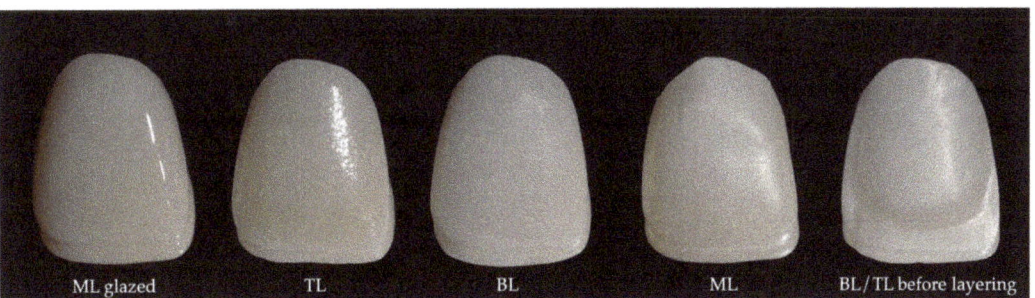

**Figure 2.** The appearance of the restorations in different fabrication steps.

The layered group was further divided into two groups according to the ceramic layers applied: bi-layer group with 0.6 mm enamel layer (BL) and tri-layer group with 0.3 mm dentin and 0.3 mm enamel layers (TL). For the BL group, a 0.8 mm thick enamel veneering ceramic (CZR Cerabien Zr Enamel A1, Kuraray Noritake Dental Inc., Tokyo, Japan) was applied to the labial surface and sintered (VITA Vacumat 6000, VITA Zahnfabrik, Bad Säckingen, Germany). After sintering at 940 °C for 1 min under vacuum, the restorations were finished to achieve a 1 mm thickness on the labial surface. The thickness was verified using a caliper.

For the TL group, a 0.5 mm dentin ceramic (CZR Cerabien Zr Dentin A1, Kuraray Noritake Dental Inc., Tokyo, Japan) was applied to the labial surface and sintered. The labial surface was finished using diamond burs, and a uniform space of 0.3 mm was created for the enamel ceramic. The enamel layer (the same as for the BL group) was applied in a 0.5 mm thickness and sintered at 940 °C for 1 min under vacuum. After the firing procedure, the labial surfaces of the crowns were finished to achieve a thickness of 1 mm.

All crowns were cleaned using a steamer and air-dried. Then, a thin glaze layer (CZR Cerabien Glaze Paste Clear, Kuraray Noritake Dental Inc., Tokyo, Japan) was applied, covering the entire surface of the crowns, and they were fired at 930 °C. Stains or ceramic effects were not used for any of the crown groups. One experienced master dental technician performed all laboratory procedures (Figure 2).

The following zirconia crown groups resulted in: monolithic (ML, n = 5), bi-layer (BL, n = 5), and tri-layer groups (TL, n = 5) all having 1 mm labial and 1.5 mm incisal thickness.

## 2.2. Substrate Fabrication

A polyethylene foil was heated until soft using a Bunsen burner and adapted over the prepared tooth. After cooling, the plastic mold was detached, and composite resin (IPS Natural Die Material, Ivoclar Vivadent, Schaan, Liechtenstein) was densely packed to obtain the duplicate resin dies. The resin was polymerized for 40 s using a light-curing lamp (1200 mW/cm$^2$, Halo, Translux Wave, Kulzer, Hanau, Germany). Nine tooth-colored resin substrates were obtained: ND1, ND2, ND3, ND4, ND5, ND6, ND7, ND8, ND9.

To fabricate the zirconia and the metal dies, the prepared tooth was scanned, and the three-dimensional model of the die was digitally processed using CAD software (InLab 15, Sirona Dentsply Gmbh, Bensheim, Germany) for preparing the virtual die for milling and additive manufacturing. For the milling process of the zirconium oxide die, the virtual die was imported in a generic CAM software (SUM3D, CIMsystem, Cinisello Balsamo, Italy), the milling strategy was configured, and the milling process was performed by using a 5-axis milling machine (Coritec 250i, Imes iCore Gmbh, Eiterfeld, Germany) using a translucent zirconia pre-colored disk (Vita YZ T color, LLL2 medium, VITA Zahnfabrik, Bad Säckingen, Germany). To produce the metal die, selective laser melting (SLM) was employed, which required the importation of the virtual die into a specific CAM software (CAMbridge, 3Shape A/S, Copenhagen, Denmark) and the exportation of the three-dimensional printing strategy to the SLM printer (MySint 100, Sisma, Piovene Rocchette, Italy). A cobalt–chromium alloy was used for the metal die fabrication process (Mediloy S-Co, BEGO Medical GmbH, Bremen, Germany) (Figure 3).

## 2.3. Color Measurements

Each of the eleven substrates was successively placed into the phantoms' head dental arch for color measurements. The crowns were seated on the die using a transparent try-in paste (Try-in paste, neutral, Ivoclar Vivadent, Schaan, Liechtenstein), and three color measurements were executed for each crown by a trained operator. The color measurements were performed using a non-contact dental spectrophotometer (Spectroshade Micro, MHT, Niederhasli, Switzerland), and the instrument was calibrated before each measurement using the white and green calibration tiles. The instrument has a CIE 45°/0° illumination/measurement geometry and converts spectral data using the CIE 2° standard observer and a CIE D65 illuminant. The recorded images were transferred to the software's database, and CIE L*, a*, b*, C*, and h° color coordinates were extracted from three areas (3 mm diameter) of the crown: cervical, middle, incisal. A template was used to ensure the same extraction area for each crown (Figure 4).

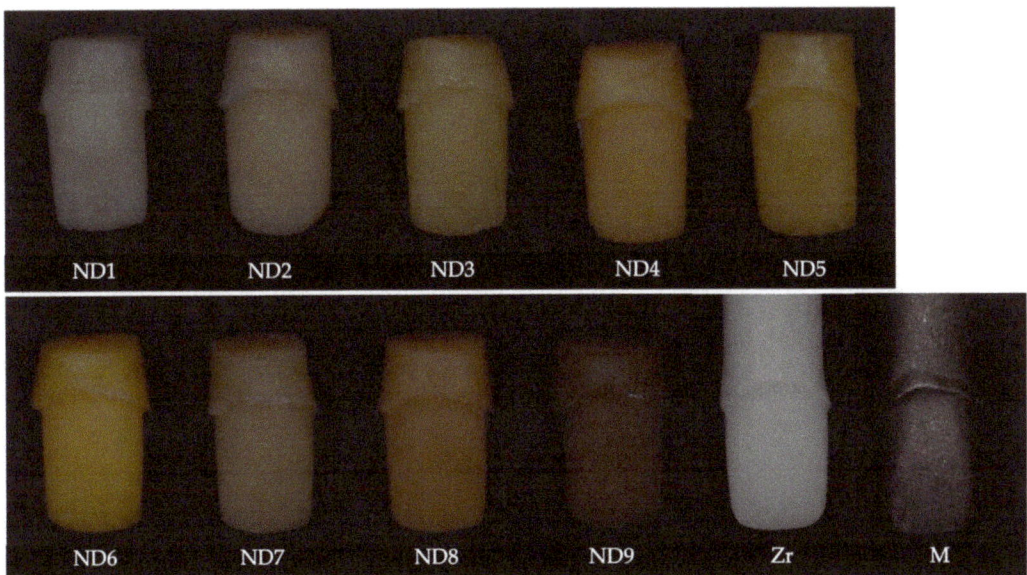

**Figure 3.** The eleven substrates made of resin composite (ND1–ND9), zirconia, and metal.

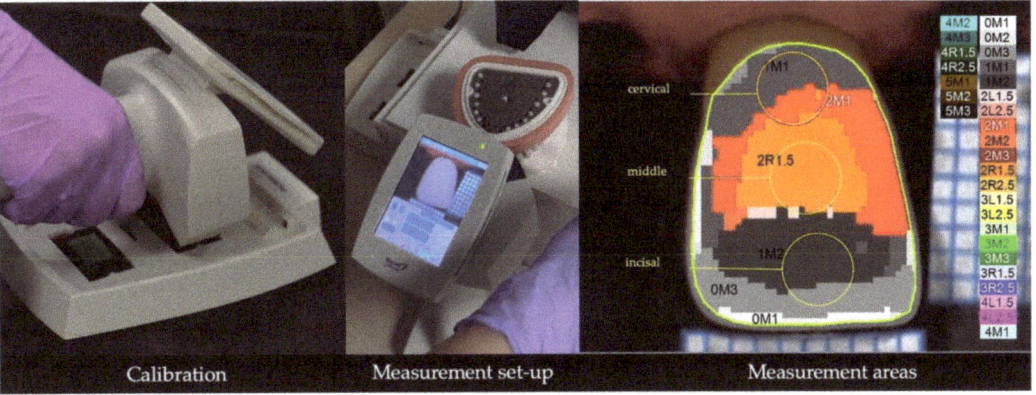

**Figure 4.** The measurement set-up for the dental spectrophotometer and the data extraction.

*2.4. Color Differences and Masking Ability*

The masking ability was expressed as the color difference between a crown seated on the ND1 substrate (the control substrate) and the same crown placed over each of the other ten substrates (the test substrates ND2–ND9, Zr, M) [13,33]. The color differences were computed for each measurement area. The CIEDE2000 color difference formula was used for all calculations:

$$\Delta E_{00} = \left[ \left( \frac{\Delta L'}{k_L S_L} \right)^2 + \left( \frac{\Delta C'}{k_C S_C} \right)^2 + \left( \frac{\Delta H'}{k_H S_H} \right)^2 + R_T \left( \frac{\Delta C'}{k_C S_C} \right) \left( \frac{\Delta H'}{k_H S_H} \right) \right]^{\frac{1}{2}}$$

where $\Delta L'$, $\Delta C'$, and $\Delta H'$ are the differences in lightness, chroma, and hue, respectively, for the same crown measured over two different substrates. The parametric factors $k_L$, $k_C$, and $k_H$ are correction terms for experimental conditions and were set to 1 in the present study. $S_L$, $S_C$, and $S_H$ refer to the weighting functions that adjust the total color difference considering the location variation of the color difference pair in $L'$, $a'$, and $b'$ coordinates. Finally, the parameter $R_T$ is a function (rotation function) that accounts for the interaction between chroma and hue differences in the blue region [20,21].

The masking ability effectiveness was clinically interpreted according to the visual 50:50% perceptibility ($PT_{00}$ = 0.8 $\Delta E_{00}$ units) and acceptability ($AT_{00}$ = 1.8 $\Delta E_{00}$ units) color thresholds for dentistry [23], recommended and standardized within ISO/TR 28642:2016 [22]. Furthermore, to evaluate the $\Delta E_{00}$ above the $AT_{00}$, a recent grading system [24] was used. It describes five intervals, where grades 5 and 4 correspond with the $PT_{00}$ and $AT_{00}$, showing an excellent (EM) and acceptable match (AM), respectively. Grades 3, 2, and 1 refer to different mismatch types: moderately unacceptable (MU) when $\Delta E_{00}$ was >1.8 and ≤3.6 $\Delta E_{00}$ units, clearly unacceptable (CU) when $\Delta E_{00}$ was > 3.6 and ≤ 5.4 $\Delta E_{00}$ units, and extremely unacceptable (EU) when $\Delta E_{00}$ was >5.4 $\Delta E_{00}$ units.

The total color difference CIEDE2000 can be divided into the three components: lightness ($\Delta L_{00}$), chroma ($\Delta C_{00}$), and hue ($\Delta H_{00}$) differences, which can be defined as follows [39]:

$$\Delta L_{00} = \frac{\Delta L'}{k_L S_L} \; ; \; \Delta C_{00} = \frac{\Delta C'}{k_C S_C} \; ; \; \Delta H_{00} = \frac{\Delta H'}{k_H S_H}$$

*2.5. Statistical Analysis*

After performing the Levene's test of homogeneity of variance ($\alpha = 0.05$) and verifying that equal variances could not be assumed for all CIE color coordinates L*, a*, b*, C*, and h° groups, a Kruskal–Wallis one-way analysis of variance by ranks were applied to evaluate the changes on chromatic coordinates between the different crown groups. The Mann–Whitney U test was applied for the pair-wise comparisons with a Bonferroni correction (level of significance, $p < 0.001$). Contrasts were made between the three crown groups for the same third using the same substrate. The statistical software package used to perform the statistical analysis was SPSS Statistics 20.0.0 (IBM Armonk, New York, NY, USA).

## 3. Results

*3.1. Color Coordinates*

The distribution of mean CIE L*, a*, and b* values of the substrates are shown in Figure 5. The Zr and M substrates were the brightest and the darkest, respectively. Among the tooth-shaded substrates, ND2 was the brightest and the least chromatic, while ND9 was the darkest, and ND6 was the most chromatic. ND2–ND6 substrates had a comparable lightness to ND1.

CIE L*, a*, b*, C*, and h° color coordinates of the three crown groups measured over different discolored substrates are presented in Tables 1–3.

For ML crowns, the color coordinates ranged between 73.26–84.67 for L*, −2.0–1.28 for a*, 6.74–16.23 for b*, 7.01–16.27 for C*, and 85.33–105.97° for h°.

For BL crowns, the color coordinates ranged between 71.00–86.24 for L*, −1.71–1.84 for a*, 2.71–14.35 for b*, 2.98–14.42 for C*, and 82.58–116.04° for h°.

For TL crowns, the color coordinates ranged between 71.51–86.18 for L*, −1.64–1.95 for a*, 4.22–16.05 for b*, 4.41–16.14 for C*, and 83.45–107.06° for h°.

The L* coordinate did not differ statistically significantly between BL and TL crowns, irrespective of the measurement area or substrate ($p \geq 0.001$). In the middle area, the L* coordinate of the ML group was statistically different from the BL and TL groups only for Zr and M substrates, while in the incisal area, only for ND7 and M substrates.

The a* coordinate was statistically different between ML crowns and layered crowns (BL and TL) for all measurement areas and substrates, except the Zr abutment. In the cervical area, the b* and C* coordinates differed significantly between the three groups of crowns ($p < 0.001$). However, in the middle and incisal areas, the ML and the TL groups showed similar behavior. The h° coordinate of the ML group differed significantly from layered groups for ND2–ND9 substrates in the cervical area, while in the middle and incisal areas, the BL and TL groups generally showed statistically significant differences among them.

### 3.2. Masking Ability

ML had better masking ability than layered crowns regardless of the measurement area or the substrate (Figures 6–8). For these crowns, the color differences were below the $AT_{00}$ only for ND2, ND3, and ND7 substrates in the cervical and middle areas and below $PT_{00}$ for the incisal area. A moderately unacceptable color mismatch (MU) was found for ML crowns on ND4, ND5, ND8, and Zr substrates and layered crowns on ND3, ND5, and ND7 substrates for both cervical and middle areas. Nevertheless, for the incisal areas, some of these color differences were acceptable ($<AT_{00}$) (Figure 8).

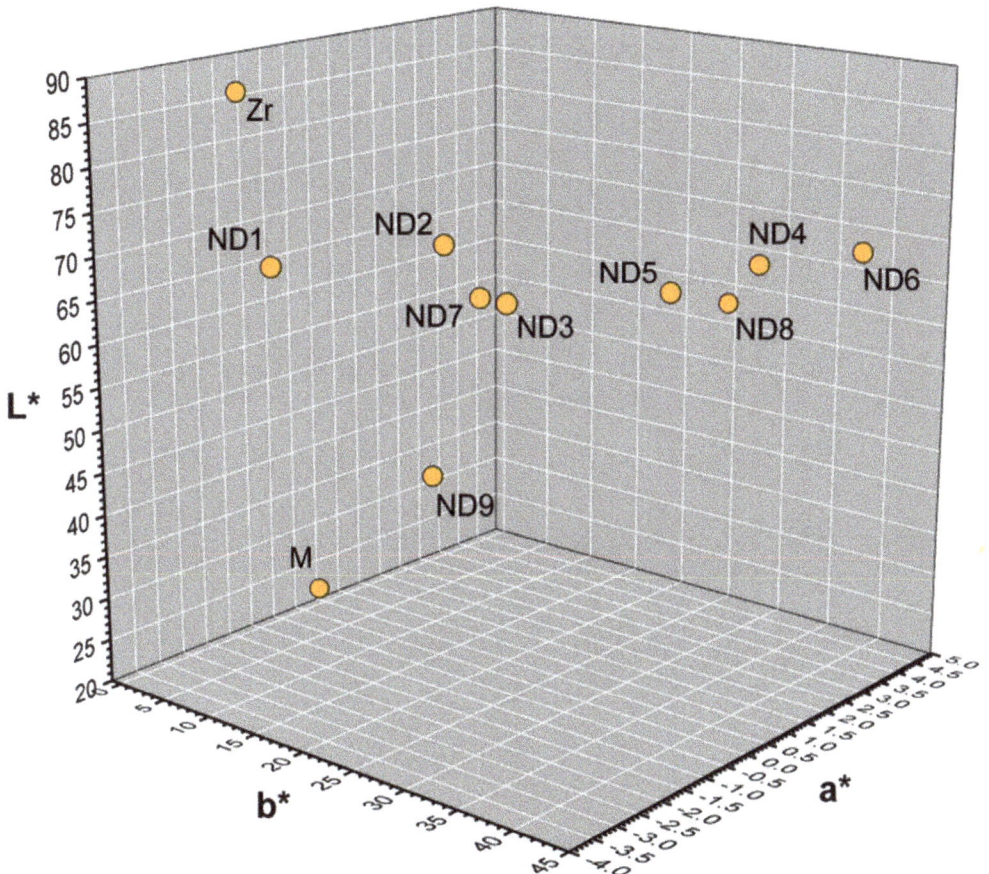

**Figure 5.** Mean CIELAB values of the eleven substrates.

Table 1. Mean values and standard deviation of CIE L*, a*, b*, C*, and h° color coordinates of zirconia crowns on different substrates evaluated for the cervical area.

| Cervical | ML | | | | | BL | | | | | TL | | | | |
|---|---|---|---|---|---|---|---|---|---|---|---|---|---|---|---|
| | L* | a* | b* | C* | h° | L* | a* | b* | C* | h° | L* | a* | b* | C* | h° |
| ND1 | 79.84 ± 0.15 [a] | −1.38 ± 0.04 | 12.24 ± 0.13 | 12.32 ± 0.14 | 96.43 ± 0.13 [c] | 79.89 ± 0.17 [a] | −1.03 ± 0.11 [b] | 8.96 ± 0.41 | 9.02 ± 0.42 | 96.53 ± 0.50 [cd] | 79.79 ± 0.29 [a] | −1.02 ± 0.18 [b] | 10.27 ± 0.33 | 10.33 ± 0.33 | 95.67 ± 0.98 [d] |
| ND2 | 79.78 ± 0.15 [a] | −0.47 ± 0.04 | 13.35 ± 0.12 | 13.35 ± 0.12 | 92.02 ± 0.18 | 79.47 ± 0.17 [b] | −0.03 ± 0.10 [c] | 10.62 ± 0.27 | 10.62 ± 0.27 | 90.15 ± 0.55 [d] | 79.56 ± 0.39 [ab] | 0.06 ± 0.13 [c] | 11.62 ± 0.29 | 11.62 ± 0.29 | 89.69 ± 0.63 [d] |
| ND3 | 78.67 ± 0.20 | −0.34 ± 0.05 | 13.38 ± 0.21 | 13.38 ± 0.21 | 91.45 ± 0.20 | 78.13 ± 0.29 [a] | 0.03 ± 0.06 [b] | 11.19 ± 0.27 | 11.19 ± 0.27 | 89.84 ± 0.33 [c] | 77.93 ± 0.35 [a] | 0.10 ± 0.09 [b] | 12.14 ± 0.27 | 12.14 ± 0.27 | 89.52 ± 0.41 [c] |
| ND4 | 78.54 ± 0.27 | 0.83 ± 0.07 | 13.89 ± 0.25 | 13.91 ± 0.26 | 86.57 ± 0.25 | 77.77 ± 0.26 [a] | 1.52 ± 0.05 [b] | 12.16 ± 0.37 | 12.25 ± 0.37 | 82.86 ± 0.24 | 77.93 ± 0.21 [a] | 1.47 ± 0.11 [b] | 12.84 ± 0.21 | 12.92 ± 0.22 | 83.45 ± 0.43 |
| ND5 | 78.53 ± 0.25 [a] | 0.15 ± 0.02 | 14.20 ± 0.16 | 14.20 ± 0.16 | 89.39 ± 0.10 | 78.02 ± 0.23 [b] | 0.66 ± 0.08 | 12.48 ± 0.38 | 12.50 ± 0.37 | 86.98 ± 0.45 [c] | 78.17 ± 0.46 [ab] | 0.75 ± 0.13 | 13.33 ± 0.34 | 13.35 ± 0.35 | 86.80 ± 0.50 [d] |
| ND6 | 79.39 ± 0.35 | 1.28 ± 0.06 | 15.64 ± 0.21 | 15.70 ± 0.21 | 85.33 ± 0.16 | 78.74 ± 0.33 [a] | 1.84 ± 0.07 [b] | 14.18 ± 0.40 | 14.30 ± 0.40 | 82.58 ± 0.35 [c] | 78.66 ± 0.35 [a] | 1.95 ± 0.17 [b] | 14.90 ± 0.41 | 15.03 ± 0.43 | 82.54 ± 0.44 [c] |
| ND7 | 77.90 ± 0.19 [a] | −0.57 ± 0.02 | 12.02 ± 0.16 | 12.04 ± 0.16 | 92.69 ± 0.08 | 77.16 ± 0.34 [b] | −0.09 ± 0.12 [c] | 9.46 ± 0.31 | 9.46 ± 0.31 | 90.53 ± 0.69 [d] | 77.63 ± 0.73 [ab] | 0.00 ± 0.10 [c] | 10.49 ± 0.34 | 10.49 ± 0.34 | 90.03 ± 0.55 [c] |
| ND8 | 76.51 ± 0.22 | 0.32 ± 0.08 | 11.44 ± 0.13 | 11.44 ± 0.13 | 88.39 ± 0.41 | 75.16 ± 0.46 [a] | 1.12 ± 0.08 [b] | 9.26 ± 0.30 | 9.33 ± 0.30 | 83.06 ± 0.61 [c] | 75.67 ± 0.55 [a] | 1.09 ± 0.16 [b] | 10.21 ± 0.33 | 10.27 ± 0.34 | 83.90 ± 0.74 [c] |
| ND9 | 73.26 ± 0.28 | −1.61 ± 0.03 | 7.68 ± 0.13 | 7.85 ± 0.12 | 101.85 ± 0.34 | 71.56 ± 0.47 [a] | −0.87 ± 0.13 [b] | 4.93 ± 0.24 | 5.01 ± 0.25 | 100.02 ± 0.98 | 72.23 ± 0.72 [a] | −0.86 ± 0.08 [b] | 6.14 ± 0.33 | 6.20 ± 0.32 | 97.99 ± 1.03 |
| Zr | 84.67 ± 0.09 | −1.48 ± 0.11 [b] | 12.66 ± 0.18 | 12.75 ± 0.19 | 96.64 ± 3.42 [d] | 85.58 ± 0.38 [a] | −1.35 ± 0.21 [bc] | 8.18 ± 0.51 | 8.30 ± 0.53 | 99.35 ± 0.99 | 85.77 ± 0.34 [a] | −1.30 ± 0.09 [c] | 9.98 ± 0.58 | 10.06 ± 0.57 | 97.43 ± 0.71 [d] |
| M | 73.69 ± 0.52 | −1.93 ± 0.04 | 6.74 ± 0.27 | 7.01 ± 0.26 | 105.97 ± 3.69 [c] | 71.00 ± 0.43 [a] | −1.24 ± 0.08 [b] | 2.71 ± 0.25 | 2.98 ± 0.26 | 114.67 ± 1.08 | 71.51 ± 0.62 [a] | −1.28 ± 0.11 [b] | 4.22 ± 0.45 | 4.41 ± 0.43 | 107.06 ± 2.17 [c] |

Same superscript letter in the same row indicates no statistical significance ($p \geq 0.001$)—comparison between crown groups for the same measurement area.

**Table 2.** Mean values and standard deviation of CIE L*, a*, b*, C*, and h° color coordinates of zirconia crowns on different substrates evaluated for the middle area.

| Middle | ML | | | | | BL | | | | | TL | | | | |
|---|---|---|---|---|---|---|---|---|---|---|---|---|---|---|---|
| | L* | a* | b* | C* | h° | L* | a* | b* | C* | h° | L* | a* | b* | C* | h° |
| ND1 | 79.65 ± 0.24 [a] | −1.34 ± 0.03 | 13.01 ± 0.10 | 13.08 ± 0.10 | 95.86 ± 0.15 [c] | 80.67 ± 0.27 | −1.22 ± 0.05 [b] | 9.20 ± 0.35 | 9.28 ± 0.35 | 97.58 ± 0.17 | 80.06 ± 0.49 [a] | −1.14 ± 0.12 [b] | 10.99 ± 0.44 | 11.05 ± 0.43 | 95.93 ± 0.80 [c] |
| ND2 | 80.12 ± 0.15 [a] | −0.44 ± 0.03 | 14.41 ± 0.08 | 14.41 ± 0.08 | 91.74 ± 0.12 [c] | 80.89 ± 0.26 [b] | −0.28 ± 0.05 | 11.21 ± 0.44 | 11.22 ± 0.44 | 91.45 ± 0.25 [c] | 80.35 ± 0.55 [ab] | −0.08 ± 0.16 | 12.89 ± 0.60 | 12.90 ± 0.60 | 90.39 ± 0.68 |
| ND3 | 78.94 ± 0.20 [a] | −0.32 ± 0.03 | 14.33 ± 0.07 [b] | 14.33 ± 0.07 [c] | 91.27 ± 0.11 [d] | 79.49 ± 0.39 [a] | −0.23 ± 0.02 | 11.77 ± 0.50 | 11.77 ± 0.50 | 91.13 ± 0.15 [d] | 78.82 ± 0.58 [a] | −0.04 ± 0.16 | 13.31 ± 0.70 [b] | 13.31 ± 0.70 [c] | 90.19 ± 0.64 |
| ND4 | 78.79 ± 0.35 [a] | 0.77 ± 0.12 | 14.65 ± 0.10 [b] | 14.67 ± 0.11 [c] | 86.99 ± 0.45 | 78.98 ± 0.36 [a] | 1.19 ± 0.09 | 12.38 ± 0.64 | 12.44 ± 0.65 | 84.51 ± 0.18 [d] | 78.57 ± 0.41 [a] | 1.40 ± 0.17 | 14.02 ± 0.59 [b] | 14.09 ± 0.60 [c] | 84.30 ± 0.45 [d] |
| ND5 | 78.96 ± 0.17 [a] | 0.20 ± 0.03 | 15.04 ± 0.08 [b] | 15.04 ± 0.08 [c] | 89.22 ± 0.12 | 79.26 ± 0.23 [a] | 0.38 ± 0.05 | 12.77 ± 0.53 | 12.77 ± 0.53 | 88.28 ± 0.20 | 78.80 ± 0.51 [a] | 0.63 ± 0.18 | 14.29 ± 0.74 [b] | 14.30 ± 0.75 [c] | 87.50 ± 0.55 |
| ND6 | 79.62 ± 0.48 [a] | 1.09 ± 0.06 | 16.23 ± 0.14 [b] | 16.27 ± 0.14 [c] | 86.17 ± 0.20 | 80.06 ± 0.43 [a] | 1.33 ± 0.11 | 14.35 ± 0.63 | 14.42 ± 0.63 | 84.70 ± 0.23 | 79.51 ± 0.48 [a] | 1.69 ± 0.18 | 16.05 ± 0.67 [b] | 16.14 ± 0.68 [c] | 84.00 ± 0.37 |
| ND7 | 78.43 ± 0.22 [a] | −0.56 ± 0.03 | 12.97 ± 0.07 | 12.98 ± 0.07 | 92.48 ± 0.14 [b] | 78.70 ± 0.37 [a] | −0.34 ± 0.07 | 9.85 ± 0.33 | 9.86 ± 0.33 | 91.97 ± 0.43 [b] | 78.23 ± 0.67 [a] | −0.12 ± 0.14 | 11.50 ± 0.57 | 11.51 ± 0.57 | 90.65 ± 0.70 |
| ND8 | 76.87 ± 0.32 [a] | 0.41 ± 0.12 | 12.23 ± 0.10 [c] | 12.24 ± 0.10 [d] | 88.07 ± 0.58 | 76.75 ± 0.58 [a] | 1.00 ± 0.10 [b] | 9.74 ± 0.40 | 9.79 ± 0.41 | 84.13 ± 0.37 [e] | 76.36 ± 0.67 [a] | 1.15 ± 0.18 [b] | 11.27 ± 0.61 [c] | 11.33 ± 0.62 [c] | 84.21 ± 0.59 [e] |
| ND9 | 73.83 ± 0.33 [a] | −1.44 ± 0.02 | 8.73 ± 0.09 | 8.85 ± 0.09 | 99.40 ± 0.15 [c] | 72.96 ± 0.98 [a] | −0.88 ± 0.09 [b] | 5.60 ± 0.17 | 5.67 ± 0.18 | 98.95 ± 0.84 [c] | 73.00 ± 1.05 [a] | −0.84 ± 0.07 [b] | 7.19 ± 0.44 | 7.24 ± 0.43 | 96.71 ± 0.86 |
| Zr | 84.64 ± 0.29 | −1.59 ± 0.11 [bc] | 14.27 ± 0.10 | 14.36 ± 0.10 | 96.35 ± 0.42 [d] | 86.24 ± 0.27 [a] | −1.70 ± 0.09 [b] | 8.81 ± 0.47 | 8.97 ± 0.48 | 100.92 ± 0.48 | 86.18 ± 0.40 [c] | −1.48 ± 0.14 [c] | 11.28 ± 0.48 | 11.37 ± 0.46 | 97.50 ± 0.97 [d] |
| M | 74.76 ± 0.54 | −2.03 ± 0.05 | 7.95 ± 0.28 | 8.21 ± 0.27 | 104.36 ± 0.72 [c] | 72.92 ± 0.88 [a] | −1.50 ± 0.09 [b] | 3.09 ± 0.34 | 3.44 ± 0.34 | 116.04 ± 1.29 | 72.81 ± 1.33 [b] | −1.52 ± 0.11 [b] | 5.21 ± 0.21 | 5.43 ± 0.20 | 106.26 ± 1.41 [c] |

Same superscript letter in the same row indicates no statistical significance ($p \geq 0.001$)—comparison between crown groups for the same measurement area.

Table 3. Mean values and standard deviation of CIE L*, a*, b*, C*, and h° color coordinates of zirconia crowns on different substrates evaluated for the incisal area.

| Incisal | ML | | | | | BL | | | | | TL | | | | |
|---|---|---|---|---|---|---|---|---|---|---|---|---|---|---|---|
| | L* | a* | b* | C* | h° | L* | a* | b* | C* | h° | L* | a* | b* | C* | h° |
| ND1 | 77.84 ± 0.30 $^{ab}$ | −1.56 ± 0.04 | 11.40 ± 0.14 $^d$ | 11.51 ± 0.14 $^e$ | 97.79 ± 0.26 | 78.08 ± 0.39 $^a$ | −1.37 ± 0.05 $^c$ | 8.18 ± 0.32 | 8.29 ± 0.32 | 99.52 ± 0.21 | 77.57 ± 0.27 $^b$ | −1.38 ± 0.03 $^c$ | 11.08 ± 0.69 $^d$ | 11.16 ± 0.68 $^e$ | 97.10 ± 0.41 |
| ND2 | 78.12 ± 0.08 $^a$ | −1.21 ± 0.04 | 11.91 ± 0.16 $^d$ | 11.97 ± 0.16 $^d$ | 95.80 ± 0.28 $^e$ | 78.28 ± 0.20 $^a$ | −0.95 ± 0.03 $^b$ | 9.07 ± 0.34 | 9.12 ± 0.34 | 96.00 ± 0.17 | 77.67 ± 0.36 | −0.89 ± 0.04 $^b$ | 11.79 ± 0.68 $^c$ | 11.83 ± 0.68 $^d$ | 94.35 ± 0.39 $^e$ |
| ND3 | 77.44 ± 0.25 $^a$ | −1.10 ± 0.05 | 11.90 ± 0.13 $^b$ | 11.95 ± 0.13 $^c$ | 95.31 ± 0.27 $^d$ | 77.70 ± 0.29 $^a$ | −0.89 ± 0.02 | 9.41 ± 0.38 | 9.45 ± 0.38 | 95.39 ± 0.27 $^d$ | 77.30 ± 0.26 $^a$ | −0.78 ± 0.02 | 12.15 ± 0.77 $^b$ | 12.18 ± 0.77 $^c$ | 93.68 ± 0.29 |
| ND4 | 76.89 ± 0.18 $^a$ | −0.69 ± 0.08 | 11.73 ± 0.16 | 11.75 ± 0.16 | 93.35 ± 0.45 | 77.14 ± 0.24 $^a$ | −0.24 ± 0.04 | 9.64 ± 0.38 | 9.64 ± 0.38 | 91.41 ± 0.24 | 77.08 ± 0.16 $^a$ | −0.09 ± 0.06 | 12.52 ± 0.79 | 12.52 ± 0.79 | 90.41 ± 0.28 |
| ND5 | 77.61 ± 0.15 $^a$ | −0.83 ± 0.01 | 12.33 ± 0.10 $^c$ | 12.36 ± 0.10 $^d$ | 95.85 ± 0.03 $^e$ | 77.28 ± 0.22 $^b$ | −0.61 ± 0.06 | 9.78 ± 0.36 | 9.80 ± 0.36 | 93.54 ± 0.36 $^e$ | 77.10 ± 0.69 $^{ab}$ | −0.45 ± 0.05 | 12.37 ± 0.88 $^c$ | 12.38 ± 0.88 $^d$ | 92.12 ± 0.35 |
| ND6 | 77.80 ± 0.19 $^a$ | −0.63 ± 0.05 | 12.53 ± 0.23 | 12.54 ± 0.22 | 92.89 ± 0.30 | 77.91 ± 0.27 $^a$ | −0.28 ± 0.06 | 10.48 ± 0.57 | 10.48 ± 0.57 | 91.57 ± 0.40 | 77.96 ± 0.32 $^a$ | −0.13 ± 0.05 | 13.24 ± 0.64 | 13.24 ± 0.64 | 90.56 ± 0.22 |
| ND7 | 77.72 ± 0.15 | −1.20 ± 0.03 | 11.48 ± 0.04 $^b$ | 11.54 ± 0.04 $^c$ | 95.95 ± 0.16 | 77.35 ± 0.27 $^a$ | −1.01 ± 0.07 | 8.39 ± 0.26 | 8.45 ± 0.26 | 96.83 ± 0.43 | 77.04 ± 0.30 $^a$ | −0.82 ± 0.03 | 11.32 ± 0.72 $^b$ | 11.35 ± 0.72 $^c$ | 94.16 ± 0.30 |
| ND8 | 76.54 ± 0.20 $^a$ | −0.80 ± 0.03 | 10.85 ± 0.16 $^b$ | 10.88 ± 0.16 $^c$ | 94.24 ± 0.16 | 76.28 ± 0.18 $^a$ | −0.23 ± 0.03 | 8.45 ± 0.35 | 8.45 ± 0.35 | 91.54 ± 0.26 | 76.24 ± 0.26 $^a$ | −0.16 ± 0.04 | 11.27 ± 0.75 $^b$ | 11.27 ± 0.75 $^c$ | 90.82 ± 0.25 |
| ND9 | 74.73 ± 0.14 $^a$ | −1.70 ± 0.02 | 8.99 ± 0.13 $^c$ | 9.15 ± 0.13 | 100.70 ± 0.26 $^d$ | 74.28 ± 0.80 $^a$ | −1.23 ± 0.05 | 6.33 ± 0.28 | 6.45 ± 0.28 | 101.00 ± 0.38 $^d$ | 74.47 ± 0.37 $^a$ | −1.12 ± 0.04 | 9.10 ± 0.70 $^b$ | 9.17 ± 0.69 $^c$ | 97.06 ± 0.50 |
| Zr | 80.21 ± 0.16 $^a$ | −1.55 ± 0.11 $^{bc}$ | 12.36 ± 0.14 $^d$ | 12.46 ± 0.14 $^e$ | 97.15 ± 0.48 $^f$ | 80.57 ± 0.32 $^a$ | −1.61 ± 0.03 $^c$ | 8.14 ± 0.23 | 8.30 ± 0.23 | 101.20 ± 0.22 | 80.19 ± 0.36 $^a$ | −1.46 ± 0.06 $^b$ | 11.38 ± 0.74 $^d$ | 11.47 ± 0.73 $^d$ | 97.35 ± 0.66 $^f$ |
| M | 76.70 ± 0.25 | −1.99 ± 0.04 | 9.56 ± 0.11 | 9.77 ± 0.11 | 101.77 ± 0.30 | 74.80 ± 0.69 $^a$ | −1.71 ± 0.10 $^b$ | 4.96 ± 0.49 | 5.25 ± 0.49 | 109.06 ± 0.99 | 75.03 ± 1.00 $^a$ | −1.64 ± 0.06 $^b$ | 8.61 ± 0.31 | 8.77 ± 0.30 | 100.78 ± 0.76 |

Same superscript letter in the same row indicates no statistical significance ($p \geq 0.001$)—comparison between crown groups for the same measurement area.

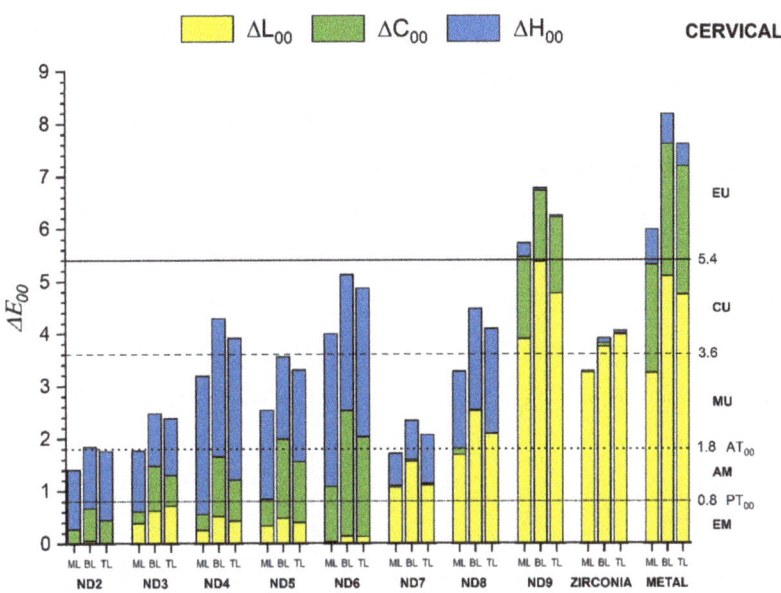

**Figure 6.** Masking ability of crown groups on different substrates evaluated for the cervical area.

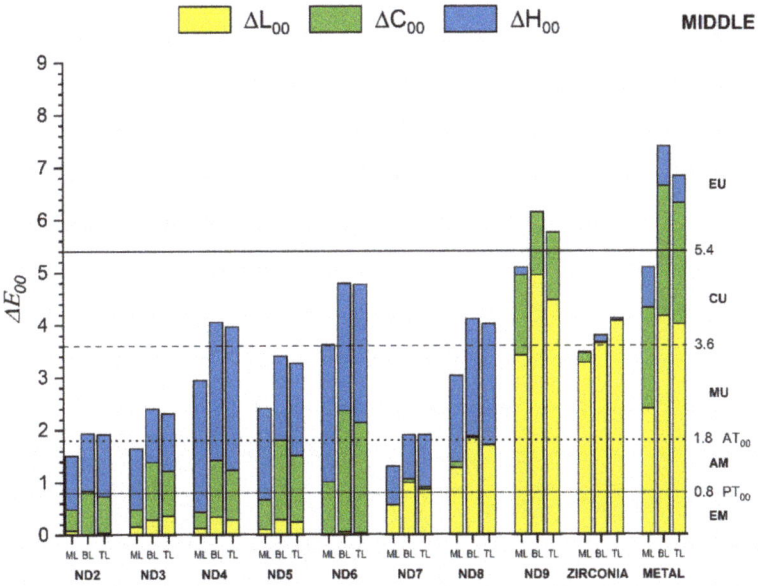

**Figure 7.** Masking ability of crown groups on different substrates evaluated for the middle area.

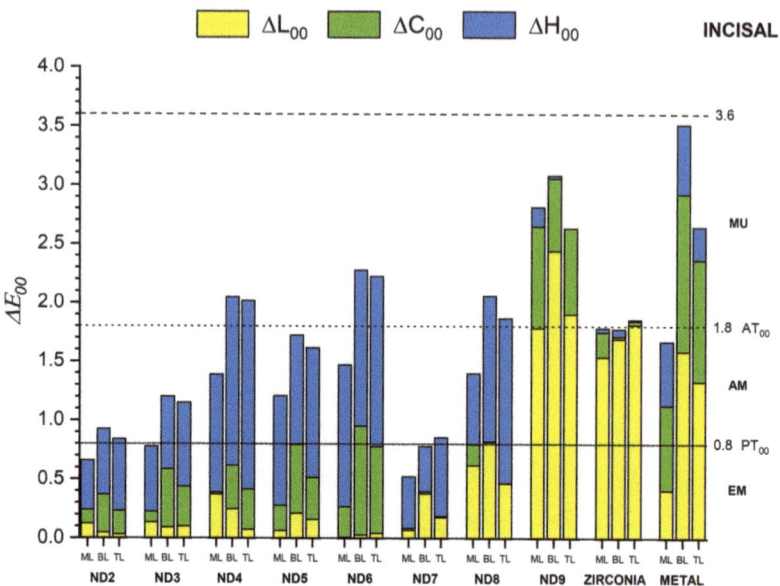

**Figure 8.** Masking ability of crown groups on different substrates evaluated for the incisal area.

The lowest masking ability was found for ND9 and M substrates in all areas. In this case, the color differences were extremely unacceptable (EU) in the cervical and middle areas (Figures 6 and 7). For substrates ND2–ND6, the differences in hue ($\Delta H_{00}$) and chroma ($\Delta C_{00}$) from the ND1 substrate contributed the most to the total color difference. For ND7 and ND8, the differences in lightness ($\Delta L_{00}$) and hue ($\Delta H_{00}$) had the most significant influence, while for ND9, Zr, and M substrates, the lightness ($\Delta L_{00}$) and chroma ($\Delta C_{00}$) differences contributed to the most to the color difference. This behavior was found in all three areas of the crowns.

Color differences for the cervical and middle areas were similar and considerably higher than for the incisal area for all crown groups and substrates.

## 4. Discussion

Treatment of localized tooth discoloration is challenging and requires knowledge about the etiology of the lesion and a good understanding of material properties used for treating the tooth defect. The success of the treatment relies on how well the material can hide the discolored substrate and, at the same time, match the color of surrounding dental structures or neighboring teeth [40]. Most esthetic materials (resin composite, dental ceramics) are translucent, and their masking ability (hiding power) of a discolored substrate depends on the severity of the discoloration, the thickness of the restoration, and the level of translucency of the restorative material [12,13,15,16].

The present study evaluated the masking ability of monolithic and layered zirconia crowns on eleven different discolored substrates. The design of the study aimed to reproduce the clinical conditions and challenges faced during shade matching of ceramic restorations placed over abutments and tooth preparations of different colors. Comparing the masking ability of crowns fabricated with different technologies (monolithic, layered with enamel, layered with enamel, and dentine ceramics) gave an insight into the colorimetric behavior of these restorations.

In addition, nine tooth-shaded resin dies (ND1–ND9) and two abutment materials (zirconia and metal) were used to simulate various discolorations of prepared teeth. ND1 and ND2 represent the shade of natural dentin; ND3, ND4, and ND5 were more chromatic but comparable in lightness to ND1 and ND2, simulating mild or moderate discolorations. ND6 substrate was the most chromatic, with the highest b* values (the yellowest). ND7 was almost similar to ND2 but less bright, while ND8 and ND9 substrates were the darkest, simulating severe dyschromia.

Moreover, due to the irregular form of the labial dental surface, the capacity to hide the dyschromic substrate was studied separately along the crown, in the cervical, middle, and incisal thirds.

The CIE L*, a*, b*, C*, and h° color coordinates were statistically significantly different between the three crown groups generally, regardless of the measurement area or the substrate. Therefore, the first null hypothesis was rejected. However, some similarities in the color coordinates were found. In the cervical area, no statistically significant differences in L*, a*, and h° coordinates were found between BL and TL crowns in general. For the middle and incisal areas, the L* coordinate showed statistically similar values among the three groups of crowns for most substrates, while b* and C* coordinates of ML and TL crowns were statistically similar only in the incisal area.

We found a masking capacity higher than the $AT_{00}$ in the cervical and middle areas, except for the ML groups on ND2, ND3, and ND7 substrates. Therefore, the second null hypothesis was also rejected. However, the incisal area showed smaller color differences as expected due to the partial influence of the substrate and the consequent increase in translucency. In this area, values above the acceptability threshold (MU) were found for the three groups of crowns only for ND9 and for the BL and TL groups in ND4, ND6, N8, and M substrates, obtaining for the rest of the cases an AM or EM masking ability. Nevertheless, the interpretation of these results should be made with caution since the substrate had a smaller influence in this area.

The darkest substrates (ND9 and M) and the most chromatic substrate (ND6) produced the highest color differences, which were completely or extremely unacceptable (CU or EU) for cervical and middle areas and moderately unacceptable (MU) for incisal areas. It is important to note that as the substrate was darker (Figure 5), the total color difference was mainly influenced by the lightness shift, whereas when it was more chromatic, the hue and chroma shifts were higher, increasing in both cases the total color difference in the three areas evaluated. This again highlights the significant influence that the substrate has on the masking capacity [13,14,17,37].

The best masking effect of the crowns was achieved for ND2, ND3, and ND7 substrates in all thirds, since these substrates were the closest to ND1 (Figure 5), requiring a lower masking ability. The masking ability was acceptable (AM) for the ML crowns and moderately unacceptable (MU) for BL and TL crowns for the cervical and middle areas. The color match was excellent (EM) for ML crowns in the incisal area. For ND7 substrate, the lightness had the most significant influence in the color difference, while for ND2 and ND3, the hue; yet this behavior was not observed in the incisal area of the crowns. Although the color differences calculated for these substrates were almost similar, their visual perception by human observers might be judged differently. A previous study [41] showed that observers preferred shades with lower chroma and/or hue difference rather than lower lightness difference when matching shade guide tabs to natural teeth.

ML crowns showed better masking ability than BL and TL crowns. This result could be explained by the higher opacity of the monolithic crown. Layered crowns were stratified with glass ceramics, which had considerably higher translucency than 3Y-TZP zirconia.

One study evaluated the masking ability of indirect restorative systems on tooth-colored resin substrates [13]. The authors concluded that 1.5 mm thick samples of veneered 3Y-TZP zirconia (ceramic layering over zirconia) had a better masking effect than monolithic lithium disilicate, translucent zirconia, hybrid ceramic, or heat-pressed ceramic over translucent zirconia samples. In our study, 1 mm thick restorations were fabricated, and the same 3Y-TZP zirconia was used for the monolithic and the layered crowns. Differences between the results could have been generated by the difference in thickness and type of samples but also because the study of Basegio et al. used different zirconia for the monolithic samples than for the layered samples.

Another study [17] also concluded that bi-layer samples produced significantly lower color differences than monolithic samples on discolored substrates. However, the authors included in the monolithic group materials with higher translucency than 3Y-TZP zirconia (4Y-TZP translucent zirconia, lithium disilicate, leucite-reinforced glass-ceramic, feldspathic ceramic).

The color differences obtained in our study were higher than the $AT_{00}$ in the cervical and middle areas of the crowns, with few exceptions (monolithic crowns on typical dentin-like substrates or with mild discolorations). This result suggests that 1 mm thick zirconia crowns have insufficient masking ability of moderately or severely discolored substrates at this thickness and in combination with a transparent try-in paste.

In a study evaluating the effect of the direct layering of substrates with high-value composite resins on the masking ability of CAD-CAM materials, the authors concluded that the layering with 0.25 mm opaque resins reduced the color differences for veneered zirconia [37]. However, the authors used 1.8 mm thick restorations, which might involve excessive tooth preparation.

One study [38] evaluated the effect of external surface treatments and abutment shades on the color of high translucency self-gazed zirconia crowns. The authors concluded that the abutment's color had a more significant influence on the final color of the crown than the type of surface finishing. The darker the abutment tooth, the higher was the color difference. Our results are in agreement with these findings; however, we also observed that when the crowns were evaluated on a zirconia abutment which is very bright, the color differences were also very high, leading to a moderately or clearly unacceptable match.

Our results showed that the color differences calculated for the incisal area of the crowns were lower than in the other two areas evaluated. This can be explained by the lower influence of the discolored substrate in the incisal area since a 1.5 mm tooth reduction was performed.

As a limitation of the present study, only 1 mm thick restorations were evaluated using an instrumental method. More configurations of the preparations should be analyzed; in addition, the results of our study should be validated by studies including human observers to judge the color differences and to relate these results with visual perception.

## 5. Conclusions

Within the limitations of the present study, it was concluded that:
1. Color coordinates of monolithic and layered crowns differed significantly on all substrates.
2. ML crowns showed better masking ability than BL and TL crowns, regardless of the substrate or the tooth area. However, an acceptable match for ML crowns was only found for ND2, ND3, and ND7 substrates in the three areas.
3. ML and layered 3Y-TZP zirconia crowns have insufficient masking ability on moderately or severely discolored substrates at 1 mm thickness.

**Author Contributions:** Conceptualization, C.G., M.M.M. and D.D.; methodology, C.G., M.M.M. and A.V.B.; software, J.R.-L.; validation, C.G., M.M.M., A.V.B., J.R.-L., S.B. and D.D.; formal analysis, C.G. and J.R.-L.; investigation, C.G., M.M.M. and A.V.B.; resources, M.M.M. and S.B.; data curation, M.M.M., C.G. and J.R.-L.; writing—original draft preparation, C.G.; writing—review and editing, M.M.M., J.R.-L., S.B. and D.D.; visualization, C.G., M.M.M., A.V.B., J.R.-L., S.B. and D.D.; supervision, D.D.; project administration, C.G. and D.D.; funding acquisition, C.G and D.D. All authors have read and agreed to the published version of the manuscript.

**Funding:** This work was supported by a grant of the Romanian Ministry of Education and Research, CCCDI-UEFISCDI, project number PN-III-P2-2.1-PED-2019-2953, 334 PED/2020.

**Institutional Review Board Statement:** Not applicable.

**Informed Consent Statement:** Not applicable.

**Data Availability Statement:** The data presented in this study are available on request from the corresponding author.

**Conflicts of Interest:** The authors declare no conflict of interest.

# References

1. Ramos, J.C.; Palma, P.J.; Nascimento, R.; Caramelo, F.; Messias, A.; Vinagre, A.; Santos, J.M. 1-year In Vitro Evaluation of Tooth Discoloration Induced by 2 Calcium Silicate-based Cements. *J. Endod.* **2016**, *42*, 1403–1407. [CrossRef]
2. Bosenbecker, J.; Barbon, F.J.; de Souza Ferreira, N.; Morgental, R.D.; Boscato, N. Tooth discoloration caused by endodontic treatment: A cross-sectional study. *J. Esthet. Restor. Dent.* **2020**, *32*, 569–574. [CrossRef]
3. Zhang, Y.; Lawn, B.R. Novel Zirconia Materials in Dentistry. *J. Dent. Res.* **2018**, *97*, 140–147. [CrossRef] [PubMed]
4. Güth, J.F.; Stawarczyk, B.; Edelhoff, D.; Liebermann, A. Zirconia and its novel compositions: What do clinicians need to know? *Quintessence Int.* **2019**, *50*, 512–520. [CrossRef] [PubMed]
5. Erdelt, K.; Pinheiro Dias Engler, M.L.; Beuer, F.; Güth, J.F.; Liebermann, A.; Schweiger, J. Computable translucency as a function of thickness in a multi-layered zirconia. *J. Prosthet. Dent.* **2019**, *121*, 683–689. [CrossRef]
6. Cho, Y.E.; Lim, Y.J.; Han, J.S.; Yeo, I.L.; Yoon, H.I. Effect of Yttria Content on the Translucency and Masking Ability of Yttria-Stabilized Tetragonal Zirconia Polycrystal. *Materials* **2020**, *13*, 4726. [CrossRef] [PubMed]
7. Baldissara, P.; Wandscher, V.F.; Marchionatti, A.M.E.; Parisi, C.; Monaco, C.; Ciocca, L. Translucency of IPS e.max and cubic zirconia monolithic crowns. *J. Prosthet. Dent.* **2018**, *120*, 269–275. [CrossRef]
8. Alp, G.; Subaşı, M.G.; Seghi, R.R.; Johnston, W.M.; Yilmaz, B. Effect of shading technique and thickness on color stability and translucency of new generation translucent zirconia. *J. Dent.* **2018**, *73*, 19–23. [CrossRef]
9. Juntavee, N.; Attashu, S. Effect of sintering process on color parameters of nano-sized yttria partially stabilized tetragonal monolithic zirconia. *J. Clin. Exp. Dent.* **2018**, *10*, e794–e804. [CrossRef]
10. Attachoo, S.; Juntavee, N. Role of sintered temperature and sintering time on spectral translucence of nano-crystal monolithic zirconia. *J. Clin. Exp. Dent.* **2019**, *11*, e146–e153. [CrossRef]
11. Subaşı, M.G.; Alp, G.; Johnston, W.M.; Yilmaz, B. Effects of fabrication and shading technique on the color and translucency of new-generation translucent zirconia after coffee thermocycling. *J. Prosthet. Dent.* **2018**, *120*, 603–608. [CrossRef] [PubMed]
12. Tabatabaian, F.; Javadi Sharif, M.; Massoumi, F.; Namdari, M. The color masking ability of a zirconia ceramic on the substrates with different values. *J. Dent. Res. Dent. Clin. Dent. Prospect.* **2017**, *11*, 7–13. [CrossRef] [PubMed]
13. Basegio, M.M.; Pecho, O.E.; Ghinea, R.; Perez, M.M.; Della Bona, A. Masking ability of indirect restorative systems on tooth-colored resin substrates. *Dent. Mater.* **2019**, *35*, e122–e130. [CrossRef]
14. Sonza, Q.N.; Della Bona, A.; Pecho, O.E.; Borba, M. Effect of substrate and cement on the final color of zirconia-based all-ceramic crowns. *J. Esthet. Restor. Dent.* **2021**, *33*, 891–898. [CrossRef] [PubMed]
15. Tabatabaian, F.; Karimi, M.; Namdari, M. Color match of high translucency monolithic zirconia restorations with different thicknesses and backgrounds. *J. Esthet. Restor. Dent.* **2020**, *32*, 615–621. [CrossRef]
16. Manziuc, M.M.; Gasparik, C.; Burde, A.V.; Dudea, D. Color and masking properties of translucent monolithic zirconia before and after glazing. *J. Prosthodont. Res.* **2021**, *65*, 303–310. [CrossRef]
17. Bacchi, A.; Boccardi, S.; Alessandretti, R.; Pereira, G.K.R. Substrate masking ability of bilayer and monolithic ceramics used for complete crowns and the effect of association with an opaque resin-based luting agent. *J. Prosthodont. Res.* **2019**, *63*, 321–326. [CrossRef]
18. Ayash, G.; Osman, E.; Segaan, L.; Rayyan, M.; Joukhadar, C. Influence of resin cement shade on the color and translucency of zirconia crowns. *J. Clin. Exp. Dent.* **2020**, *12*, e257–e263. [CrossRef]
19. Dai, S.; Chen, C.; Tang, M.; Chen, Y.; Yang, L.; He, F.; Chen, B.; Xie, H. Choice of resin cement shades for a high-translucency zirconia product to mask dark, discolored or metal substrates. *J. Adv. Prosthodont.* **2019**, *11*, 286–296. [CrossRef]
20. The International Commission on Illumination. *CIE 015:2018 Colorimetry*, 4th ed.; CIE Central Bureau: Vienna, Austria, 2018.
21. Luo, M.R.; Cui, G.; Rigg, B. The Development of the CIE 2000 Colour-Difference Formula: CIEDE2000. *Color Res. Appl.* **2001**, *26*, 340–350. [CrossRef]
22. International Organization for Standardization. *ISO/TR 28642; Dentistry—Guidance on Colour Measurement.* ISO: Geneva, Switzerland, 2016.
23. Paravina, R.D.; Ghinea, R.; Herrera, L.J.; Della Bona, A.; Igiel, C.; Linninger, M.; Sakai, M.; Takahashi, H.; Tashkandi, E.; Perez, M.M. Color Difference Thresholds in Dentistry. *J. Esthet. Restor. Dent.* **2015**, *27*, S1–S9. [CrossRef] [PubMed]
24. Paravina, R.D.; Pérez, M.M.; Ghinea, R. Acceptability and perceptibility thresholds in dentistry: A comprehensive review of clinical and research applications. *J. Esthet. Restor. Dent.* **2019**, *31*, 103–112. [CrossRef] [PubMed]
25. Dos Santos, R.B.; Collares, K.; Brandeburski, S.B.N.; Pecho, O.E.; Della Bona, A. Experimental methodologies to evaluate the masking ability of dental materials: A systematic review. *J. Esthet. Restor. Dent.* **2021**. [CrossRef] [PubMed]
26. Iravani, M.; Shamszadeh, S.; Panahandeh, N.; Sheikh-Al-Eslamian, S.M.; Torabzadeh, H. Shade reproduction and the ability of lithium disilicate ceramics to mask dark substrates. *Restor. Dent. Endod.* **2020**, *45*, e41. [CrossRef] [PubMed]

27. Ellakany, P.; Madi, M.; Aly, N.M.; Al-Aql, Z.S.; AlGhamdi, M.; AlJeraisy, A.; Alagl, A.S. Effect of CAD/CAM Ceramic Thickness on Shade Masking Ability of Discolored Teeth: In Vitro Study. *Int. J. Environ. Res. Public Health* **2021**, *18*, 13359. [CrossRef]
28. Durães, I.; Cavalcanti, A.; Mathias, P. The Thickness and Opacity of Aesthetic Materials Influence the Restoration of Discolored Teeth. *Oper. Dent.* **2021**, *118*, 517–523. [CrossRef]
29. Jung, J.; Roh, B.D.; Kim, J.H.; Shin, Y. Masking of High-Translucency Zirconia for Various Cores. *Oper. Dent.* **2021**, *46*, 54–62. [CrossRef]
30. Porojan, L.; Vasiliu, R.D.; Porojan, S.D. Masking Abilities of Dental Cad/Cam Resin Composite Materials Related to Substrate and Luting Material. *Polymers* **2022**, *14*, 364. [CrossRef]
31. Basso, G.R.; Kodama, A.B.; Pimentel, A.H.; Kaizer, M.R.; Bona, A.D.; Moraes, R.R.; Boscato, N. Masking Colored Substrates Using Monolithic and Bilayer CAD-CAM Ceramic Structures. *Oper. Dent.* **2017**, *42*, 387–395. [CrossRef]
32. Miotti, L.L.; Santos, I.S.; Nicoloso, G.F.; Pozzobon, R.T.; Susin, A.H.; Durand, L.B. The Use of Resin Composite Layering Technique to Mask Discolored Background: A CIELAB/CIEDE2000 Analysis. *Oper. Dent.* **2017**, *42*, 165–174. [CrossRef]
33. Skyllouriotis, A.L.; Yamamoto, H.L.; Nathanson, D. Masking properties of ceramics for veneer restorations. *J. Prosthet. Dent.* **2017**, *118*, 517–523. [CrossRef] [PubMed]
34. Tabatabaian, F.; Taghizade, F.; Namdari, M. Effect of coping thickness and background type on the masking ability of a zirconia ceramic. *J. Prosthet. Dent.* **2018**, *119*, 159–165. [CrossRef] [PubMed]
35. Șoim, A.; Strimbu, M.; Burde, A.V.; Culic, B.; Dudea, D.; Gasparik, C. Translucency and masking properties of two ceramic materials for heat-press technology. *J. Esthet. Restor. Dent.* **2018**, *30*, E18–E23. [CrossRef] [PubMed]
36. Dalmolin, A.; Perez, B.G.; Gaidarji, B.; Ruiz-López, J.; Lehr, R.M.; Pérez, M.M.; Durand, L.B. Masking ability of bleach-shade resin composites using the multilayering technique. *J. Esthet. Restor. Dent.* **2021**, *33*, 807–814. [CrossRef]
37. Dotto, L.; Soares Machado, P.; Slongo, S.; Rocha Pereira, G.K.; Bacchi, A. Layering of discolored substrates with high-value opaque composites for CAD-CAM monolithic ceramics. *J. Prosthet. Dent.* **2021**, *126*, 128.e1–128.e6. [CrossRef]
38. Li, S.; Wang, Y.; Tao, Y.; Liu, Y. Effects of surface treatments and abutment shades on the final color of high-translucency self-glazed zirconia crowns. *J. Prosthet. Dent.* **2021**, *126*, 795.e1–795.e8. [CrossRef]
39. Nobbs, J.H. A lightness, chroma and hue splitting approach to CIEDE2000 colour differences. *Adv. Colours Sci. Technol.* **2002**, *5*, 46–53.
40. Lo Giudice, R.; Lipari, F.; Puleio, F.; Alibrandi, A.; Lo Giudice, F.; Tamà, C.; Sazonova, E.; Lo Giudice, G. Spectrophotometric Evaluation of Enamel Color Variation Using Infiltration Resin Treatment of White Spot Lesions at One Year Follow-Up. *Dent. J.* **2020**, *8*, 35. [CrossRef]
41. Pecho, O.E.; Pérez, M.M.; Ghinea, R.; Della Bona, A. Lightness, chroma and hue differences on visual shade matching. *Dent. Mater.* **2016**, *32*, 1362–1373. [CrossRef]

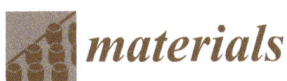

*Article*

# Cross-Contamination Risk of Dental Tray Adhesives: An In Vitro Study

Isabel Paczkowski [1], Catalina S. Stingu [2], Sebastian Hahnel [1], Angelika Rauch [1] and Oliver Schierz [1,*]

[1] Department of Prosthodontics and Materials Science, University of Leipzig, Liebigstrasse 12, D-04103 Leipzig, Germany; Isabel.paczkowski@medizin.uni-leipzig.de (I.P.); sebastian.hahnel@medizin.uni-leipzig.de (S.H.); angelika.rauch@medizin.uni-leipzig.de (A.R.)

[2] Institute for Medical Microbiology and Virology, University Hospital of Leipzig, Liebigstrasse 21, D-04103 Leipzig, Germany; catalinasuzana.stingu@medizin.uni-leipzig.de

* Correspondence: oliver.schierz@medizin.uni-leipzig.de; Tel.: +49-341-9721310

**Abstract:** Background: The aim of this study was to investigate the risk of cross-contamination in dental tray adhesives with reusable brush systems. Methods: Four dental tray adhesives with different disinfectant components were examined for risk as a potential transmission medium for *Staphylococcus aureus*, *Escherichia coli*, *Pseudomonas aeruginosa*, *Streptococcus oralis*, and *Candida albicans*. Bacterial and fungal strains were mixed with artificial saliva. The contaminated saliva was intentionally added to tray adhesive liquid samples. At baseline and up to 60 min, 100 microliters of each sample were collected and cultivated aerobically on Columbia and Sabouraud agar for 24 or 48 h, respectively. Results: At baseline, contamination with *Staphylococcus aureus* and *Candida albicans* could be identified in three out of four adhesives. In the subsequent samples, low counts of up to 20 colony-forming units per milliliter could be observed for *Staphylococcus aureus*. All other strains did not form colonies at baseline or subsequently. Adhesives with isopropanol or ethyl acetate as disinfectant additives were most effective in preventing contamination, while adhesives with hydrogen chloride or acetone as a disinfectant additive were the least effective. Conclusion: Within 15 min, the tested adhesives appeared to be sufficiently bactericidal and fungicidal against all microorganisms tested.

**Keywords:** dental tray adhesive; reusable brush; disinfectant additive; cross-contamination risk; disinfection

## 1. Introduction

Numerous guidelines and hygiene recommendations outline proper aseptic handling and corresponding workflows in everyday dentistry [1,2], which not only protect patients but also ensure workplace safety for medical healthcare providers [3]. In recent years, disposable products have gained importance, whereas reusable materials have become less frequently used in direct patient contact. However, monetary and ecological aspects play a relevant role in the decision-making process. Therefore, reusable materials may stay relevant in routine dental practice [4].

Since approximately 1.2 million impressions are billed annually in Germany alone [5], conventional impression-taking is still state of the art despite the availability of digital impression-taking procedures [6,7]. Impression tray adhesives provide a chemical adhesion of impression materials to the tray, prevent distortion, and ensure dimensional stability of the impression after removal from the mouth. The adhesive is usually delivered in a reusable glass flask with a screw cap. On the inside of the cap, a brush is fixed for applying the adhesive liquid. The use of the brush may lead to contamination of the adhesive reservoir in the glass flask if there is no proper intermediate disinfection of the impression tray after intraoral try-in. Lasting contamination of the reservoir could pose a risk to all subsequently treated patients [3,8–10]. This would expose risk to patients who are suffering from severe primary disease and immunosuppression as well as the increasing number of multimorbid elderly. Exacerbating this issue, the current COVID-19 pandemic has further underlined the relevance of proper hygiene measures.

Manufacturers assume sufficient disinfectant activity through additives such as isopropanol, ethyl acetate, hydrogen chloride, acetone, toluene, or trichloroethane. The first scientific considerations addressing the risk of cross-contamination in the impression-taking process were published in 1987 [9]. Six years later, the disinfectant effects of different tray adhesives in three in vitro cultured bacterial strains (*Staphylococcus aureus*, *Salmonella* Choleraesuis, and *Pseudomonas aeruginosa*) were investigated. Only the Express adhesive, with additives trichloroethane and toluene, showed small deficits in antibacterial effect [8]. In the recent literature, a publication contradicted the hypothesis that adhesives disinfect sufficiently [10]. None of the adhesive systems tested revealed sufficient disinfectant activity when using the Kirby–Bauer zone of inhibition method. Apart from some in vitro bacterial strains (*Pseudomonas aeruginosa*, *Escherichia coli*, *Streptococcus mutans*, and *Staphylococcus aureus*), the study also investigated bacterial cultures from twenty saliva samples. Driven by these results, the contamination of an impression tray adhesive in glass flasks with repeated-use brushes was investigated under clinical conditions. While no quantitative analysis was performed, the qualitative analysis showed bacterial contamination in 6 out of 400 agar plates [11].

Against this background, the current in vitro study aimed to observe the disinfecting effect of four commercially available tray adhesives with reusable brush systems that had been deliberately contaminated with potentially pathogenic bacteria and fungi of the oral microbiome. The null hypothesis was that no microorganisms could be cultivated in the dental impression tray adhesive liquid.

## 2. Materials and Methods

Four common adhesive systems with different disinfectant additives were investigated, including an adhesive with the disinfecting additive isopropanol (FA: Fix Adhesive; Dentsply DeTrey GmbH, Konstanz, Germany; charge: 2001000870/1905000723); an adhesive with ethyl acetate (UA: Universal Adhesive; Kulzer GmbH, Hanau, Germany; charge: K01005-4/-8/-6), an adhesive with hydrogen chloride, isopropanol, and ethyl acetate (PA: Polyether Adhesive; 3M GmbH, Neuss, Germany; charge: 5386594); and one with ethyl acetate and acetone (PCTA: Polyether Contact Tray Adhesive; 3M GmbH, Neuss, Germany; charge: 4581863) (Figure 1). All adhesives were tested for sterility before use by inoculating the tested adhesive liquid onto Columbia and Chocolate agar and examining the agar plates after a 24 h incubation time.

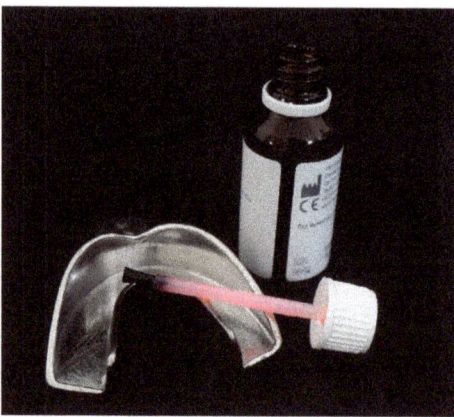

**Figure 1.** Impression tray, reusable brush, and adhesive flask (sample).

Clinically common and potentially pathogenic bacteria and fungi (freeze-dried bacterial and fungal strains from American Type Culture Collection (ATCC) and German Collection of Microorganism and Cell Cultures (DSM)) were selected as test strains, including

- Staphylococcus aureus (ATCC 29213);
- Escherichia coli (ATCC 25922);
- Pseudomonas aeruginosa (ATCC 29213);
- Streptococcus oralis (DSM 20627);
- Candida albicans (ATCC 90028).

Reference strains were cultivated aerobically on Columbia agar for 24 h and on Sabouraud agar for 48 h. Artificial saliva was prepared in the laboratory according to the recipe of Rosentritt et al. [12,13] and stored in a refrigerator at −20 degrees Celsius (°C). Prior to use, the artificial saliva was brought to room temperature and tested for sterility. In order to verify the sterility, 100 microliters (µL) of the saliva was placed onto Columbia and Chocolate agar and examined after an incubation time of 24 h.

Growing colonies of the reference strains were isolated and added to the artificial saliva in a starting concentration of $1 \times 10^9$ for bacteria and $1 \times 10^5$ colony-forming units per milliliter (CFU/mL) for fungi according to the average occurrence of bacteria and fungi in the oral cavity [14–16]. The bacterial count was photometrically verified by three subsequent measurements using an optical density of 0.85 for bacteria and 0.125 for fungi at a wavelength of 580 nanometers (Ultraspec 2000 UV-VIS spectrophotometer, Pharmacia Biotech, Waldkirch, Germany). The fungal strain was diluted 1:100 in order to obtain a final fungal concentration of $1 \times 10^5$ CFU/mL.

Prior to initiating the growth inhibition test, the contaminated saliva samples were examined regarding bacterial and fungal purity. The purity was verified by inoculating the samples onto agar plates. After incubation, the plates were visually inspected, and the colonies were identified using the matrix-assisted laser desorption–ionization time-of-flight mass spectrometry (MALDI-TOF; VITEK® MS, bioMérieux, Lyon, France). Twenty microliters of the contaminated saliva was added to 2 mL of the respective adhesive liquid (ratio of 1:100) and mixed for five seconds (IKA VF2 Vortex Mixer, IKA®-Werke GmbH & Co. KG, Staufen, Germany). Twenty microliters corresponds to the average amount of saliva adhering to an impression tray after try-in. This amount was determined by using a precision scale (Cubis®, Sartorius AG, Goettingen, Germany) and 20 impression tray samples.

At baseline and in 15 min intervals up to 60 min, 100 µL of each sample was inoculated onto Columbia and Sabouraud agar using a pipette system (Multipette® (4780)); Eppendorf Combitips advanced®, Eppendorf AG, Hamburg, Germany) and a sterile disposable spatula. The agar plates were incubated aerobically for 24 or 48 h at 37 °C and 5 percent (%) $CO_2$ (Heracell 150i $CO_2$ Incubator, Thermo Fisher Scientific, Dreieich, Germany), and the bacterial count was documented (Figure 2).

Initially, 10 samples per bacterium or fungus in combination with each adhesive were examined (5 strains × 4 adhesives × 10 test rows × 5 timeslots). Due to a relevant number of positive results after the initial test series, *Staphylococcus aureus* was tested with a further 10 samples to allow statistical demarcation between the various adhesives. In total, 1200 agar plates were screened.

The counting was repeated three times for an exact determination of the bacterial or fungal count, and the results were averaged. In addition, agar plates with a bacterial count of more than 50 colonies were divided into quarters, more than 100 colonies into eighths, and more than 200 colonies into sixteen parts to facilitate the counting process. If the number of colonies exceeded 300, proper counting was no longer possible. These counts were defined as "confluent culture". For statistical evaluation, confluent cultures were included with 300 CFU per agar.

The statistical software package STATA was used for descriptive analysis and statistical evaluation of the results (Stata Statistical Software: Release 15.1. StataCorp LP, College

Station, TX, USA). The Wilcoxon rank-sum test and the Kruskal–Wallis test were performed for statistical analysis. Level of significance was set to $p = 0.05$, and for compensation of multiple testing, Bonferroni correction was applied.

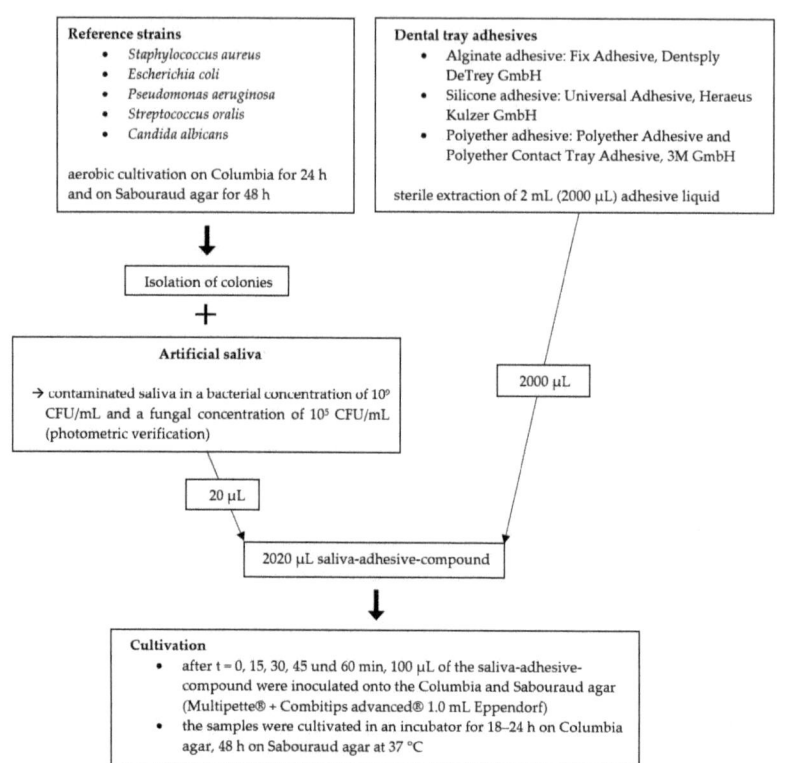

Figure 2. Overview of the materials and method.

## 3. Results

At baseline, in three out of four adhesives (UA, PA, PCTA), positive bacterial growth of Staphylococcus aureus was detected. The bacterial count varied significantly depending on the examined adhesive, with PA and PCTA showing the greatest deficits in instant disinfectant efficiency, allowing bacterial growth on all agar plates (100%). UA showed growth of Staphylococcus aureus in 65 % of all samples. FA allowed no growth at all (Figure 3).

In 75% of the PCTA samples, confluent cultures of Staphylococcus aureus were detected. Additionally, fungal growth was identified in 5% of PA cultures. Except for PA, all adhesives inhibited fungal growth completely. A statistical significance could be proven when comparing the different adhesives at baseline using the Kruskal–Wallis test ($p = 0.002$). FA proved to have the best disinfectant properties compared to all other tested adhesives (Wilcoxon, all $p = 0.001$) for Staphylococcus aureus at baseline. UA's disinfectant properties proved to be superior to PCTA (UA vs. PA $p = 0.057$; UA vs. PCTA $p = 0.026$) in Staphylococcus aureus. No statistically significant difference could be detected between PA and PCTA ($p = 0.311$).

After an incubation time of 15 min, 15% of PA showed growth of Staphylococcus aureus, with an average bacterial count of 13.3 CFU/mL (standard deviation of 4.71). No growth was identified for all other strains and adhesives. After a period of 30 min, 5% of PCTA showed Staphylococcus aureus counts of 10 CFU/mL (Figure 4, Table 1). No growth was identified on all other samples. No bacterial or fungal cultures were detected at either 45 or 60 min.

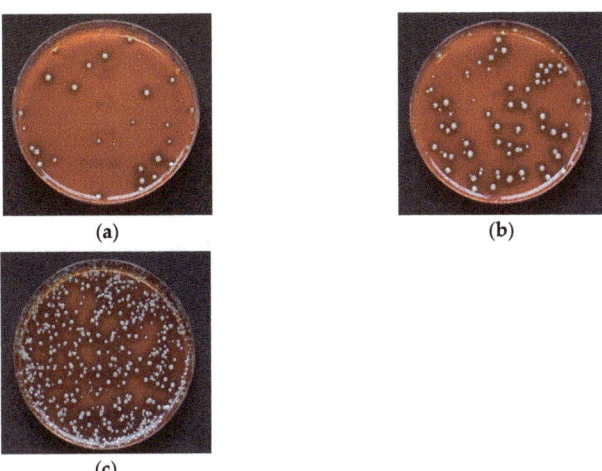

**Figure 3.** Examples for *Staphylococcus aureus* on Columbia agar at baseline after 0 min incubation. (**a**) Universal Adhesive (UA); (**b**) Polyether Adhesive (PA); (**c**) Polyether Contact Tray Adhesive (PCTA). In Fix adhesive (FA), no colonies of *Staphylococcus aureus* could be detected.

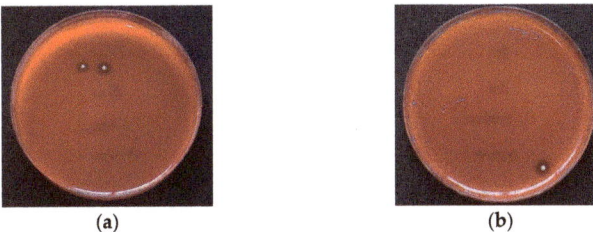

**Figure 4.** Examples of *Staphylococcus aureus* on Columbia agar. (**a**) Polyether Adhesive (PA) after 15 min incubation; (**b**) Polyether Contact Tray Adhesive (PCTA) after 30 min incubation. In Universal Adhesive (UA) and Fix Adhesive (FA), no colonies could be detected at both times.

**Table 1.** Agar probes of *Staphylococcus aureus* and *Candida albicans* up to 30 min incubation. All other strains showed no viable bacteria or fungi at any time.

| Microorganism | $t_0$ | | $t_{15}$ | | $t_{30}$ | | $t_0$ vs. $t_{15}$ | $t_{15}$ vs. $t_{30}$ |
|---|---|---|---|---|---|---|---|---|
| | Median in CFU/mL | Min; Max | Median in CFU/mL | Min; Max | Median in CFU/mL | Min; Max | $p$-Value [1] | $p$-Value [1] |
| *Staphylococcus aureus* | | | | | | | | |
| Fix | 0 | 0; 0 | 0 | 0; 0 | 0 | 0; 0 | n.a. | n.a. |
| Universal | 15 | 0; 1887 | 0 | 0; 0 | 0 | 0; 0 | <0.001 | <0.001 |
| Polyether | 328 | 10; 2223 | 0 | 0; 20 | 0 | 0; 0 | <0.001 | <0.001 |
| Polyether Contact Tray | 3000 | 220; 3000 | 0 | 0; 0 | 0 | 0; 10 | <0.001 | <0.001 |
| *Candida albicans* | | | | | | | | |
| Fix | 0 | 0; 0 | 0 | 0; 0 | 0 | 0; 0 | n.a. | n.a. |
| Universal | 0 | 0; 0 | 0 | 0; 0 | 0 | 0; 0 | n.a. | n.a. |
| Polyether | 0 | 0; 10 | 0 | 0; 0 | 0 | 0; 0 | 0.317 | n.a. |
| Polyether Contact Tray | 0 | 0; 0 | 0 | 0; 0 | 0 | 0; 0 | n.a. | n.a. |

[1] Wilcoxon rank-sum test; n.a. = not applicable.

## 4. Discussion

The bacterial and fungal cultures detected after an incubation of 15 min or longer were not clinically relevant since no more bacterial and fungal growth could be identified in the current study. However, compared to the initial bacteria count of $10^9$ CFU/mL in the contaminated saliva, bacteria were detected in 15% of PA samples after 15 min and in 5% of PCTA samples after 30 min. These samples revealed a small colony count of up to 20 CFU/mL. Therefore, the risk of cross-contamination with reusable brushes is highly unlikely, and the null hypothesis has to be accepted.

Intermediate disinfection of the impression trays after try-in seems unnecessary since the adhesives' additives feature a sufficient disinfecting effect. However, it should be noted that significant differences exist in the disinfectant potency of the examined adhesives. In the current study, only FA could suppress any growth of bacteria and fungi due to its effective additive isopropanol. Isopropanol has an optimum bactericidal concentration between 60 and 90 % and can kill resistant *Staphylococcus aureus* within 10 s [17]. Even at baseline, no positive bacterial or fungal growth could be detected. PA and PCTA, which contain hydrogen chloride, isopropanol, acetone, and ethyl acetate as additives, showed the lowest antimicrobial effect. Different statements regarding the disinfectant efficiency of tray adhesives have led to increasing insecurities about reusable adhesive systems. In 1993, Herman [8] assumed a sufficient disinfectant effect of tray adhesives, while following publications by Pollak [10] and Schierz [11] contradicted the results and documented a potential cross-contamination risk for patients. The Kirby–Bauer method, as applied by Pollak [10], is to be evaluated critically, as it causes evaporation of the additives in the adhesive liquid, leading to a loss of disinfecting components and a corresponding distortion of test results. In addition, the specified amount of adhesive and saliva is not clinically relevant, which explains why the procedures do not allow any practical conclusions for a dental practice. Schierz et al. documented viable bacteria in 1.5% of investigated samples [11]; this should, however, be interpreted with caution, as several dermal bacteria were detected, and no quantification of the bacteria was performed.

In the current study, artificial saliva was combined with clinically relevant bacteria and fungi to optimize the informative value. While natural saliva shows individual variations in bacteria quantity and species [18], artificial saliva is produced according to a fixed recipe, can be reproduced in sufficient quantities, and has consistent quality. In addition, the possibility of adding individual bacterial and fungal species to the artificial saliva, as shown in this study, can avoid the competition between them regarding nourishment and habitat [19–21], which allows a reliable statement and reproducible results.

To guarantee sterile saliva, individual components were sterilized before merging. The mucin (Mucin from a porcine stomach; Sigma-Aldrich, St. Louis, MO, USA) was decontaminated according to the manufacturer's recommendation by placing the powder in 95% ethanol and heating the covered mucin at 70 °C for 24 h. Phosphate-buffered saline (PBS; Sigma Aldrich, St. Louis, MO, USA) was filtered (0.2 µm) before use.

To simulate clinical conditions, common and potentially pathogenic bacteria and fungi were chosen for the present investigation. *Staphylococcus aureus* is known as the main pathogen for bacterial endocarditis and osteomyelitis [22–25]. *Escherichia coli* is the most frequent enteric intestinal bacterium [26]. *Pseudomonas aeruginosa* is a hospital pathogen with increasing resistance, responsible for severe pneumonia and persistent urinary tract infections [27]. *Streptococcus oralis* can be assumed as a reference resident bacterium of the oral microflora. *Candida albicans* was included as the most common fungus in the oral environment and trigger of candidiasis [28,29].

The strengths of this study include the reproducibility of the testing approach, the clinically relevant chosen observation time with 15 min intervals, and the inclusion of common pathogens. However, the bacterial and fungal selection was not completely representative, and—particularly in the contemporary pandemic context—viruses should also be subjects of further investigation [30]. Within a period of 15 min, all products showed a sufficient disinfectant effect. Using reusable brush systems in adhesive systems is less likely to create a critical risk for patients due to contamination of the adhesive reservoir with the tested bacteria and fungi.

The current COVID-19 pandemic has underlined the relevance of proper hygiene standards and has increased awareness regarding adequate protective equipment in everyday dentistry. The use of disposable utensils to safeguard dental professionals and patients has gained in importance. Companies offer alternative forms of application to minimize transmission risks, such as single-use brush systems or adhesive liquid in spray form. However, economic and environmental aspects also play a relevant role. Further studies concerning potential cross-contamination risk should include viruses.

## 5. Conclusions

The tested impression tray adhesives and the corresponding additives appear to be sufficiently bactericidal and fungicidal. Since only a low count of *Staphylococcus aureus*, up to 20 CFU/mL, could be identified after baseline, the cross-contamination risk among patients is extremely low. Furthermore, compared to the initial bacteria count of $10^9$ CFU/mL, the remaining amount of 20 CFU/mL proves the tray adhesives' extremely high disinfectant capacity.

The pandemic has provoked an increasing awareness in patients regarding possible transmissions of microorganisms and hygiene standards. This investigation underlines that the clinical use of the tested tray adhesives is safe.

**Author Contributions:** All authors contributed to the study's conception and design. Material preparation and data collection were performed by I.P. under the supervision of C.S.S., I.P., O.S., S.H. completed the study design and draft of the manuscript, and A.R. supported the study realization and improved the manuscript. All authors commented on previous versions of the manuscript. All authors have read and agreed to the published version of the manuscript.

**Funding:** The work was supported by the Department of Prosthodontics and Materials Science and the Institute for Medical Microbiology and Epidemiology of Infectious Diseases in Leipzig, Germany.

**Institutional Review Board Statement:** Not applicable.

**Informed Consent Statement:** Not applicable.

**Data Availability Statement:** Data available on request.

**Acknowledgments:** We thank the companies producing the tested products for providing samples without cost.

**Conflicts of Interest:** The authors declare no competing interests.

## References

1. Centers for Disease Control and Prevention. *Summary of Infection Prevention Practices in Dental Settings: Basic Expectations for Safe Car*; Centers for Disease Control and Prevention, US Dept of Health and Human Services: Atlanta, GA, USA, 2021. Available online: https://www.cdc.gov/oralhealth/infectioncontrol/pdf/safe-care2.pdf (accessed on 8 July 2021).
2. Centers for Disease Control and Prevention. *Guidelines for Infection Control in Dental Health Care Settings*; 2003. Available online: https://www.cdc.gov/mmwr/PDF/rr/rr5217.pdf (accessed on 8 July 2021).
3. Cristina, M.L.; Spagnolo, A.M.; Sartini, M.; Dallera, M.; Ottria, G.; Perdelli, F.; Orlando, P. Investigation of organizational and hygiene features in dentistry: A pilot study. *J. Prev. Med. Hyg.* **2009**, *50*, 175–180. [CrossRef]
4. Puttaiah, R.; Cederberg, R.; Youngblood, D. A pragmatic approach towards single-use-disposable devices in dentistry. *Bull. Group. Int. Rech. Sci. Stomatol. Odontol.* **2006**, *47*, 18–26. [PubMed]
5. Bundeszahnärztekammer. *Statistisches Jahrbuch 2019/2020*; Kassenzahnärztliche Bundesvereinigung: Cologne, Germany, 2019.
6. Ahlholm, P.; Sipilä, K.; Vallittu, P.; Jakonen, M.; Kotiranta, U. Digital Versus Conventional Impressions in Fixed Prosthodontics: A Review. *J. Prosthodont.* **2018**, *27*, 35–41. [CrossRef] [PubMed]
7. Sivaramakrishnan, G.; Alsobaiei, M.; Sridharan, K. Patient preference and operating time for digital versus conventional impressions: A network meta-analysis. *Aust. Dent. J.* **2020**, *65*, 58–69. [CrossRef] [PubMed]
8. Herman, D.A. A study of the antimicrobial properties of impression tray adhesives. *J. Prosthet. Dent.* **1993**, *69*, 102–105. [CrossRef]
9. White, J.T.; Jordan, R.D. Infection control during elastomeric impressions. *J. Prosthet. Dent.* **1987**, *58*, 711–712. [CrossRef]
10. Bensel, T.; Pollak, R.; Stimmelmayr, M.; Hey, J. Disinfection effect of dental impression tray adhesives. *Clin. Oral Investig.* **2013**, *17*, 497–502. [CrossRef] [PubMed]

11. Schierz, O.; Müller, H.; Stingu, C.S.; Hahnel, S.; Rauch, A. Dental tray adhesives and their role as potential transmission medium for microorganisms. *Clin. Exp. Dent. Res.* **2021**. [CrossRef]
12. Nabert-Georgi, C.; Rodloff, A.C.; Jentsch, H.; Reissmann, D.R.; Schaumann, R.; Stingu, C.S. Influence of oral bacteria on adhesion of Streptococcus mutans and Streptococcus sanguinis to dental materials. *Clin. Exp. Dent. Res.* **2018**, *4*, 72–77. [CrossRef]
13. Rosentritt, M.; Behr, M.; Bürgers, R.; Feilzer, A.J.; Hahnel, S. In vitro adherence of oral streptococci to zirconia core and veneering glass-ceramics. *J. Biomed. Mater. Res. B Appl. Biomater.* **2009**, *91*, 257–263. [CrossRef]
14. Zhou, X.; Li, Y. *Atlas of Oral Microbiology: From Healthy Microflora to Disease*; Elsevier: Amsterdam, The Netherlands; Academic Press: Amsterdam, The Netherlands; New York, NY, USA, 2015; ISBN 978-0-12-802234-4.
15. Krishnan, K.; Chen, T.; Paster, B.J. A practical guide to the oral microbiome and its relation to health and disease. *Oral Dis.* **2017**, *23*, 276–286. [CrossRef]
16. Rupf, S.; Jentsch, H.; Eschrich, K. Lebensraum Mundhöhle: Mikroorganismen und orale Erkrankungen. *Biol. Unserer Zeit* **2007**, *37*, 51–59. [CrossRef]
17. Rutala, W.; Weber, D.; The Healthcare Infection Control Practices Advisory Committee. Guideline for Disinfection and Sterilization in Healthcare Facilities. Available online: https://www.cdc.gov/infectioncontrol/pdf/guidelines/disinfection-guidelines-H.pdf (accessed on 8 July 2021).
18. Renson, A.; Jones, H.E.; Beghini, F.; Segata, N.; Zolnik, C.P.; Usyk, M.; Moody, T.U.; Thorpe, L.; Burk, R.; Waldron, L.; et al. Sociodemographic variation in the oral microbiome. *Ann. Epidemiol.* **2019**, *35*, 73–80.e2. [CrossRef]
19. Hibbing, M.E.; Fuqua, C.; Parsek, M.R.; Peterson, S.B. Bacterial competition: Surviving and thriving in the microbial jungle. *Nat. Rev. Microbiol.* **2010**, *8*, 15–25. [CrossRef] [PubMed]
20. Fujikawa, H.; Munakata, K.; Sakha, M.Z. Development of a competition model for microbial growth in mixed culture. *Biocontrol Sci.* **2014**, *19*, 61–71. [CrossRef] [PubMed]
21. Basson, N.J. Competition for glucose between Candida albicans and oral bacteria grown in mixed culture in a chemostat. *J. Med. Microbiol.* **2000**, *49*, 969–975. [CrossRef] [PubMed]
22. Asgeirsson, H.; Thalme, A.; Weiland, O. Staphylococcus aureus bacteraemia and endocarditis—Epidemiology and outcome: A review. *Infect. Dis.* **2018**, *50*, 175–192. [CrossRef] [PubMed]
23. Muthukrishnan, G.; Masters, E.A.; Daiss, J.L.; Schwarz, E.M. Mechanisms of Immune Evasion and Bone Tissue Colonization That Make Staphylococcus aureus the Primary Pathogen in Osteomyelitis. *Curr. Osteoporos. Rep.* **2019**, *17*, 395–404. [CrossRef]
24. Foster, T.J. Antibiotic resistance in Staphylococcus aureus. Current status and future prospects. *FEMS Microbiol. Rev.* **2017**, *41*, 430–449. [CrossRef] [PubMed]
25. Oliveira, D.; Borges, A.; Simões, M. Staphylococcus aureus Toxins and Their Molecular Activity in Infectious Diseases. *Toxins* **2018**, *10*, 252. [CrossRef] [PubMed]
26. Gomes, T.A.T.; Elias, W.P.; Scaletsky, I.C.A.; Guth, B.E.C.; Rodrigues, J.F.; Piazza, R.M.F.; Ferreira, L.C.S.; Martinez, M.B. Diarrheagenic Escherichia coli. *Braz. J. Microbiol.* **2016**, *47* (Suppl. 1), 3–30. [CrossRef] [PubMed]
27. Azam, M.W.; Khan, A.U. Updates on the pathogenicity status of Pseudomonas aeruginosa. *Drug Discov. Today* **2019**, *24*, 350–359. [CrossRef] [PubMed]
28. Gow, N.A.R.; Yadav, B. Microbe Profile: Candida albicans: A shape-changing, opportunistic pathogenic fungus of humans. *Microbiology* **2017**, *163*, 1145–1147. [CrossRef] [PubMed]
29. Bertolini, M.; Dongari-Bagtzoglou, A. The Relationship of Candida albicans with the Oral Bacterial Microbiome in Health and Disease. *Adv. Exp. Med. Biol.* **2019**, *1197*, 69–78. [CrossRef] [PubMed]
30. Sabino-Silva, R.; Jardim, A.C.G.; Siqueira, W.L. Coronavirus COVID-19 impacts to dentistry and potential salivary diagnosis. *Clin. Oral Investig.* **2020**, *24*, 1619–1621. [CrossRef] [PubMed]

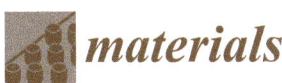 

*Review*

# Calcium Silicate-Based Root Canal Sealers: A Narrative Review and Clinical Perspectives

Germain Sfeir [1], Carla Zogheib [1], Shanon Patel [2], Thomas Giraud [3], Venkateshbabu Nagendrababu [4] and Frédéric Bukiet [3,*]

1 Department of Endodontics, Faculty of Dental Medicine, Saint Joseph University of Beirut, Beirut 17-5208, Lebanon; germain.sfeir@usj.edu.lb (G.S.); carla.zogheibmoubarak@usj.edu.lb (C.Z.)
2 King's College London Dental Institute, Guy's Tower, Guy's Hospital, St. Thomas' Street, London SE1 9RT, UK; shanonpatel@gmail.com
3 Assistance Publique des Hôpitaux de Marseille, 13005 France; Aix Marseille Univ, CNRS, ISM, Inst Movement Sci, 13288 Marseille, France; thomas.giraud@univ-amu.fr
4 Department of Preventive and Restorative Dentistry, College of Dental Medicine, University of Sharjah, Sharjah 27272, United Arab Emirates; hivenkateshbabu@yahoo.com
* Correspondence: frederic.bukiet@univ-amu.fr; Tel.: +33-(0)6-4395-2183

**Citation:** Sfeir, G.; Zogheib, C.; Patel, S.; Giraud, T.; Nagendrababu, V.; Bukiet, F. Calcium Silicate-Based Root Canal Sealers: A Narrative Review and Clinical Perspectives. *Materials* **2021**, *14*, 3965. https://doi.org/10.3390/ma14143965

Academic Editors: Laura-Cristina Rusu and Lavinia Cosmina Ardelean

Received: 12 June 2021
Accepted: 8 July 2021
Published: 15 July 2021

**Publisher's Note:** MDPI stays neutral with regard to jurisdictional claims in published maps and institutional affiliations.

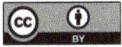

**Copyright:** © 2021 by the authors. Licensee MDPI, Basel, Switzerland. This article is an open access article distributed under the terms and conditions of the Creative Commons Attribution (CC BY) license (https://creativecommons.org/licenses/by/4.0/).

**Abstract:** Over the last two decades, calcium silicate-based materials have grown in popularity. As root canal sealers, these formulations have been extensively investigated and compared with conventional sealers, such as zinc oxide–eugenol and epoxy resin-based sealers, in in vitro studies that showed their promising properties, especially their biocompatibility, antimicrobial properties, and certain bioactivity. However, the consequence of their higher solubility is a matter of debate and still needs to be clarified, because it may affect their long-term sealing ability. Unlike conventional sealers, those sealers are hydraulic, and their setting is conditioned by the presence of humidity. Current evidence reveals that the properties of calcium silicate-based sealers vary depending on their formulation. To date, only a few short-term investigations addressed the clinical outcome of calcium silicate-based root canal sealers. Their use has been showed to be mainly based on practitioners' clinical habits rather than manufacturers' recommendations or available evidence. However, their particular behavior implies modifications of the clinical protocol used for conventional sealers. This narrative review aimed to discuss the properties of calcium silicate-based sealers and their clinical implications, and to propose rational indications for these sealers based on the current knowledge.

**Keywords:** calcium silicate-based root canal sealer; hydraulic root canal sealer; root canal obturation; root canal treatment

## 1. Introduction

Despite numerous technological leaps, the purpose of root canal treatment is still prevention and healing of apical periodontitis by achieving proper disinfection and three-dimensional filling of the root canal space [1]. Root canal filling prevents diffusion of microorganisms and their byproducts and has been subject to various modifications from the use of solid material to gutta-percha cones in association with root canal sealers [2]. Various types of root canal sealers have been developed, such as zinc oxide–eugenol, epoxy resin, glass ionomer, and silicone-based sealers [3]. In the last decade, calcium silicate-based sealers (CSBS), often called "bioceramic" sealers, have been released and extensively investigated by comparing their properties to those of zinc oxide–eugenol-based and epoxy resin-based sealers [4,5]. Many formulations are available on the market. Unlike conventional root canal sealers, CSBS are hydraulic and hygroscopic with a particular setting process [6]. CSBS exhibit several interesting properties, especially biocompatibility, antimicrobial properties, and bioactivity [7–12]. Nevertheless, the dimensional stability of CSBS showed contradicting results among studies; while some studies showed no shrinkage upon setting, other demonstrated a slight expansion [3,4]. Mineral layer formation during setting induces a chemical bond with dentin walls in biological environment, which contributes to their sealing ability [4–6].

To date, if laboratory studies showed favorable results regarding CSBS' physico-chemical and biological properties [13–18], only a few short-term investigations addressing the clinical outcome of CSBS have been published [19–21]. Moreover, a recent survey demonstrated that the methods of using CSBS in clinical practice were variable and based on practitioners' habits rather than manufacturers' recommendations or available evidence on these sealers [22]. This highlights the possible inappropriate use of CSBS, which may negatively impact the obturation, and thus the outcome of the root canal treatment. Moreover, this exposes a knowledge gap between the fundamental research on CSBS and their clinical application, justifying the need to better connect these two aspects. The number of CSBS formulations is strongly increasing over time, so it is of prime importance to better understand their specificities and their clinical perspectives.

Hence, the current review aimed to discuss the properties of CSBS and their clinical implications, and to propose rational indications based on the current knowledge and CSBS specificities.

*1.1. Literature Search Methodology*

Two independent reviewers (G.S., C.Z.) performed a comprehensive literature search to identify related studies in PubMed, Scopus, Web of Science, and Cochrane Library databases, between 1 January 2010 and 15 May 2021. The following search strategy was used to find relevant studies: (bioceramic sealer OR bioceramic root canal sealer) OR (hydraulic sealer OR hydraulic root canal sealer) OR (calcium silicate-based sealer OR calcium silicate-based root canal sealer) AND (root canal OR endodontics OR root canal treatment) OR (root canal filling OR root canal obturation). The references list of the included studies and previously published reviews were searched. Laboratory and clinical studies investigating at least one of the CSBS' properties/outcome were included in the review. The studies performed in training simulated resin teeth or animal teeth were excluded.

*1.2. Terminology*

Rheological properties of calcium silicate-based materials such as ProRoot® Mineral trioxide aggregate (MTA) (Denstply Sirona, Ballaigues, Switzerland) or Biodentine (Septodont, Saint-Maur-des-Fossés, France) were not appropriate to be used as a root canal sealer in association with gutta-percha for obturation. Therefore, in the past 10 years, specific root canal sealer formulations intended for this purpose were developed. These sealers are usually called "bioceramics" by most manufacturers for marketing purpose. This term is not accurate enough [6]. Indeed, chemically, bioceramics represent a large family of biomaterials in terms of composition, and further involve a sintering step in their implementation [23]. Therefore, this new family of root canal sealers should rather be identified as "calcium silicate-based sealers" (CSBS) or "hydraulic calcium silicate-based sealers", due to their hydrophilic nature, chemical composition, and setting reaction [24]. CSBS are usually formulated from synthetic calcium silicate or from Portland/MTA. It is of prime importance to highlight that CSBS' properties can strongly vary depending on the additives included in each formulation [25], and potentially influence their indications and clinical application.

## 2. Review
*2.1. Physico-Chemical Properties*
2.1.1. Setting Reaction and Setting Time

Unlike conventional sealers, CSBS are hydraulic and need water to trigger the setting process (Figure 1). In the presence of water, calcium silicates form a calcium silicate hydrate gel (CSH, $CaO \cdot SiO \cdot H_2O$), which leads to calcium hydroxide ($CaOH_2$) formation [26], as shown in Figure 1. Ion exchanges, predominantly silicon ($Si^{4+}$) from CSH, and calcium

($Ca^{2+}$) and hydroxyl ($OH^-$) ions from calcium hydroxide dissociation, contribute to CSBS' biological properties [7,8,10,12]. These ions provide different effects; $Si^{4+}$ and $Ca^{2+}$ promote biomineralization, while $OH^-$ ions increase pH environment and provide antimicrobial properties. Finally, in the presence of phosphate, microscopic investigations showed that CSBS formed an interfacial layer at the dentin wall known as the "mineral infiltration zone" due to calcium phosphate formation inducing apatite precursors and hydroxyapatite precipitation on the surface of the material [24,27,28].

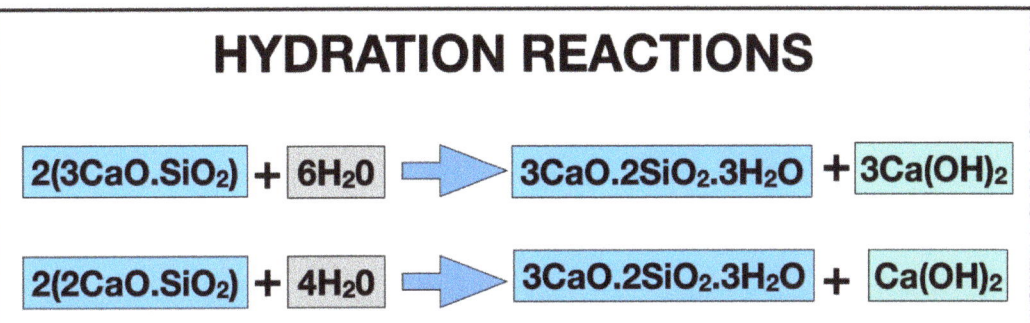

**Figure 1.** Setting reaction of CSBS consisting of two hydration reactions.

Setting time is evaluated by analyzing created indentations on a material sample's surface; when indentations cease to be visible, setting time can be recorded [29,30]. CSBS overall reported a shorter setting time compared to conventional formulations such as AH Plus® (Dentsply Sirona, York, PA, USA) [3,31]. However, prolonged setting times were also highlighted [32], depending not only on formulation, but also on root canal moisture, as it has been noted that when the root canal is dry, setting time tends to increase [18]. This explains why setting times vary between clinical trials and laboratory studies, and small amounts of fluids in contact with sealers may affect the latter [33]. For instance, it has been demonstrated in vitro that BioRoot™ RCS (Septodont, Saint-Maur-des-Fossés, France) had a setting time inferior to 6 h, while MTA Fillapex® (Angelus, Londrina, Brazil) did not completely set within one week [34]. This lack of setting was also reported by another study [35] also investigating BioRoot™ RCS that indicated an influence of contact media (culture media) on the observed setting times. By contrast, when simulating different conditions (with an increased fluid intake), the setting time for both EndoSequence® BC Sealer™ (Brasseler USA, Savannah, GA, USA) and MTA Fillapex® was inferior to 3 h, which is much shorter than epoxy or zinc oxide–eugenol-based sealers [3]. Another study comparing EndoSequence® BC Sealer™ and EndoSequence® BC Sealer™ HiFlow (Brasseler USA, Savannah, GA), reported comparable initial setting times of 4 h for both formulations [36]. Although variable, these values remain generally lower than those of conventional sealers (zinc oxide–eugenol and resin-based). Finally, it was shown that applying heat during root canal filling resulted in an extended setting time for premixed CSBS such as HiFlow® and Endosequence® BC Sealer™, while the setting process was faster for BioRoot™ RCS, highlighting again the influence of the formulation on sealer properties [37].

2.1.2. Flowability

Unlike the first calcium silicate-based materials, with inappropriate flowability/consistency for root canal filling [38], CSBS flowability should allow good sealer distribution into the ramifications/irregularities of the root canal space. The flow values are studied by placing a sample of mixed material between two glass plates with the application of a mass on top. At the end of the assay, the sample diameter is determined and used to assess the material flow capacity and must be superior or at least 17 mm [29,30]

(ANSI/ADA, 2000; ISO 6876, 2012). Among available studies, it has been demonstrated that MTA Fillapex®, EndoSequence® BC Sealer™, and Endoseal MTA® (Maruchi, Wonju, Korea) [3,27,35,39,40] met the minimum expected values, and the highest values for MTA Fillapex® were generally reported. However, while BioRoot™ RCS was characterized by results slightly below the minimum standard (16 mm) [13], it was also characterized as meeting the standard requirements with values above 21 mm [35], but decreasing with heat application [41]. HiFlow® formulation exhibited the highest flow as compared to EndoSequence® BC Sealer™, although it decreased with heat application [36]. Overall, based on the available literature, CSBS flowability should be considered as overall comparable to the conventional sealers, especially epoxy resin-based sealers such as AH Plus®.

2.1.3. Wettability

Root canal sealers should have a good wetting ability and adhesion to dentinal walls [42]. Wettability reflects the spreading ability and the capability of sealers to penetrate into both the main and lateral canals, as well as into the dentinal tubules [43]. Since CSBS are hydrophilic, this might induce a good spreading ability on wet root canal walls [4]. This was confirmed by a recent study showed the best wetting ability and adhesion for EndoSequence® BC Sealer™ and EndoSeal MTA® compared to AH Plus® [42].

2.1.4. Film Thickness

Film thickness of tested material is determined under stress by placing the sample of the sealer between two glass slides and a load application. According to ISO6876/2012 and ANSI/ADA no 57, film thickness must not exceed 50 µm for sealers, as an end result of the test conditions [29,30]. This property is respected by various formulations such as EndoSequence® BC Sealer™ HiFlow®, Endoseal MTA®, and MTA Fillapex® [3,35,36], presenting overall higher values compared to AH Plus®. Moreover, BioRoot™ RCS exhibited the highest values of film thickness [35], and other studies described this property as slightly above the standard values [13,41]. Here too, film thickness values were reported to be increased by heat application for BioRoot™ RCS, EndoSequence® BC Sealer™, and EndoSequence® BC Sealer™ HiFlow® [36,41]. Moreover, it can be considered that this characteristic for CSBS should be put in perspective with their better dimensional stability and their use with sealer-based obturation techniques such as cold hydraulic condensation (CHC).

2.1.5. Dimensional Stability

CSBS dimensional stability is overall better than the one of conventional sealers, especially zinc oxide–eugenol-based sealers, which tend to shrink upon setting, especially if sealer film thickness increases [44–46]. It should be mentioned that this parameter is no longer present in the latest ISO standard. As initially demonstrated for MTA-based formulations, CSBS may present a slight hygroscopic expansion up to 0.2%, but this was not highlighted for all formulations [44].

Lee et al. (2017) compared dimensional stability between AH Plus®, AD Seal® (Meta Biomed, Cheongju, Korea), and Radic-Sealer® (Seoul, Korea) and the CSBS formulation Endoseal MTA®. It was shown that AH Plus® and Endoseal MTA® revealed the least dimensional changes, especially for Endoseal MTA®, which remained lower than AH Plus® 30 days later. The other two resin-based formulations had higher values than recommended [39]. In another study, no significant difference in volumetric change between AH Plus® and TotalFill BC sealer was reported [27]. On the other hand, MTA Fillapex® showed a slight shrinkage upon setting (which might have been due to the presence of resin in this formulation), while EndoSequence® BC Sealer™ demonstrated an expansion, but inferior to 0.1% [3]. The expansion of EndoSequence® BC Sealer™ might be influenced by direct contact of CSBS with enzymes [47]. By contrast, using micro-CT, a higher volumetric loss also was reported [32], but to a lesser extent with the use of PBS [26]. The better dimensional stability of CSBS is often highlighted as the main reason for allowing their use with cold hydraulic condensation, especially the single-cone (SC) technique (Figure 2). This aspect must also take into account the solubility of CSBS.

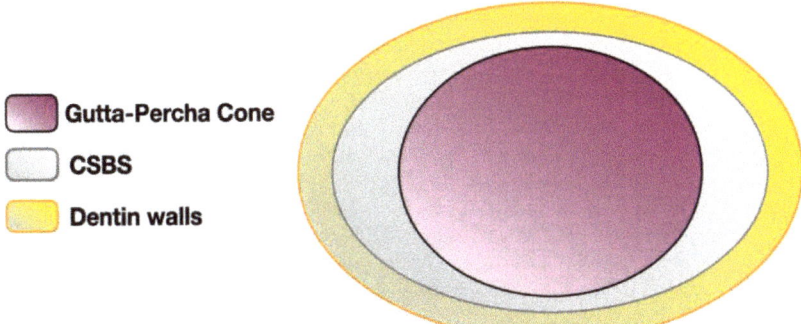

Figure 2. Updated single-cone technique with CSBS (sealer-based obturation) considering their enhanced dimensional stability.

### 2.1.6. Solubility of CSBS

Overall, CSBS solubility indicated higher values than those of conventional sealers without necessarily respecting the specifications of the standards (less than 3%) [29,30]. Systematically, studies reported that CSBS present higher solubility compared to epoxy resin-based sealers [3,26,27,32,34–36,47,48]. However, while some studies reported values of solubility with respect to ISO 6876/2012 and ANSI/ADA recommendations, others did not. Indeed, although the standard recommends using water, solubility values may strongly differ depending on experimental conditions such as setting conditions and contact liquid (water, PBS, culture media); for example, solubility reported for BioRoot™ RCS and MTA Fillapex® fulfilled the standard recommendations (inferior to 3%), and the use of PBS lowered BioRoot™ RCS solubility [34]. This was also the case for MTA Fillapex® and EndoSequence® BC Sealer™ in the study of Zhou et al. (2013), which used a modified sample setting method and fulfilled the weight-loss requirements [3]. Another study indicated low solubility rates for EndoSequence® BC Sealer™ and EndoSequence® BC Sealer™ HiFlow formulations [36]. Moreover, solubility of EndoSequence® BC Sealer™ was higher when in contact with biological fluids such as the Esterase enzyme as compared to PBS but remained in compliance with the ISO standard requirement in both conditions [47]. On the other hand, other studies have reported values much higher than the standard requirements (frequently above 10%), also using classical or various assay conditions, and concerned the previously mentioned CSBS formulations [26,27,32,35,48].

Investigation of CSBS' solubility is a major matter of debate. Indeed, higher solubility of CSBS might lead to jeopardize their long-term sealing ability [5]. However, microscopic analysis has demonstrated mineral deposition and an infiltration zone into the dentin [26], which might call into question the above concern. Indeed, it must be pointed out that CSBS' biological properties can be explained by their solubility and related release of ions [49], which leads to specific interaction between CSBS and the dentin walls (mineral infiltration zone). Furthermore, solubility may be overestimated due to the chemical class of CSBS, which could explain the discrepancies sometimes found between the high solubility values and the relatively lower ones concerning dimensional variations [27,32]. These contradictory results might be explained by the bias in the solubility of CSBS due to their hydrophilic nature. Moreover, since fluid environments (use of culture media) might strongly influence solubility results [35], it can be hypothesized that in vivo application of endodontic sealer should be relatively different with notably limited contact with aqueous fluids compared to in vitro test conditions.

### 2.1.7. Adhesion–Interaction with Dentin Walls

CSBS adhesion and interaction with dentin walls were investigated by push-out test, filtration assays, or microscopy analysis. As mentioned previously, CSBS form a specific interfacial layer at the dentin walls known as the mineral infiltration zone [49]. The sealer's hydration products alter the collagen of the interfacial dentin due to their alkaline effects [50]. This alteration leads to the formation of a porous structure promoting the diffusion of high concentrations of $Ca^{2+}$, $OH^-$, and $CO_3^{2-}$ ions, favoring mineralization in this area [18]. This chemical and micromechanical interaction (tag-like structures) represents the main reason for assessment of the adhesion between CSBS and dentin [49,51].

Laboratory studies found higher push-out bond strength (POBS) values for AH Plus® when compared to MTA Fillapex®, TotalFill® BC Sealer™, and BioRoot™ RCS [52,53]. On the other hand, Tuncel et al. (2015) compared the POBS of AH Plus® to iRoot SP® (IBC, Burnaby, BC, Canada), and found that iRoot SP® had significantly better results [54]. CSBS and conventional sealers showed variable results regarding bond strength and adhesion to the dentin walls; however, only one study showed no difference between CSBS and resin-based sealers [55]. Some variations have also been demonstrated between different CSBS formulations and depending on the root canal filling technique used; Delong et al. (2015) demonstrated that the lowest adhesion was found with MTA Plus® (Prevest, Jammu, India) when warm obturation techniques were used. However, BC Sealer® had higher bond-strength values than MTA Plus® when both were used with the SC technique [56].

### 2.1.8. Adhesion between the Gutta-Percha and the Sealer

CSBS are hydrophilic materials and the surface of gutta-percha cones is hydrophobic, which is why this interface remains questionable regarding potential micro-organism leakage [22]. Some manufacturers have proposed different strategies to enhance the adhesion between CSBS and gutta-percha. The use of specific pre-impregnated gutta-percha cones with "bioceramic" nanoparticles has been suggested with premixed formulations, while Septodont claimed the inclusion of an organic polymer (povidone) in their BioRoot™ RCS formulation. The only available study showed that the interface between these specific gutta-percha cones and the corresponding CSBS was not satisfactory [57]. Moreover, the contact between gutta-percha and sodium hypochlorite for disinfection before any obturation technique has been shown to degrade the gutta-percha cones [58]. This led us to wonder if specific coated gutta-percha cones may lose the claimed benefit when immersed in sodium hypochlorite. To our knowledge, there is no available scientific evidence supporting the use of specific pre-impregnated gutta-percha cones. Likewise, the effect of the povidone included in BioRoot™ RCS has not been investigated yet.

### 2.1.9. Microhardness

Microhardness reflects the resistance of materials to deformation under a specific load. This property is not a part of the ISO/ADA requirements, and so it has been rarely investigated. Microhardness can be used as an indirect measurement of material setting [59]. The Vickers hardness test is used to assess the microhardness of sealers. Microhardness may impact CSBS removal when a non-surgical retreatment is indicated [22,59].

### 2.1.10. Radiopacity

The ISO 6876 standard establishes 3 mm of aluminum (Al) as the minimum radiopacity for 1 mm root canal sealer sample thickness, as is the case of ANSI/ADA specification No. 57 [29,30]. Two main radio-opacifiers are generally included in CSBS formulations: Portland/MTA based-formulations most often contain bismuth oxide [60,61], whereas other CSBS generally include zirconium oxide in their formulations [38]. Overall, the standard specifications are respected in all CSBS formulations [62]. Different formulations of CSBS demonstrated higher radiopacity compared to the ISO standards. This was demonstrated for BioRoot™ RCS [13], EndoSequence® BC Sealer™, EndosealMTA®, and MTA Fillapex® [39]. TotalFill® BC Sealer HiFlow™ might exhibit an additional radiopacity of 20% compared to standard TotalFill® BC Sealer™ according to the manufacturer's instructions (FKG Dentaire catalogue, La Chaux-De-Fonds, Switzerland).

## 2.2. Biological Properties

As previously presented, CSBS' biological properties rely on a hydration reaction leading to CSH and calcium hydroxide formation. Indeed, hydration byproducts, $OH^-$, $Ca^{+2}$, and $Si^{+4}$ ions are involved in modulating environment alkalization and cell metabolism, especially cell differentiation and tissue mineralization [63–65]. As a biomaterial, CSBS formulations must notably be non-genotoxic and non-cytotoxic, while also exhibiting antimicrobial properties and inducing appropriate host response in their specific use. These capacities, which rely on biocompatibility, are, among others, framed and evaluated through the ISO standard series 10993 [66]. Moreover, it is important to highlight that these studied properties, mostly in vitro, vary according to the protocols used. Indeed, biomaterial state (freshly mixed/set), type of contact (direct/extracts and associated dilutions), and targeted organisms chosen (cell lines/primary cell culture, planktonic bacterial strains/organized biofilms) will more or less accurately reflect the clinical use.

### 2.2.1. Genotoxicity and Cytotoxicity

Genotoxicity is assessed using various protocols to study DNA breaks or nucleus division anomalies. In a study using a $\gamma$-H2AX foci assay, no difference in genotoxicity was highlighted between unset formulations of CSBS (BioRoot™ RCS, iRoot SP®, MTA Fillapex®) in comparison to conventional sealers (epoxy- and methacrylate-based), except a slight increase for iRoot SP®, while BioRoot™ RCS was revealed to be less genotoxic on periodontal ligament (PDL) cells [67]. However, when compared to a zinc oxide–eugenol formulation (Tubliseal), iRoot SP® and EndoSequence® BC Sealer ™ were shown to be the least genotoxic using a comet assay (DNA breaks) on L929 murine fibroblasts [68]. Furthermore, when human gingival fibroblast cultures were submitted to unset EndoSequence® BC Sealer™, it led to a reduced genotoxicity potential as compared to AH Plus using a micronucleus assay [69]. Finally, set formulations of MTA Fillapex® and AH Plus®, although depending on the concentration and the incubation time used, were shown to be more genotoxic by micronucleus assay on V79 fibroblasts as compared to classical MTA formulation [70].

In parallel, cytotoxicity was studied on PDL cells using unset biomaterial samples, and demonstrated a reduced effect of BioRoot™ RCS, iRootSP®, and MTA Fillapex® as compared to other resin-based sealers such as AH Plus®. However, MTA Fillapex® was revealed to be three times more cytotoxic than BioRoot™ RCS [67]. In another study, evaluating both freshly mixed and set sealer sample on human PDL cells, it was shown that BioRoot RCS was the least cytotoxic in both set and freshly mixed conditions, even allowing cell proliferation [71]. By contrast AH Plus® was revealed to be cytotoxic in a freshly mixed condition, but not after setting, while MTA Fillapex and Pulp Canal Sealer (PCS) were characterized as cytotoxic in both fresh and set states [71]. Close results were obtained while comparing AH Plus MTA Fillapex® and EndoSequence® BC Sealer™ on gingival fibroblasts, indicating higher cell viabilities for EndoSequence® BC Sealer™ in fresh/set conditions [72]. Conversely, AH Plus® was more cytotoxic when freshly mixed, while MTA Fillapex® was reported to be cytotoxic in both conditions [72]. Using set biomaterial samples, it was demonstrated on L929 murine fibroblasts by MTT assay that the zinc oxide–eugenol formulation was the more cytotoxic as compared to EndoSequence® BC Sealer™ and iRoot SP® [68]. Using direct contact with set biomaterial on isolated PDL cells, a much greater number of present cells for BioRoot™ RCS were demonstrated compared to a zinc oxide–eugenol (PCS) [12]. This has also been demonstrated on cell proliferation using sealer extracts, leading to a greater decrease with the use of PCS [12]. These results were confirmed in another study that used sealer extract on human PDL fibroblasts, and which demonstrated an increase of cell proliferation with the use of BioRoot™ RCS extracts as compared to PCS [73]. Moreover, a much lower CSBS cytotoxicity was also highlighted using an adenosine triphosphate luminescence assay on a murine osteoblast precursor cell line [74]. Indeed, AH Plus® was revealed to be cytotoxic at concentrations a hundred times lower than EndoSequence® BC Sealer™ and ProRoot ES (Dentsply Tulsa Dental Specialties, Tulsa, OK, USA) [74]. Cytotoxicity was also investigated in human PDL stem cells (PDLSCs) in two works by Collado-Gonzalez et al. that evaluated set biomaterial sample effects and indicated an overall cytotoxicity of MTA Fillapex®, Endoseal MTA®, and AH Plus®, while BioRoot™ RCS was characterized as highly biocompatible [7,75]. Similar findings have been reported in human PDLSCs by Rodríguez-Lozano et al., who concluded that TotalFill® BC Sealer™ induced a lower cytotoxicity as compared to MTA Fillapex® and AH Plus® [76]. Finally, it was recently also demonstrated using sealer eluates from set biomaterials on PDLSCs that EndoSequence® BC Sealer™ and EndoSequence® BC Sealer™ HiFlow formulations were not cytotoxic, conversely to AH Plus® [77].

2.2.2. Antimicrobial Activity

CSBS' antimicrobial activity is mostly linked to their ability to increase pH, as presented before, consecutive to hydroxyl ion releasing. Indeed, a pH increase was highlighted by many studies, in comparison to conventional sealer formulations [3,13,14,40,78,79]. Unlike the latter, CSBS induced an alkalization lasting in time, although this property was sometimes reported as reduced in the case of MTA Fillapex®. Evaluation of CSBS' antimicrobial activity was also widely studied, using various protocols, micro-organism strains, and types of contact/micro-organism organization. Indeed, using set material sample for a direct-contact test on planktonic micro-organisms and a biofilm model on dentin, it was shown that TotalFill BC Sealer® was more efficient against both *E. faecalis* and *C. albicans* [80]. In comparison with many other formulations, a fast and significant effectiveness of iRoot SP® was shown just after mixing against *E. faecalis*, even after 3 days, conversely to AH Plus® using a direct-contact test [81]. Regarding the antibacterial effect of CSBS, Candeiro et al. (2016) found a similar antibacterial effect of EndoSequence® BC Sealer™ and AH Plus® against *E. faecalis* using a direct-contact test up to 7 days [69]. Assessment against multiple bacterial strains in both a planktonic state and in simulated mono-specie biofilms, it was reported that TotalFill BC Sealer® and AH Plus® possessed antibacterial activity [82]. However, while AH Plus® presented high antibacterial activity against all planktonic and biofilm bacteria strains during the first day, this property was drastically reduced for longer times. TotalFill BC Sealer® use showed an antibacterial effect on planktonic strains up to 7 days, while its effect was lower on mono-specie biofilms, especially against *S. aureus* and *E. faecalis* [82]. Using an 8-week-old biofilm of *E. faecalis* in an infected root model, Bukhari and Karabucak demonstrated a superior antibacterial effect of EndoSequence® BC Sealer™ after 1 day and up to 2 weeks, in comparison to AH Plus® [83]. Antibacterial property was also studied depending on final irrigant use by an agar diffusion test and an intratubular infection model for BioRoot™ RCS, MTA Fillapex®, and AH Plus® against *E. faecalis*. It was concluded that the formulations exhibited higher antimicrobial effects after EDTA use as compared to PBS, and that BioRoot™ RCS exhibited the highest activity [84].

Overall, CSBS presented similar or even higher antimicrobial properties than conventional sealers. However, a lack of standardization for assessment of antimicrobial properties has been highlighted [85]. Moreover, it must be pointed out that the clinician should rely on the root canal disinfection/cleaning procedure instead of the antibacterial properties of endodontic sealers.

2.2.3. Bioactivity

Although a biomaterial can be characterized as biocompatible, its bioactivity qualification implies an ability to stimulate metabolic/cellular-specific events, leading to tissue healing, whether through regenerative step induction, inflammation control, or both. In the case of endodontic sealers, events such mesenchymal stem cell migration, growth factor secretion, and cell differentiation are implicated in periapical healing, just as the modulation of pro-inflammatory factor cell secretion/expression or immune cells recruitment are related to periapical inflammation resolution.

Jung et al. (2018) showed in two studies that in comparison to PCS, AH Plus®, and MTA Fillapex, only the BioRoot™ RCS had a positive influence on cell metabolism of both PDL cells and osteoblasts [71,86]. Furthermore, human PDLSC activity and migration were evaluated using a scratch wound healing assay and adhesion to collagen type I with set sealer eluates of TotalFill BC Sealer®, MTA Fillapex®, and AH Plus® [76]. Results indicated the most-favorable responses with the use of TotalFill BC Sealer®, while the use of MTA Fillapex® resulted in the least-favorable responses, even compared to AH Plus® [76]. All of these previously mentioned cell populations are essential in periapical tissue regeneration, and alteration of their metabolism/activity may impact this latter. Evaluating PDL lipopolysaccharides (LPS)-stimulated fibroblast implication in both regeneration and inflammation events, it was demonstrated that BioRoot™ RCS, conversely to PCS, did not alter PDL stem cell migration while controlling immune cell (THP-1 model) migration and activation. Furthermore, this study highlighted that BioRoot™ RCS induced PDL fibroblast growth factor (TGF-β1) secretion and reduced pro-inflammatory cytokine (IL-6) secretion by ELISA [73]. It has also been shown that the use of BioRoot™ RCS did not alter the cell mesenchymal character and migration ability of human PDLSCs [7]. Moreover, PDL cell angiogenic/osteogenic growth factor secretions (VEGF, FGF, BMP-1) were shown to be increased by the use of BioRoot™ RCS extracts [12]. In addition to their secretion, it has also been shown that the expression of osteogenic factor by murine osteoblast precursor cell line was increased by EndoSequence® BC Sealer™ and ProRoot ES, using fluorescence and RT-PCR (DMP-1, ALP), while the use of AH Plus® impaired this osteogenic potential [74]. However, using diluted material extracts of EndoSequence® BC Sealer™, MTA Fillapex® and AH Plus® both increased the cell osteogenic potential of an osteoblast cell line after an LPS-induced inflammation state [87]. Moreover, in addition to an osteogenic potential, it has also been demonstrated by qPCR that the EndoSequence® BC Sealer™ and HiFlow formulations were able to stimulate human PDLSC mineralization and cementogenic marker expressions (ALP, CEMP, RUNX2, and CAP), while AH Plus® did not [77]. Concerning the inflammation process, the effect of iRoot® SP use was studied on macrophage viability, cytokine expression, and macrophage polarization [88,89]. Indeed, the inflammatory reaction is a complex process, and while often considered to be deleterious, is necessary for the implementation of the regeneration steps, and macrophage polarization plays an important role. Indeed, the macrophage M1 phenotype is recognized as pro-inflammatory, while shifting to the M2 phenotype acts as anti-inflammatory [90]. Zhu et al. demonstrated that iRoot® SP was not cytotoxic for a model of macrophage (RAW 264.7) and induced both pro- and anti-inflammatory cytokine expressions (IL-1b, TNF-a, IL-10, IL-12p40). Moreover, use of this CSBS formulation induced an increase of M1 and M2 macrophage marker expression and reduced the balance of M1/M2 macrophage phenotypes, indicating that this sealer could promote healing processes [89]. Close results were obtained by Yuan et al., who studied iRoot® SP's effects on the same events after an LPS-induced inflammatory state simulation. This work also found a potential effect of iRoot® SP on mRNA inflammation factor expressions and M1/M2 macrophage phenotype balance [88].

Taken together, the whole of these in vitro studies, clearly demonstrated that CSBS, presented promising biological properties, when compared to conventional sealers. It may hypothesize that, in addition to an adequate endodontic clinical protocol, CSBS could promote the healing process in case of apical periodontitis due to their enhanced biocompatibility and certain bioactivity. However, it must be pointed out that additive in formulations can alter these properties. Indeed, more inconsistent results in the literature were obtained with MTA Fillapex® formulation. This is often explained by the presence of resinous compounds of the salicylic type in their formulations and substance leaching [72,91,92], just as a silicate hydration reaction alteration and reduced or absent calcium hydroxide formation [25].

*2.3. Obturation Quality*

The main objective of obturation is to prevent leakage and reinfection of the root canal system [93]; microleakage can occur due to gaps or voids occurrence [94,95]. While the postoperative radiograph helps in assessing the obturation quality in a clinical approach, many laboratory methods can value the root canal filling quality in vitro: dye penetration, dye diffusion, bacterial and endotoxin infiltration, electrochemical, microscopy, or 3D evaluation [62]. Voids are often investigated because they represent some spaces where residual bacteria might re-grow and release their byproducts, thus jeopardizing the long-term success of the root canal treatment [96,97].

A study evaluating apical sealing ability using apical linear dye penetration and comparing AH Plus®, Endosequence BC® Sealer™, and MTA Fillapex ® showed the lowest apical leakage value for the SC technique used with the EndoSequence BC® Sealer™ [98]. As already shown in the literature, results for the dye techniques remain contradictory, inducing a wide variability. An important consideration in relation to dye penetration studies is that air trapped in voids within the root canal obturation material might interfere with fluid movement [62,99].

One study evaluated the microleakage of different types of sealer, demonstrating that the Endosequence BC® Sealer™ group showed the least dye leakage, while the highest leakage was observed in zinc oxide–eugenol-based sealer [100].

Nevertheless, many factors may influence voids' proportion, including the root canal filling technique (Figure 3), film thickness, flowability, and wettability.

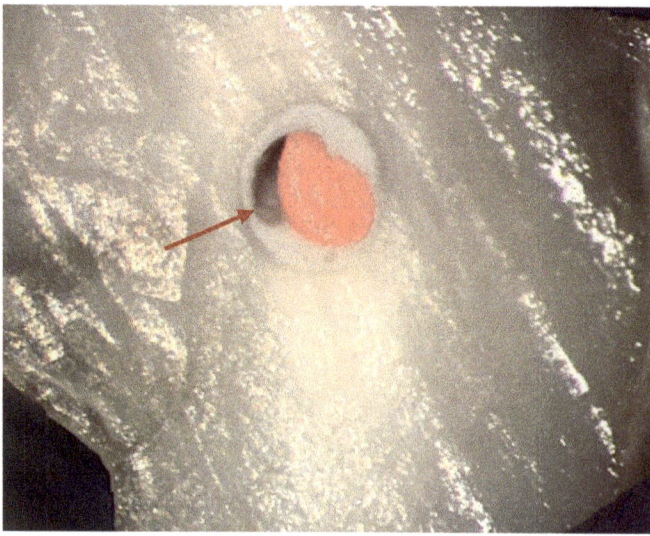

**Figure 3.** Large void following root canal obturation with single cone technique.

Void incidence has been reported to be greater within oval root canals, especially when this space was filled with CHC and especially when using the SC technique or cold lateral compaction [101,102]. Another study assessed the filling quality of five obturation techniques in oval-shaped root canals by using an optical numeric microscope, SEM, and energy-dispersive X-rays (EDX) [103]. This study investigated the proportions of gutta-percha-filled areas, sealer-filled areas, void areas, and the sealer/gutta tags into dentinal tubules. Obturation quality was overall better when using a warm gutta-percha obturation technique compared to the use of the SC technique, regardless of the type of sealer. A recent study based on confocal microscopic evaluation showed that the use of warm vertical compaction enhanced the penetration of CSBS into the dentinal tubules in comparison with the SC technique [104]. The inherent limitations of the SC technique even using CSBS was demonstrated in a micro-CT study [105].

Micro-CT has been suggested to be the most reliable technique to investigate the filling quality differentiating gutta-percha, sealer, and voids. This technique allows the evaluation of void/porosity incidence (apical, middle, or coronal thirds), and the identification of their type (internal, external, or combined) [106,107]. A study assessed the remaining voids after obturation between Endosequence® BC Sealer™ and AH Plus® using the SC technique. EndoSequence® BC Sealer™ showed a lower ratio of voids compared to AH Plus® in the apical third, but it was highlighted by the authors that this difference was likely due to root canal anatomy variations [108]. A recent study showed that the proportion of open and closed porosity can change over time [107]. Initially, significantly greater open and total porosity were found for MTA Fillapex® than for AH Plus®. After 6 months, the percentage of open and total porosity increased in BioRoot™ RCS and MTA Fillapex®, and decreased in AH Plus® and Endosequence® BC Sealer™. These findings were explained by the greater solubility of BioRoot™ RCS and MTA Fillapex® compared to AH Plus®. The better ability of EndoSequence® BC Sealer™ to create apatite formation compared to BioRoot™ RCS might explain the reduction of porosity for EndoSequence® BC Sealer™ 6 months after storage [107].

When compared to conventional sealers, CSBS have overall shown comparable results when evaluating void incidence using micro-CT [109]. However, void incidence should be always put in perspective with the root canal anatomy and the obturation technique used.

*2.4. Retreatability*

Non-surgical retreatment implies removal of root canal filling material in order to re-establish apical patency, then clean and fill the entire root canal system (AAE 2012). Therefore, retreatability is one of the requested properties of filling materials [110,111]. Currently there is no technique allowing complete removal of filling materials from a root canal system [111]. In addition, several factors may influence the retreatability, such as the filling technique implemented, and the type of sealer used with gutta-percha [110,111].

CSBS are known to be hard upon setting [112] and to create hydroxyapatite crystals upon their interface with dentin [113]. In addition to that, they are capable of penetrating into the dentinal tubule. These properties may render retreatment procedures difficult [114]. To study removal of filling materials, different methods have been used such as micro-computed tomography (micro-CT), cone-beam computed tomography (CBCT), radiography, tooth splitting and direct visualization by SEM, confocal microscopy, stereomicroscopy or digital cameras, and rendering the teeth transparent [110,114–117]. As it has already shown to be reliable for evaluation of the quality of the root canal filling, micro-CT is non-invasive and allows for the comparison of the remaining volume of the filling material to the initial volume. In addition to visualizing and measuring the remaining filling material, SEM and confocal microscopy can also be used to assess the degree of penetration of the sealer inside dentinal tubules, or to quantify the number of open tubules [114,116].

Ersev et al. (2012) compared the retreatability of four root canal sealers (Hybrid Root SEAL, EndoSequence® BCSealer™, the Activ GP system, and AH Plus®) and found no significant differences between the different sealers, or between the techniques used [118]. As demonstrated in many investigations, no technique allowed the complete removal of the filling material. Simsek et al. (2014) compared the number of opened tubules using SEM after the removal of iRoot® SP, AH Plus®, and MM Seal® in straight premolars filled with the lateral compaction technique after the use of R-endo rotary instruments or ESI ultrasonic tips. Likewise, no group showed complete removal of the filling material, with greatest leftover in the apical third [116].

Kim et al. (2015) also did not find any significant differences between Endosequence® BC Sealer™ and AH Plus® when comparing the amount of residual material using SEM analysis [114]. According to Uzunoglu et al. (2015), more remaining filling material was observed following the SC technique with iRoot® SP compared to SC with AH-26® or lateral compaction with AH-26® (DeTrey, Dentsply Maillefer, USA), when assessed with SEM [110]. In addition, Suk et al. (2017) did not find any significant differences in the removability of EndoSequence® BC Sealer™ and AH Plus®. In this study, MTA Fillapex® was found to be the easiest to remove [117].

Hess et al. (2011) noted better removability of AH Plus® compared to Endosequence® BC Sealer™ in canals of less than 20 degrees of curvature [119]. More remnants of this CSBS were found in the apical third upon SEM analysis, and patency was not re-established in 20% of samples with BC Sealer and master cone to the WL, or in 70% of samples with BC Sealer and master cone short of the WL. Agrafioti et al. (2015) compared the retreatability of Total Fill® BC Sealer™, MTA Fillapex®, and AH Plus® in straight canals [113]. Authors have demonstrated that WL and apical patency were re-established in 100% of cases, when the gutta-percha cones were placed at WL. Oltra et al. (2017) compared the retreatability of BC Sealer and AH Plus® using micro-CT imaging and found that the latter was associated with less residual filling materials, and that the use of chloroform may help BC Sealer removal [120]. On the other hand, Donnermeyer et al. (2018) found that AH Plus® was associated with more remnants when compared to Bio Root™ RCS, MTA Fillapex®, and Endo CPM (Egeo, Buenos Aires, Argentina) [112].

Contradicting results between studies [112,120] could be related to the application of different methodologies, especially the length of adjustment of the gutta-percha cone and the dental sample anatomy. In the study conducted by Hess et al. (2011), gutta-percha cones were intentionally placed short of the apical foramen. It must be pointed out that this method represented the most realistic scenario of a non-surgical retreatment. This could clearly compromise retreatment outcome [119]. In other studies, gutta-percha cones were placed at full WL This different protocol could strongly influence the ability to re-establish the apical patency after removal of root canal filling material. Indeed, with the gutta-percha cone being introduced to the full working length, the apical patency could easily be re-established following easy removal of the latter. However, these situations did not correspond to the vast majority of retreatment indications. Indeed, it is well known that apical periodontitis is usually diagnosed in the case of poor quality and short obturation [121].

On the other hand, root canal anatomy, such as canal curvature and cross-section, may also impact retreatability. Hess et al. (2011) used mesial canals of mandibular molars, while in Agrafioti et al. (2015), straight canals from anterior teeth were evaluated [113,119].

In addition, the obturation technique used can influence the results. Manufacturers usually recommend CSBS with the SC technique, and some studies demonstrated that the use of these sealers with continuous wave condensation may decrease their bond strength [56]. This may explain the absence of differences between CSBS and resin-based sealers in the studies conducted by Agrafioti et al. (2015) and Kim et al, (2015) [113,114].

Contradictory results were also obtained regarding the retreatment time. Simsek et al. (2014) did not find a statistical difference in the time to reach WL when removing iRoot® SP, MM Seal, and AH Plus® [116]. Similar findings were obtained by Kim et al. (2015) when comparing time for removal of EndoSequence® BC Sealer™ and AH Plus® [114]. Uzunoglu et al. (2015) reported a faster retreatment when the filling material consisted of gutta-percha and MTA Fillapex® compared to AH Plus® and iRoot® SP, which showed similar results [110]. Donnermeyer et al. (2018) found that the removal of CSBS (BioRoot™ RCS and Endo CPM) was faster than for AH Plus® [112].

In conclusion, most ex vivo studies showed possible CSBS removal, and an ability to regain apical patency in the majority of cases. However, methodological bias could be observed in many studies, and further studies better simulating retreatment indications and conditions are needed.

## 3. A Proposal for Clinical Perspectives on CSBS with Cold Hydraulic Condensation

### 3.1. Root Canal Anatomy

CHC and cold lateral compaction are known to increase void occurrence compared to warm gutta-percha obturation techniques, especially in large and oval canals regardless of the type of sealer [103,105,122,123]. However, in case of narrow, long, and curved canals, the use of warm vertical compaction can be questionable, since penetration of the heat plugger at the appropriate level (4 mm short of the working length) can sometimes be impossible. Thus, the gutta-percha is not heated and melted in the apical third, and the obturation of this area behaves as a SC technique [124]. Using CHC with CSBS in these types of anatomy makes root canal obturation easier and faster while taking advantage of CSBS' physico-chemical and biological properties.

### 3.2. Operative Accessibility

It is common sense to highlight that CHC and CSBS should make the obturation procedure easier and faster when dealing with a restricted access (limited mouth opening/posterior teeth) compared to the use of thermoplasticized gutta-percha obturation techniques. Indeed, by using CHC, the technical difficulties are limited to the intracanal sealer placement and the insertion of the gutta-percha cones (Figure 4).

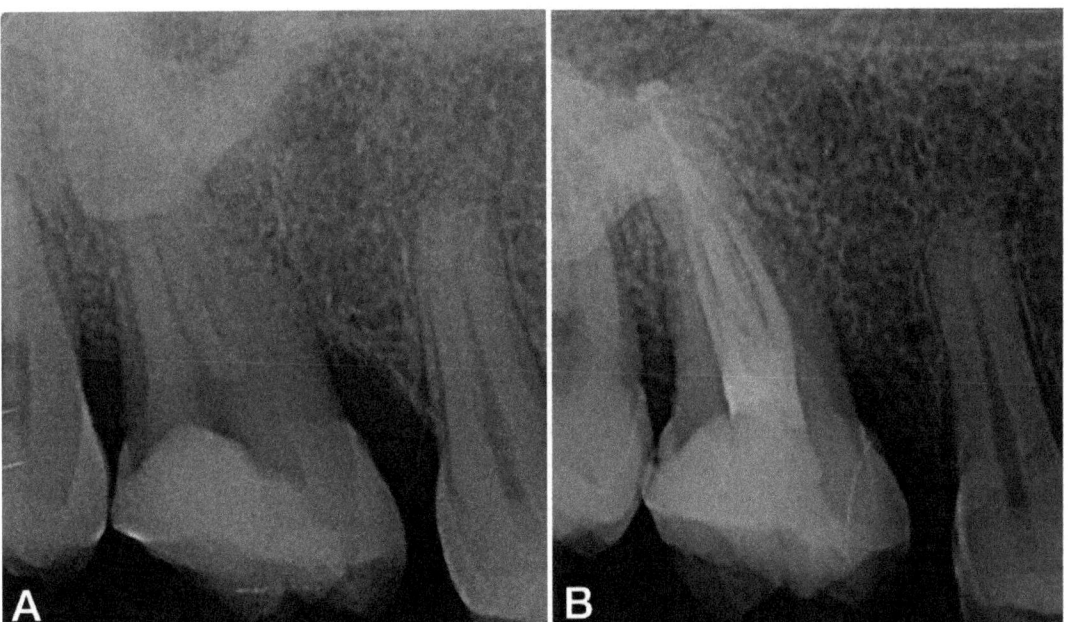

**Figure 4.** Example of indication of the single-cone technique with CSBS. (**A**) Preoperative periapical radiograph of a necrotic maxillary molar with long roots, sinus proximity, and patient's limited mouth opening. (**B**) Postoperative periapical radiograph of root canal obturation using CSBS.

### 3.3. Biological Aspects

As mentioned previously, their biological properties are the main advantages of CSBS over conventional sealers. A recent international survey showed that this has been claimed to be the most-frequent reason to justify their clinical use [22]. Based on the findings of in vitro studies, CSBS antibacterial activity and biomineralization ability might have the potential to stimulate and improve the periapical healing, and thus should be suitable in the case of apical periodontitis. Likewise, CSBS alkalization ability and calcium hydroxide formation might make them interesting to use in the case of external inflammatory root resorptions.

Finally, even if sealer extrusion in the periapical area is not suitable and should remain inadvertent, a sealer "puff" during obturation can be difficult to predict and control [125]. Taking into consideration better CSBS biological properties over the ones of conventional sealers highlighted in this narrative review, CSBS might be preferable to use in the following situations:

- Connection between the roots and the maxillary sinus, especially for immunocompromised patients for whom zinc oxide–eugenol-based and formaldehyde-based sealers are not recommended [22].
- Connection between the roots and inferior alveolar nerve: CSBS are more biocompatible, and their use with CHC avoids thermal nerve injuries.
- Middle or apical root canal perforations, consequences of a false canal: the use of CSBS with CHC allows the filling of the root canal and the perforation at the same time while also taking advantage of their biological properties.
- Patients with high risks of osteonecrosis connected to treatments such as radiotherapy or anti-resorptive drugs such as bisphosphonates, because it is suitable to reduce bone aggression factors in these situations.

However, it must be highlighted that regarding the biological aspects, a direct translation from the findings of in vitro studies to clinical outcome is not relevant. Indeed, the healing of the periapical area is not only related to the sealer's choice, but involves numerous complex mechanisms, including the patient's immune system [126].

## 4. Clinical Application of CSBS

### 4.1. Can CSBS Be Used with Any Type of Gutta-Percha?

Based on our review of the literature investigating the interface between gutta-percha and CSBS, there is no available evidence supporting the use of specific pre-impregnated gutta-percha cones with CSBS. However, a different interface quality between CSBS and the gutta-percha cone might be observed, depending on the type of gutta-percha and related chemical composition [22,57,127].

### 4.2. Do CSBS Usage Impact the Final Irrigation Protocol and the Root Canal Drying Technique?

Intracanal moisture negatively influences the setting process of conventional sealers and their adhesion to dentinal walls [128]. Unlike them, CSBS need water to initiate the hydration reaction that conditions their setting process, and also their biological properties [4]. According to the manufacturers, the dentinal tubules' moisture initiates the setting of premixed formulations [4]. Therefore, intracanal dentin desiccation should be avoided, leading to gently dry the root canal before obturation [129]. This procedure is difficult to control, as it was shown in restorative dentistry in a wet-bonding procedure [130]. The use of intracanal micro-suction to empty the canal before the use of one sterile paper point could help preventing over-dehydration [129]. On this basis, a final rinse with ethanol is contra-indicated when using CSBS [22,129].

Finally, since the canal has to remain slightly wet, potential interactions between the final irrigant and CSBS should be taken into account. Indeed, several studies showed that most of the available irrigants (NaOCl, CHX, EDTA) may negatively affect CSBS [52,84,131]. So far, the clinical significance of such interactions remains unclear. However, it seems suitable to perform a final rinse with sterile water to flush out the last irrigant before root canal drying.

### 4.3. How to Reduce Voids Occurrence When Using CSBS with CHC?

As mentioned previously, the presence of open porosity occurring at the interface between the sealer and dentinal wall/gutta-percha may constitute a space for residual micro-organisms to regrow and leak toward the periapical area [107,132].

SC obturation induces a higher void ratio compared to warm obturation techniques, especially in oval or wide root canals [103]. However, as reported in the literature, all the filling techniques investigated are never "void-free" regardless of the type of sealer used [133,134]. When dealing with CHC, especially the SC technique, more emphasis is put on the sealer than the gutta-percha (sealer-based obturation concept). Although the intracanal sealer placement technique might impact void incidence, the latter is rarely specified in most publications. Many techniques can be used to place CSBS into the root canal system, depending on the formulation and the anatomy:

- Coating the master cone with CSBS followed by its slow insertion to the full working length. This technique might be insufficient when dealing with oval or wide canals. Accessory cones can also be used to complete the sealer distribution.
- Lentulo spiral usage at low speed (around 700–800 rpm) or flexible injection tip before master cone insertion.

Applying sonic/ultrasonic activation and other sealer activation/agitation procedures may also contribute to improve CSBS distribution in the root canal space [135], but the level of evidence on these points is still weak.

### 4.4. Can CSBS Be Used with Thermoplasticized Gutta-Percha Obturation Techniques?

As stated previously, the SC technique being associated with greater void incidence, using CSBS with thermoplasticized gutta-percha obturation could make sense, as this would combine the advantages of these techniques already used by many endodontic specialists with the improved properties of CSBS. However, this leads us to question the impact of heat on CSBS' properties, which have been addressed in several studies showing different findings according to the formulations tested [25,37,136,137]. A temperature rise (especially above 100 °C) may lead to a change in CSBS' physical properties, especially their flowability, setting time, and adhesion to dentin walls [104,136]. Based on the available knowledge, Endosequence® BC Sealer™ HiFlow® and EndoSequence® BC Sealer™ formulations could be used with heat [104], but not all CSBS can. For instance, BioRoot™ RCS is contra-indicated with warm gutta-percha obturation [25,37]. Therefore, there is a need for additional studies to clarify the impact of heat on each CSBS formulation. These considerations should also take into account the real temperature delivered by the heater plugger, which has been reported to be much lower than the one displayed on the device screen [137]. Finally, conventional sealers have also been reported to be negatively impacted by heat application in laboratory studies [37], while they have been used widely for decades with thermoplasticized gutta-percha obturation techniques and with satisfactory clinical outcome. This points out the gap existing between the findings of in vitro studies and the complexity of parameters involved in the clinical outcome.

### 4.5. Does Use of CSBS Make Non-Surgical Retreatment More Difficult?

The literature showed that CSBS may be removed with difficulty in the case of retreatments [119]. No specific solvent is available for removing CSBS during retreatments, even if formic acid and chloroform may help the endodontist. As stated previously, studies assessing CSBS retreatability have shown that apical patency could be properly achieved when the obturation of the previous treatment reached the full working length [112,118,138,139]. Nevertheless, non-surgical retreatments are mainly indicated when the obturation is short. Good flowability of CSBS may result in CSBS penetration beyond the gutta-percha cone tip. The presence of CSBS only and its hardness may make apical patency much more challenging to achieve, especially in curved root canals [119] blocking the access to the apical third and resulting in possible procedural errors such as ledges. Furthermore, retreatments also aim to remove all previous materials and disinfect the root canal system before filling it again. Nevertheless, the complete removal of the obturation material remains impossible, and all the techniques shown in the literature were only able to partially remove CSBS from the root canal [114,117] as demonstrated with any filling material.

## 5. Conclusions

This narrative review aimed to discuss the properties of CSBS and their clinical implications, and to propose rational indications based on the current knowledge. This work may help practitioners in selecting the appropriate sealer and pave the way for reasoned CSBS usage. CSBS have shown good all-around performance when compared to conventional sealers, but significant differences could be observed between the different CSBS formulations. Their particularity remains in their interesting biological properties, which were proven to be better than those of conventional sealers. However, the clinical impact of CSBS solubility must be clarified in the future. Likewise, available CSBS formulations can present specificities that have to be considered by the practitioner for proper clinical usage. Finally, the usual clinical endodontic protocol has to be slightly revised to consider CSBS specific behavior.

**Author Contributions:** Conceptualization, G.S., F.B. and C.Z.; methodology, F.B., C.Z. and V.N.; validation, F.B., C.Z. and V.N.; literature search and data extraction, G.S., C.Z. and F.B.; writing—original draft preparation, G.S., F.B. and C.Z.; writing—review and editing, G.S., C.Z., S.P., T.G., V.N. and F.B.; supervision, C.Z. and F.B.; funding acquisition, G.S. and C.Z. All authors have read and agreed to the published version of the manuscript.

**Funding:** This research was funded by the University of Saint-Joseph, Beirut, Lebanon.

**Institutional Review Board Statement:** Not Applicable.

**Informed Consent Statement:** Not Applicable.

**Data Availability Statement:** No new data were created or analyzed in this study. Data sharing is not applicable to this article.

**Conflicts of Interest:** The authors have stated explicitly that there are no conflicts of interest in connection with this article.

## References

1. Ng, Y.-L.; Mann, V.; Rahbaran, S.; Lewsey, J.; Gulabivala, K. Outcome of primary root canal treatment: Systematic review of the literature—Part 2. Influence of clinical factors. *Int. Endod. J.* **2007**, *41*, 6–31. [CrossRef]
2. Rossi-Fedele, G.; Ahmed, H.M.A. Assessment of Root Canal Filling Removal Effectiveness Using Micro–computed Tomography: A Systematic Review. *J. Endod.* **2017**, *43*, 520–526. [CrossRef]
3. Zhou, H.; Shen, Y.; Zheng, W.; Li, L.; Zheng, Y.; Haapasalo, M. Physical Properties of 5 Root Canal Sealers. *J. Endod.* **2013**, *39*, 1281–1286. [CrossRef] [PubMed]
4. Silva Almeida, L.H.; Moraes, R.R.; Morgental, R.D.; Pappen, F.G. Are Premixed Calcium Silicate–based Endodontic Sealers Comparable to Conventional Materials? A Systematic Review of In Vitro Studies. *J. Endod.* **2017**, *43*, 527–535. [CrossRef] [PubMed]
5. Camilleri, J. Will Bioceramics be the Future Root Canal Filling Materials? *Curr. Oral Health Rep.* **2017**, *4*, 228–238. [CrossRef]
6. Lim, M.; Jung, C.; Shin, D.-H.; Cho, Y.-B.; Song, M. Calcium silicate-based root canal sealers: A literature review. *Restor. Dent. Endod.* **2020**, *45*, e35. [CrossRef] [PubMed]
7. Collado-González, M.; García-Bernal, D.; Oñate-Sánchez, R.E.; Ortolani-Seltenerich, P.S.; Lozano, A.; Forner, L.; Llena, C.; Rodríguez-Lozano, F.J. Biocompatibility of three new calcium silicate-based endodontic sealers on human periodontal ligament stem cells. *Int. Endod. J.* **2016**, *50*, 875–884. [CrossRef]
8. Mukhtar-Fayyad, D. Cytocompatibility of new bioceramic-based materials on human fibroblast cells (MRC-5). *Oral Surg. Oral Med. Oral Pathol. Oral Radiol. Endodontology* **2011**, *112*, e137–e142. [CrossRef]
9. Morgental, R.D.; Vier-Pelisser, F.V.; Oliveira, S.; Antunes, F.C.; Cogo, D.M.; Kopper, P.M.P. Antibacterial activity of two MTA-based root canal sealers. *Int. Endod. J.* **2011**, *44*, 1128–1133. [CrossRef] [PubMed]
10. Güven, E.P.; Taşlı, P.N.; Yalvac, M.E.; Sofiev, N.; Kayahan, M.B.; Sahin, F. In vitrocomparison of induction capacity and biomineralization ability of mineral trioxide aggregate and a bioceramic root canal sealer. *Int. Endod. J.* **2013**, *46*, 1173–1182. [CrossRef]
11. Singh, G.; Gupta, I.; ElShamy, F.M.M.; Boreak, N.; Homeida, H.E. In vitro comparison of antibacterial properties of bioceramic-based sealer, resin-based sealer and zinc oxide eugenol based sealer and two mineral trioxide aggregates. *Eur. J. Dent.* **2016**, *10*, 366–369. [CrossRef] [PubMed]
12. Camps, J.; Jeanneau, C.; El Ayachi, I.; Laurent, P.; About, I. Bioactivity of a Calcium Silicate–based Endodontic Cement (BioRoot RCS): Interactions with Human Periodontal Ligament Cells in Vitro. *J. Endod.* **2015**, *41*, 1469–1473. [CrossRef]
13. Khalil, I.; Naaman, A.; Camilleri, J. Properties of Tricalcium Silicate Sealers. *J. Endod.* **2016**, *42*, 1529–1535. [CrossRef]

14. Zamparini, F.; Siboni, F.; Prati, C.; Taddei, P.; Gandolfi, M.G. Properties of calcium silicate-monobasic calcium phosphate materials for endodontics containing tantalum pentoxide and zirconium oxide. *Clin. Oral Investig.* **2019**, *23*, 445–457. [CrossRef] [PubMed]
15. Borges, R.P.; Sousa-Neto, M.D.; Versiani, M.A.; Rached-Junior, F.A.; De-Deus, G.; Miranda, C.E.S.; Pécora, J.D. Changes in the surface of four calcium silicate-containing endodontic materials and an epoxy resin-based sealer after a solubility test. *Int. Endod. J.* **2011**, *45*, 419–428. [CrossRef] [PubMed]
16. Da Silva, E.J.N.L.; Zaia, A.A.; Peters, O.A. Cytocompatibility of calcium silicate-based sealers in a three-dimensional cell culture model. *Clin. Oral Investig.* **2016**, *21*, 1531–1536. [CrossRef]
17. Vouzara, T.; Dimosiari, G.; Koulaouzidou, E.A.; Economides, N. Cytotoxicity of a New Calcium Silicate Endodontic Sealer. *J. Endod.* **2018**, *44*, 849–852. [CrossRef]
18. Xuereb, M.; Vella, P.; Damidot, D.; Sammut, C.V.; Camilleri, J. In Situ Assessment of the Setting of Tricalcium Silicate–based Sealers Using a Dentin Pressure Model. *J. Endod.* **2015**, *41*, 111–124. [CrossRef]
19. Chybowski, E.A.; Glickman, G.N.; Patel, Y.; Fleury, A.; Solomon, E.; He, J. Clinical Outcome of Non-Surgical Root Canal Treatment Using a Single-cone Technique with Endosequence Bioceramic Sealer: A Retrospective Analysis. *J. Endod.* **2018**, *44*, 941–945. [CrossRef]
20. Bardini, G.; Casula, L.; Ambu, E.; Musu, D.; Mercadè, M.; Cotti, E. A 12-month follow-up of primary and secondary root canal treatment in teeth obturated with a hydraulic sealer. *Clin. Oral Investig.* **2021**, *25*, 2757–2764. [CrossRef] [PubMed]
21. Zavattini, A.; Knight, A.; Foschi, F.; Mannocci, F. Outcome of Root Canal Treatments Using a New Calcium Silicate Root Canal Sealer: A Non-Randomized Clinical Trial. *J. Clin. Med.* **2020**, *9*, 782. [CrossRef]
22. Guivarc'H, M.; Jeanneau, C.; Giraud, T.; Pommel, L.; About, I.; Azim, A.A.; Bukiet, F. An international survey on the use of calcium silicate-based sealers in non-surgical endodontic treatment. *Clin. Oral Investig.* **2020**, *24*, 417–424. [CrossRef]
23. Eliaz, N.; Metoki, N. Calcium Phosphate Bioceramics: A Review of Their History, Structure, Properties, Coating Technologies and Biomedical Applications. *Materials* **2017**, *10*, 334. [CrossRef] [PubMed]
24. Prati, C.; Gandolfi, M.G. Calcium silicate bioactive cements: Biological perspectives and clinical applications. *Dent. Mater.* **2015**, *31*, 351–370. [CrossRef] [PubMed]
25. Camilleri, J. Sealers and Warm Gutta-percha Obturation Techniques. *J. Endod.* **2015**, *41*, 72–78. [CrossRef] [PubMed]
26. Torres, F.F.E.; Zordan-Bronzel, C.L.; Guerreiro-Tanomaru, J.M.; Chávez-Andrade, G.M.; Pinto, J.C.; Tanomaru-Filho, M. Effect of immersion in distilled water or phosphate-buffered saline on the solubility, volumetric change and presence of voids within new calcium silicate-based root canal sealers. *Int. Endod. J.* **2020**, *53*, 385–391. [CrossRef]
27. Tanomaru-Filho, M.; Torres, F.F.E.; Chávez-Andrade, G.M.; de Almeida, M.; Navarro, L.G.; Steier, L.; Guerreiro-Tanomaru, J.M. Physicochemical Properties and Volumetric Change of Silicone/Bioactive Glass and Calcium Silicate–based Endodontic Sealers. *J. Endod.* **2017**, *43*, 2097–2101. [CrossRef]
28. Koutroulis, A.; Kuehne, S.A.; Cooper, P.R.; Camilleri, J. The role of calcium ion release on biocompatibility and antimicrobial properties of hydraulic cements. *Sci. Rep.* **2019**, *9*, 1–10. [CrossRef]
29. ANSI/ADA. *Specification N° 57 Endodontic Sealing Materials Reaffirmed 2012*; ADA: Chicago, IL, USA, 2000.
30. ISO. ISO 6876. In *Dental Root Canal Sealing Materials, International Standard ISO 6876:2012*, 3rd ed.; ISO: Geneva, Switzerland, 2012.
31. Mendes, A.T.; Da Silva, P.B.; Só, B.B.; Hashizume, L.N.; Vivan, R.R.; Da Rosa, R.A.; Duarte, M.A.H.; Só, M.V.R. Evaluation of Physicochemical Properties of New Calcium Silicate-Based Sealer. *Braz. Dent. J.* **2018**, *29*, 536–540. [CrossRef] [PubMed]
32. Zordan-Bronzel, C.L.; Esteves Torres, F.F.; Tanomaru-Filho, M.; Chávez-Andrade, G.M.; Bosso-Martelo, R.; Guerreiro-Tanomaru, J.M. Evaluation of Physicochemical Properties of a New Calcium Silicate–based Sealer, Bio-C Sealer. *J. Endod.* **2019**, *45*, 1248–1252. [CrossRef]
33. Al-Haddad, A.; Che Ab Aziz, Z.A. Bioceramic-Based Root Canal Sealers: A Review. *Int. J. Biomater.* **2016**, *2016*, 97532. [CrossRef] [PubMed]
34. Prüllage, R.-K.; Urban, K.; Schäfer, E.; Dammaschke, T. Material Properties of a Tricalcium Silicate–containing, a Mineral Trioxide Aggregate–containing, and an Epoxy Resin–based Root Canal Sealer. *J. Endod.* **2016**, *42*, 1784–1788. [CrossRef]
35. Kebudi Benezra, M.; Schembri Wismayer, P.; Camilleri, J. Interfacial Characteristics and Cytocompatibility of Hydraulic Sealer Cements. *J. Endod.* **2018**, *44*, 1007–1017. [CrossRef] [PubMed]
36. Chen, B.; Haapasalo, M.; Mobuchon, C.; Li, X.; Ma, J.; Shen, Y. Cytotoxicity and the Effect of Temperature on Physical Properties and Chemical Composition of a New Calcium Silicate–based Root Canal Sealer. *J. Endod.* **2020**, *46*, 531–538. [CrossRef]
37. Aksel, H.; Makowka, S.; Bosaid, F.; Guardian, M.G.; Sarkar, D.; Azim, A.A. Effect of heat application on the physical properties and chemical structure of calcium silicate-based sealers. *Clin. Oral Investig.* **2021**, *25*, 2717–2725. [CrossRef] [PubMed]
38. Torabinejad, M.; Parirokh, M.; Dummer, P.M.H. Mineral trioxide aggregate and other bioactive endodontic cements: An updated overview—Part II: Other clinical applications and complications. *Int. Endod. J.* **2018**, *51*, 284–317. [CrossRef] [PubMed]
39. Lee, J.K.; Kwak, S.W.; Ha, J.-H.; Lee, W.; Kim, H.-C. Physicochemical Properties of Epoxy Resin-Based and Bioceramic-Based Root Canal Sealers. *Bioinorg. Chem. Appl.* **2017**, *2017*, 1–8. [CrossRef]
40. Candeiro, G.T.d.M.; Correia, F.C.; Duarte, M.A.H.; Ribeiro-Siqueira, D.C.; Gavini, G. Evaluation of Radiopacity, pH, Release of Calcium Ions, and Flow of a Bioceramic Root Canal Sealer. *J. Endod.* **2012**, *38*, 842–845. [CrossRef]
41. Heran, J.; Khalid, S.; Albaaj, F.; Tomson, P.L.; Camilleri, J. The single cone obturation technique with a modified warm filler. *J. Dent.* **2019**, *89*, 103181. [CrossRef]

42. Ha, J.-H.; Kim, H.-C.; Kim, Y.K.; Kwon, T.-Y. An Evaluation of Wetting and Adhesion of Three Bioceramic Root Canal Sealers to Intraradicular Human Dentin. *Materials* **2018**, *11*, 1286. [CrossRef]
43. Mulay, S.; Ajmera, K.; Jain, H. The wetting ability of root canal sealers after using various irrigants. *J. Orofac. Sci.* **2017**, *9*, 95. [CrossRef]
44. Trope, M.; Bunes, A.; Debelian, G. Root Filling Materials and Techniques: Bioceramics a New Hope? *Endod. Top.* **2015**, *32*, 86–96. [CrossRef]
45. Georgopoulou, M.K.; Wu, M.-K.; Nikolaou, A.; Wesselink, P.R. Effect of thickness on the sealing ability of some root canal sealers. *Oral Surg. Oral Med. Oral Pathol. Oral Radiol. Endodontol.* **1995**, *80*, 338–344. [CrossRef]
46. De-Deus, G.; Gurgel-Filho, E.D.; Magalhães, K.M.; Coutinho-Filho, T. A laboratory analysis of gutta-percha-filled area obtained using Thermafil, System B and lateral condensation. *Int. Endod. J.* **2006**, *39*, 378–383. [CrossRef] [PubMed]
47. Marashdeh, M.Q.; Friedman, S.; Lévesque, C.; Finer, Y. Esterases affect the physical properties of materials used to seal the endodontic space. *Dent. Mater.* **2019**, *35*, 1065–1072. [CrossRef]
48. Poggio, C.; Dagna, A.; Ceci, M.; Meravini, M.-V.; Colombo, M.; Pietrocola, G. Solubility and pH of bioceramic root canal sealers: A comparative study. *J. Clin. Exp. Dent.* **2017**, *9*, e1189–e1194. [CrossRef] [PubMed]
49. Donnermeyer, D.; Bürklein, S.; Dammaschke, T.; Schäfer, E. Endodontic sealers based on calcium silicates: A systematic review. *Odontology* **2019**, *107*, 421–436. [CrossRef] [PubMed]
50. Pane, E.S.; Palamara, J.E.A.; Messer, H.H. Critical Evaluation of the Push-out Test for Root Canal Filling Materials. *J. Endod.* **2013**, *39*, 669–673. [CrossRef]
51. Oliveira, D.S.; Cardoso, M.L.; Queiroz, T.F.; Silva, E.J.N.L.; Souza, E.M.; Dedeus, G. Suboptimal push-out bond strengths of calcium silicate-based sealers. *Int. Endod. J.* **2016**, *49*, 796–801. [CrossRef]
52. Donnermeyer, D.; Dornseifer, P.; Schäfer, E.; Dammaschke, T. The push-out bond strength of calcium silicate-based endodontic sealers. *Head Face Med.* **2018**, *14*, 13. [CrossRef]
53. Carvalho, N.K.; Prado, M.C.; Senna, P.M.; Neves, A.A.; Souza, E.M.; Fidel, S.R.; Sassone, L.M.; Silva, E.J.N.L. Do smear-layer removal agents affect the push-out bond strength of calcium silicate-based endodontic sealers? *Int. Endod. J.* **2017**, *50*, 612–619. [CrossRef]
54. Tuncel, B.; Nagas, E.; Cehreli, Z.; Uyanik, O.; Vallittu, P.; Lassila, L. Effect of endodontic chelating solutions on the bond strength of endodontic sealers. *Braz. Oral Res.* **2015**, *29*, 1–6. [CrossRef]
55. Shokouhinejad, N.; Gorjestani, H.; Nasseh, A.A.; Hoseini, A.; Mohammadi, M.; Shamshiri, A.R. Push-out bond strength of gutta-percha with a new bioceramic sealer in the presence or absence of smear layer. *Aust. Endod. J.* **2013**, *39*, 102–106. [CrossRef] [PubMed]
56. DeLong, C.; He, J.; Woodmansey, K.F. The Effect of Obturation Technique on the Push-out Bond Strength of Calcium Silicate Sealers. *J. Endod.* **2015**, *41*, 385–388. [CrossRef] [PubMed]
57. Eltair, M.; Pitchika, V.; Hickel, R.; Kühnisch, J.; Diegritz, C. Evaluation of the interface between gutta-percha and two types of sealers using scanning electron microscopy (SEM). *Clin. Oral Investig.* **2018**, *22*, 1631–1639. [CrossRef] [PubMed]
58. Valois, C.R.; Silva, L.P.; Azevedo, R.B. Structural Effects of Sodium Hypochlorite Solutions on Gutta-Percha Cones: Atomic Force Microscopy Study. *J. Endod.* **2005**, *31*, 749–751. [CrossRef]
59. Yang, D.-K.; Kim, S.; Park, J.-W.; Kim, E.; Shin, S.-J. Different Setting Conditions Affect Surface Characteristics and Microhardness of Calcium Silicate-Based Sealers. *Scanning* **2018**, *2018*, 7136345. [CrossRef] [PubMed]
60. Chang, S.W. Chemical Composition and Porosity Characteristics of Various Calcium Silicate-Based Endodontic Cements. *Bioinorg. Chem. Appl.* **2018**, *2018*, 278432. [CrossRef]
61. Parirokh, M.; Torabinejad, M. Mineral Trioxide Aggregate: A Comprehensive Literature Review—Part I: Chemical, Physical, and Antibacterial Properties. *J. Endod.* **2010**, *36*, 16–27. [CrossRef]
62. Jafari, F.; Jafari, S. Composition and physicochemical properties of calcium silicate based sealers: A review article. *J. Clin. Exp. Dent.* **2017**, *9*, e1249–e1255. [CrossRef]
63. An, S.; Gao, Y.; Huang, Y.; Jiang, X.; Ma, K.; Ling, J. Short-term effects of calcium ions on the apoptosis and onset of mineralization of human dental pulp cells in vitro and in vivo. *Int. J. Mol. Med.* **2015**, *36*, 215–221. [CrossRef]
64. Han, P.; Wu, C.; Xiao, Y. The effect of silicate ions on proliferation, osteogenic differentiation and cell signalling pathways (WNT and SHH) of bone marrow stromal cells. *Biomater. Sci.* **2013**, *1*, 379–392. [CrossRef]
65. Shi, M.; Zhou, Y.; Shao, J.; Chen, Z.; Song, B.; Chang, J.; Wu, C.; Xiao, Y. Stimulation of osteogenesis and angiogenesis of hBMSCs by delivering Si ions and functional drug from mesoporous silica nanospheres. *Acta Biomater.* **2015**, *21*, 178–189. [CrossRef] [PubMed]
66. ISO. ISO. ISO 10993-1. In *Biological Evaluation of Medical Devices—Part 1: Evaluation and Testing within a Risk Management Process, International ISO 10993-1:2018*, 5th ed.; ISO: Geneva, Switzerland, 2018.
67. Eldeniz, A.U.; Shehata, M.; Hogg, C.; Reichl, F.X.; Rothmund, L. DNA double-strand breaks caused by new and contemporary endodontic sealers. *Int. Endod. J.* **2015**, *49*, 1141–1151. [CrossRef]
68. Nair, R.R.; Nayak, M.; Prasada, L.K.; Shetty, V.; Kumar, C.N.V.; Nair, A.V. Comparative Evaluation of Cytotoxicity and Genotoxicity of Two Bioceramic Sealers on Fibroblast Cell Line: An in vitro Study. *J. Contemp. Dent. Pract.* **2018**, *19*, 656–661. [CrossRef] [PubMed]

69. Candeiro, G.T.M.; Moura-Netto, C.; D'Almeida-Couto, R.S.; Azambuja-Júnior, N.; Marques, M.M.; Cai, S.; Gavini, G. Cytotoxicity, genotoxicity and antibacterial effectiveness of a bioceramic endodontic sealer. *Int. Endod. J.* **2016**, *49*, 858–864. [CrossRef]
70. Bin, C.V.; Valera, M.C.; Camargo, S.E.A.; Rabelo, S.B.; Silva, G.O.; Balducci, I.; Camargo, C.H.R. Cytotoxicity and Genotoxicity of Root Canal Sealers Based on Mineral Trioxide Aggregate. *J. Endod.* **2012**, *38*, 495–500. [CrossRef] [PubMed]
71. Jung, S.; Libricht, V.; Sielker, S.; Hanisch, M.R.; Schäfer, E.; Dammaschke, T. Evaluation of the biocompatibility of root canal sealers on human periodontal ligament cells ex vivo. *Odontology* **2018**, *107*, 54–63. [CrossRef] [PubMed]
72. Zhou, H.; Du, T.; Shen, Y.; Wang, Z.; Zheng, Y.; Haapasalo, M. In Vitro Cytotoxicity of Calcium Silicate–containing Endodontic Sealers. *J. Endod.* **2015**, *41*, 56–61. [CrossRef]
73. Jeanneau, C.; Giraud, T.; Laurent, P.; About, I. BioRoot RCS Extracts Modulate the Early Mechanisms of Periodontal Inflammation and Regeneration. *J. Endod.* **2019**, *45*, 1016–1023. [CrossRef]
74. Giacomino, C.M.; Wealleans, J.A.; Kuhn, N.; Diogenes, A. Comparative Biocompatibility and Osteogenic Potential of Two Bioceramic Sealers. *J. Endod.* **2019**, *45*, 51–56. [CrossRef] [PubMed]
75. Collado-González, M.; Tomás-Catalá, C.J.; Oñate-Sánchez, R.E.; Moraleda, J.M.; Rodríguez-Lozano, F.J. Cytotoxicity of GuttaFlow Bioseal, GuttaFlow2, MTA Fillapex, and AH Plus on Human Periodontal Ligament Stem Cells. *J. Endod.* **2017**, *43*, 816–822. [CrossRef]
76. Rodríguez-Lozano, F.J.; García-Bernal, D.; Oñate-Sánchez, R.E.; Ortolani-Seltenerich, P.S.; Forner, L.; Moraleda, J.M. Evaluation of cytocompatibility of calcium silicate-based endodontic sealers and their effects on the biological responses of mesenchymal dental stem cells. *Int. Endod. J.* **2017**, *50*, 67–76. [CrossRef] [PubMed]
77. Rodríguez-Lozano, F.J.; López-García, S.; García-Bernal, D.; Tomás-Catalá, C.J.; Santos, J.M.; Llena, C.; Lozano, A.; Murcia, L.; Forner, L. Chemical composition and bioactivity potential of the new Endosequence BC Sealer formulation HiFlow. *Int. Endod. J.* **2020**, *53*, 1216–1228. [CrossRef] [PubMed]
78. Siboni, F.; Taddei, P.; Zamparini, F.; Prati, C.; Gandolfi, M.G. Properties of BioRoot RCS, a tricalcium silicate endodontic sealer modified with povidone and polycarboxylate. *Int. Endod. J.* **2017**, *50* (Suppl. 2), e120–e136. [CrossRef]
79. Urban, K.; Neuhaus, J.; Donnermeyer, D.; Schäfer, E.; Dammaschke, T. Solubility and pH Value of 3 Different Root Canal Sealers: A Long-term Investigation. *J. Endod.* **2018**, *44*, 1736–1740. [CrossRef]
80. Zordan-Bronzel, C.L.; Tanomaru-Filho, M.; Rodrigues, E.M.; Chávez-Andrade, G.M.; Faria, G.; Guerreiro-Tanomaru, J.M. Cytocompatibility, bioactive potential and antimicrobial activity of an experimental calcium silicate-based endodontic sealer. *Int. Endod. J.* **2019**, *52*, 979–986. [CrossRef]
81. Zhang, H.; Shen, Y.; Ruse, N.D.; Haapasalo, M. Antibacterial Activity of Endodontic Sealers by Modified Direct Contact Test Against Enterococcus faecalis. *J. Endod.* **2009**, *35*, 1051–1055. [CrossRef]
82. Kapralos, V.; Koutroulis, A.; Ørstavik, D.; Sunde, P.T.; Rukke, H.V. Antibacterial Activity of Endodontic Sealers against Planktonic Bacteria and Bacteria in Biofilms. *J. Endod.* **2018**, *44*, 149–154. [CrossRef]
83. Bukhari, S.; Karabucak, B. The Antimicrobial Effect of Bioceramic Sealer on an 8-week Matured Enterococcus faecalis Biofilm Attached to Root Canal Dentinal Surface. *J. Endod.* **2019**, *45*, 1047–1052. [CrossRef]
84. Arias-Moliz, M.T.; Camilleri, J. The effect of the final irrigant on the antimicrobial activity of root canal sealers. *J. Dent.* **2016**, *52*, 30–36. [CrossRef]
85. Camilleri, J.; Arias Moliz, T.; Bettencourt, A.; Costa, J.; Martins, F.; Rabadijeva, D.; Rodriguez, D.; Visai, L.; Combes, C.; Farrugia, C.; et al. Standardization of antimicrobial testing of dental devices. *Dent. Mater.* **2020**, *36*, e59–e73. [CrossRef] [PubMed]
86. Jung, S.; Sielker, S.; Hanisch, M.R.; Libricht, V.; Schäfer, E.; Dammaschke, T. Cytotoxic effects of four different root canal sealers on human osteoblasts. *PLoS ONE* **2018**, *13*, e0194467. [CrossRef] [PubMed]
87. Lee, B.-N.; Hong, J.-U.; Kim, S.-M.; Jang, J.-H.; Chang, H.-S.; Hwang, Y.-C.; Hwang, I.-N.; Oh, W.-M. Anti-inflammatory and Osteogenic Effects of Calcium Silicate–based Root Canal Sealers. *J. Endod.* **2019**, *45*, 73–78. [CrossRef]
88. Yuan, Z.; Zhu, X.; Li, Y.; Yan, P.; Jiang, H. Influence of iRoot SP and mineral trioxide aggregate on the activation and polarization of macrophages induced by lipopolysaccharide. *BMC Oral Health* **2018**, *18*, 56. [CrossRef] [PubMed]
89. Zhu, X.; Yuan, Z.; Yan, P.; Li, Y.; Jiang, H.; Huang, S. Effect of iRoot SP and mineral trioxide aggregate (MTA) on the viability and polarization of macrophages. *Arch. Oral Biol.* **2017**, *80*, 27–33. [CrossRef] [PubMed]
90. Yunna, C.; Mengru, H.; Lei, W.; Weidong, C. Macrophage M1/M2 polarization. *Eur. J. Pharmacol.* **2020**, *877*, 173090. [CrossRef]
91. Assmann, E.; Böttcher, D.E.; Hoppe, C.B.; Grecca, F.S.; Kopper, P.M.P. Evaluation of Bone Tissue Response to a Sealer Containing Mineral Trioxide Aggregate. *J. Endod.* **2015**, *41*, 62–66. [CrossRef]
92. Tavares, C.O.; Böttcher, D.E.; Assmann, E.; Kopper, P.M.P.; De Figueiredo, J.A.P.; Grecca, F.S.; Scarparo, R.K. Tissue Reactions to a New Mineral Trioxide Aggregate–containing Endodontic Sealer. *J. Endod.* **2013**, *39*, 653–657. [CrossRef] [PubMed]
93. Sundqvist, G.; Figdor, D.; Persson, S.; Sjögren, U. Microbiologic analysis of teeth with failed endodontic treatment and the outcome of conservative re-treatment. *Oral Surg. Oral Med. Oral Pathol. Oral Radiol. Endodontology* **1998**, *85*, 86–93. [CrossRef]
94. Adib, V.; Spratt, D.; Ng, Y.-L.; Gulabivala, K. Cultivable microbial flora associated with persistent periapical disease and coronal leakage after root canal treatment: A preliminary study. *Int. Endod. J.* **2004**, *37*, 542–551. [CrossRef]
95. Yanpiset, K.; Banomyong, D.; Chotvorrarak, K.; Srisatjaluk, R.L. Bacterial leakage and micro-computed tomography evaluation in round-shaped canals obturated with bioceramic cone and sealer using matched single cone technique. *Restor. Dent. Endod.* **2018**, *43*, 30. [CrossRef] [PubMed]

96. Brosco, V.H.; Bernardineli, N.; Torres, S.A.; Consolaro, A.; Bramante, C.M.; de Moraes, I.G.; Ordinola-Zapata, R.; Garcia, R.B. Bacterial leakage in obturated root canals—Part 2: A comparative histologic and microbiologic analyses. *Oral Surg. Oral Med. Oral Pathol. Oral Radiol. Endodontology* **2010**, *109*, 788–794. [CrossRef]
97. Tabassum, S.; Khan, F.R. Failure of endodontic treatment: The usual suspects. *Eur. J. Dent.* **2016**, *10*, 144–147. [CrossRef] [PubMed]
98. Mohamed El Sayed, M.A.A.; Al Husseini, H. Apical dye leakage of two single-cone root canal core materials (hydrophilic core material and gutta-percha) sealed by different types of endodontic sealers: An in vitro study. *J. Conserv. Dent.* **2018**, *21*, 147–152. [CrossRef]
99. Wu, M.-K.; De Gee, A.J.; Wesselink, P.R. Leakage of four root canal sealers at different thicknesses. *Int. Endod. J.* **1994**, *27*, 304–308. [CrossRef]
100. Ballullaya, S.V.; Vinay, V.; Thumu, J.; Devalla, S.; Bollu, I.P.; Balla, S. Stereomicroscopic Dye Leakage Measurement of Six Different Root Canal Sealers. *J. Clin. Diagn. Res.* **2017**, *11*, ZC65–ZC68. [CrossRef]
101. Santos-Junior, A.O.; Tanomaru-Filho, M.; Pinto, J.C.; Tavares, K.I.M.C.; Torres, F.F.E.; Guerreiro-Tanomaru, J.M. Effect of obturation technique using a new bioceramic sealer on the presence of voids in flattened root canals. *Braz. Oral Res.* **2021**, *35*, e028. [CrossRef] [PubMed]
102. da Silva, P.J.P.; Marceliano-Alves, M.F.; Provenzano, J.C.; Dellazari, R.L.A.; Gonçalves, L.S.; Alves, F.R.F. Quality of Root Canal Filling Using a Bioceramic Sealer in Oval Canals: A Three-Dimensional Analysis. *Eur. J. Dent.* **2021**. [CrossRef]
103. Mancino, D.; Kharouf, N.; Cabiddu, M.; Bukiet, F.; Haïkel, Y. Microscopic and chemical evaluation of the filling quality of five obturation techniques in oval-shaped root canals. *Clin. Oral Investig.* **2021**, *25*, 3757–3765. [CrossRef]
104. Eid, D.; Medioni, E.; De-Deus, G.; Khalil, I.; Naaman, A.; Zogheib, C. Impact of Warm Vertical Compaction on the Sealing Ability of Calcium Silicate-Based Sealers: A Confocal Microscopic Evaluation. *Materials* **2021**, *14*, 372. [CrossRef]
105. Celikten, B.; Uzuntas, C.F.; Orhan, A.I.; Tufenkci, P.; Misirli, M.; Demiralp, K.O.; Orhan, K. Micro-CT assessment of the sealing ability of three root canal filling techniques. *J. Oral Sci.* **2015**, *57*, 361–366. [CrossRef] [PubMed]
106. Germain, S.; Meetu, K.; Issam, K.; Alfred, N.; Carla, Z. Impact of the Root Canal Taper on the Apical Adaptability of Sealers used in a Single-cone Technique: A Micro-computed Tomography Study. *J. Contemp. Dent. Pract.* **2018**, *19*, 808–815. [CrossRef] [PubMed]
107. Milanovic, I.; Milovanovic, P.; Antonijevic, D.; Dzeletovic, B.; Djuric, M.; Miletic, V. Immediate and Long-Term Porosity of Calcium Silicate–Based Sealers. *J. Endod.* **2020**, *46*, 515–523. [CrossRef] [PubMed]
108. Celikten, B.; Uzuntas, C.F.; Orhan, A.I.; Orhan, K.; Tufenkci, P.; Kursun, S.; Demiralp, K.Ö. Evaluation of root canal sealer filling quality using a single-cone technique in oval shaped canals: An In vitro Micro-CT study. *Scanning* **2016**, *38*, 133–140. [CrossRef]
109. Roizenblit, R.N.; Soares, F.O.; Lopes, R.T.; Dos Santos, B.C.; Gusman, H. Root canal filling quality of mandibular molars with EndoSequence BC and AH Plus sealers: A micro-CT study. *Aust. Endod. J.* **2020**, *46*, 82–87. [CrossRef]
110. Uzunoglu, E.; Yilmaz, Z.; Sungur, D.D.; Altundasar, E. Retreatability of Root Canals Obturated Using Gutta-Percha with Bioceramic, MTA and Resin-Based Sealers. *Iran. Endod. J.* **2015**, *10*, 93–98.
111. Yürüker, S.; Gorduysus, M.; Küçükkaya, S.; Uzunoglu, E.; Ilgın, C.; Gülen, O.; Tuncel, B.; Gördüysus, M.Ö. Efficacy of Combined Use of Different Nickel-Titanium Files on Removing Root Canal Filling Materials. *J. Endod.* **2016**, *42*, 487–492. [CrossRef]
112. Donnermeyer, D.; Bunne, C.; Schäfer, E.; Dammaschke, T. Retreatability of three calcium silicate-containing sealers and one epoxy resin-based root canal sealer with four different root canal instruments. *Clin. Oral Investig.* **2018**, *22*, 811–817. [CrossRef]
113. Agrafioti, A.; Koursoumis, A.D.; Kontakiotis, E.G. Re-establishing apical patency after obturation with Gutta-percha and two novel calcium silicate-based sealers. *Eur. J. Dent.* **2015**, *9*, 457–461. [CrossRef]
114. Kim, H.; Kim, E.; Lee, S.-J.; Shin, S.-J. Comparisons of the Retreatment Efficacy of Calcium Silicate and Epoxy Resin–based Sealers and Residual Sealer in Dentinal Tubules. *J. Endod.* **2015**, *41*, 2025–2030. [CrossRef]
115. Madani, Z.S.; Simdar, N.; Moudi, E.; Bijani, A. CBCT Evaluation of the Root Canal Filling Removal Using D-RaCe, ProTaper Retreatment Kit and Hand Files in Curved Canals. *Iran. Endod. J.* **2015**, *10*, 69–74.
116. Simsek, N.; Keles, A.; Ahmetoglu, F.; Ocak, M.S.; Yologlu, S. Comparison of different retreatment techniques and root canal sealers: A scanning electron microscopic study. *Braz. Oral Res.* **2014**, *28*, 1–7. [CrossRef] [PubMed]
117. Suk, M.; Bago, I.; Katić, M.; Snjaric, D.; Munitić, M.Š.; Anić, I. The efficacy of photon-initiated photoacoustic streaming in the removal of calcium silicate-based filling remnants from the root canal after rotary retreatment. *Lasers Med. Sci.* **2017**, *32*, 2055–2062. [CrossRef] [PubMed]
118. Ersev, H.; Yılmaz, B.; Dinçol, M.E.; Dağlaroğlu, R. The efficacy of ProTaper Universal rotary retreatment instrumentation to remove single gutta-percha cones cemented with several endodontic sealers. *Int. Endod. J.* **2012**, *45*, 756–762. [CrossRef] [PubMed]
119. Hess, D.; Solomon, E.; Spears, R.; He, J. Retreatability of a Bioceramic Root Canal Sealing Material. *J. Endod.* **2011**, *37*, 1547–1549. [CrossRef] [PubMed]
120. Oltra, E.; Cox, T.C.; LaCourse, M.R.; Johnson, J.D.; Paranjpe, A. Retreatability of two endodontic sealers, EndoSequence BC Sealer and AH Plus: A micro-computed tomographic comparison. *Restor. Dent. Endod.* **2017**, *42*, 19–26. [CrossRef]
121. Peciuliene, V.; Rimkuviene, J.; Maneliene, R.; Ivanauskaite, D. Apical periodontitis in root filled teeth associated with the quality of root fillings. *Stomatologija* **2006**, *8*, 122–126.
122. Hirai, V.H.G.; Machado, R.; Budziak, M.C.L.; Piasecki, L.; Kowalczuck, A.; Neto, U.X.D.S. Percentage of Gutta-Percha-, Sealer-, and Void-Filled Areas in Oval-Shaped Root Canals Obturated with Different Filling Techniques: A Confocal Laser Scanning Microscopy Study. *Eur. J. Dent.* **2020**, *14*, 8–12. [CrossRef]

123. Keleş, A.; Alcin, H.; Kamalak, A.; Versiani, M.A. Micro-CT evaluation of root filling quality in oval-shaped canals. *Int. Endod. J.* **2014**, *47*, 1177–1184. [CrossRef]
124. Venturi, M.; Pasquantonio, G.; Falconi, M.; Breschi, L. Temperature change within gutta-percha induced by the System-B Heat Source. *Int. Endod. J.* **2002**, *35*, 740–746. [CrossRef] [PubMed]
125. Scarparo, R.K.; Grecca, F.S.; Fachin, E.V.F. Analysis of Tissue Reactions to Methacrylate Resin-based, Epoxy Resin-based, and Zinc Oxide–Eugenol Endodontic Sealers. *J. Endod.* **2009**, *35*, 229–232. [CrossRef] [PubMed]
126. Holland, R.; Gomes, J.E.; Cintra, L.T.A.; Queiroz, Í.O.D.A.; Estrela, C. Factors affecting the periapical healing process of endodontically treated teeth. *J. Appl. Oral Sci.* **2017**, *25*, 465–476. [CrossRef] [PubMed]
127. De-Deus, G.; Oliveira, D.S.; Cavalcante, D.M.; Simões-Carvalho, M.; Belladonna, F.G.; Antunes, L.S.; Souza, E.; Silva, E.J.N.L.; Versiani, M. Methodological proposal for evaluation of adhesion of root canal sealers to gutta-percha. *Int. Endod. J.* **2021**. [CrossRef] [PubMed]
128. Zmener, O.; Pameijer, C.H.; Serrano, S.A.; Vidueira, M.; Macchi, R.L. Significance of Moist Root Canal Dentin with the Use of Methacrylate-based Endodontic Sealers: An In Vitro Coronal Dye Leakage Study. *J. Endod.* **2008**, *34*, 76–79. [CrossRef]
129. Nagas, E.; Uyanik, M.O.; Eymirli, A.; Cehreli, Z.C.; Vallittu, P.K.; Lassila, L.V.J.; Durmaz, V. Dentin Moisture Conditions Affect the Adhesion of Root Canal Sealers. *J. Endod.* **2012**, *38*, 240–244. [CrossRef]
130. Kanca, J. Improving Bond Strength Through Acid Etching of Dentin and Bonding to Wet Dentin Surfaces. *J. Am. Dent. Assoc.* **1992**, *123*, 35–43. [CrossRef]
131. Razmi, H.; Bolhari, B.; Karamzadeh Dashti, N.; Fazlyab, M. The Effect of Canal Dryness on Bond Strength of Bioceramic and Epoxy-resin Sealers after Irrigation with Sodium Hypochlorite or Chlorhexidine. *Iran. Endod. J.* **2016**, *11*, 129–133. [CrossRef]
132. Ortiz, F.G.; Jimeno, E.B. Analysis of the porosity of endodontic sealers through micro-computed tomography: A systematic review. *J. Conserv. Dent.* **2018**, *21*, 238–242. [CrossRef]
133. Zogheib, C.; Hanna, M.; Pasqualini, D.; Naaman, A. Quantitative volumetric analysis of cross-linked gutta-percha obturators. *Ann. Stomatol.* **2016**, *7*, 46–51. [CrossRef]
134. Pedullà, E.; Abiad, R.S.; Conte, G.; La Rosa, G.R.M.; Rapisarda, E.; Neelakantan, P. Root fillings with a matched-taper single cone and two calcium silicate–based sealers: An analysis of voids using micro-computed tomography. *Clin. Oral Investig.* **2020**, *24*, 4487–4492. [CrossRef] [PubMed]
135. Kim, J.-A.; Hwang, Y.-C.; Rosa, V.; Yu, M.-K.; Lee, K.-W.; Min, K.-S. Root Canal Filling Quality of a Premixed Calcium Silicate Endodontic Sealer Applied Using Gutta-percha Cone-mediated Ultrasonic Activation. *J. Endod.* **2018**, *44*, 133–138. [CrossRef]
136. Donnermeyer, D.; Ibing, M.; Bürklein, S.; Weber, I.; Reitze, M.P.; Schäfer, E. Physico-Chemical Investigation of Endodontic Sealers Exposed to Simulated Intracanal Heat Application: Hydraulic Calcium Silicate-Based Sealers. *Materials* **2021**, *14*, 728. [CrossRef] [PubMed]
137. Atmeh, A.R.; Hadis, M.; Camilleri, J. Real-time chemical analysis of root filling materials with heating: Guidelines for safe temperature levels. *Int. Endod. J.* **2020**, *53*, 698–708. [CrossRef]
138. Carpenter, M.T.; Sidow, S.J.; Lindsey, K.W.; Chuang, A.; McPherson, J.C. Regaining Apical Patency after Obturation with Gutta-percha and a Sealer Containing Mineral Trioxide Aggregate. *J. Endod.* **2014**, *40*, 588–590. [CrossRef] [PubMed]
139. Neelakantan, P.; Grotra, D.; Sharma, S. Retreatability of 2 Mineral Trioxide Aggregate–based Root Canal Sealers: A Cone-beam Computed Tomography Analysis. *J. Endod.* **2013**, *39*, 893–896. [CrossRef] [PubMed]

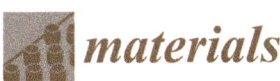 

*Article*

# Impact of Warm Vertical Compaction on the Sealing Ability of Calcium Silicate-Based Sealers: A Confocal Microscopic Evaluation

Diana Eid [1], Etienne Medioni [2], Gustavo De-Deus [3], Issam Khalil [1], Alfred Naaman [1] and Carla Zogheib [1,*]

1. Department of Endodontics, Faculty of Dentistry, Saint Joseph University, Beirut BP 17-5208, Lebanon; dianageid@gmail.com (D.E.); issamtkhalil@gmail.com (I.K.); alfrednaaman@gmail.com (A.N.)
2. Micoralis Laboratory EA7354, Faculty of Dentistry, University of Nice Sophia Antipolis, Pôle Odontologie du CHU de NICE, Hopital St. Roch, 06000 Nice, France; etienne.medioni@univ-cotedazur.fr
3. Department of Endodontics, School of Dentistry, UNIGRANRIO—Universidade Grande Rio, 1.160-jardim 25 DE Agosto, 22061-030 Rio de Janeiro, Brazil; endogus@gmail.com
* Correspondence: Carla.zogheibmoubarak@usj.edu.lb

**Citation:** Eid, D.; Medioni, E.; De-Deus, G.; Khalil, I.; Naaman, A.; Zogheib, C. Impact of Warm Vertical Compaction on the Sealing Ability of Calcium Silicate-Based Sealers: A Confocal Microscopic Evaluation. *Materials* **2021**, *14*, 372. https://doi.org/10.3390/ma14020372

Received: 16 October 2020
Accepted: 8 December 2020
Published: 14 January 2021

**Publisher's Note:** MDPI stays neutral with regard to jurisdictional claims in published maps and institutional affiliations.

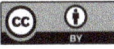

**Copyright:** © 2021 by the authors. Licensee MDPI, Basel, Switzerland. This article is an open access article distributed under the terms and conditions of the Creative Commons Attribution (CC BY) license (https://creativecommons.org/licenses/by/4.0/).

**Abstract:** The aim of this in vitro study was to evaluate the dentinal tubule penetration of two calcium silicate-based sealers used in warm vertical compaction (WVC) obturation technique in comparison with the single cone (SC) technique by confocal laser scanning microscopy (CLSM). The null hypothesis was that both obturation techniques produced similar sealer penetration depths at 1 and 5 mm from the apex. Forty-four mandibular single-rooted premolars were randomly divided into four equally experimental groups (n = 10) and two control groups (n = 2) according to the type of sealer (Bio-C Angelus, Londrína, PR, Brazil or HiFlow Brasseler, Savannah, GA, USA) with either SC or WVC. The sealers were mixed with a fluorescent dye Rhodamine B (0.1%) to enable the assessment under the CLSM. All the specimens were sectioned horizontally at 1 and 5 mm from the apex. The maximum penetration depth was calculated using the ImageJ Software (ImageJ, NIH). Data were analyzed by Mann–Whitney U and Kruskal–Wallis tests ($p < 0.05$). A significant difference was shown between the four groups at 1 mm ($p = 0.0116$), whereas similar results were observed at 5 mm ($p = 0.20$). WVC allowed better diffusion for both sealers at 1 mm ($p = 0.01$) and 5 mm ($p = 0.034$). The maximum penetration of the Bio-C and HiFlow sealers was more important at 5 mm with the two obturation techniques. Within the limitations of this study, WVC enhanced the penetration of calcium silicate-based sealers into the dentinal tubules in comparison with the SC technique at both levels.

**Keywords:** calcium silicate; confocal laser scanning microscopy; tubule penetration; warm vertical compaction

## 1. Introduction

Many obturation techniques have been investigated to seal the root canal system. A three-dimensional obturation is likely to create a fluid-tight seal and to prevent microleakage, which is one of the main causes of endodontic failure [1]. To overcome this challenge, which compromises long-term success, the sealers' deep penetration into the dentinal tubules is more implicated in producing a sufficient seal to entomb residual bacteria. Moreover, it enhances lateral and vertical sealing by filling spaces and voids [2].

Various types of sealers have been proposed to fill the spaces between the gutta-percha and the canal walls. Ideally, they should create a tight and adequate seal with the core material and dentine to reduce gaps. These requirements are affected by their physicochemical properties and their placement method. Therefore, the selection of an appropriate sealer is mandatory with the selection of the filling obturation technique [3].

Owing to their high biocompatibility, low cytotoxicity, and viscosity, tricalcium silicate-based sealers have aroused renewed interest in relation to improving filling quality [4]. According to the manufacturer, calcium silicate-based sealers such as Endosequence BC (Brasseler USA, Savannah, GA, USA) and iRoot SP (Innovative BioCeramix Inc., Vancouver, BC, Canada) are composed of calcium silicate, calcium phosphate, calcium hydroxide, zirconium oxide, and other agents [5]. They showed effective antimicrobial activity against multiple microorganisms [6]. Furthermore, they revealed a slight volume expansion while setting. These factors improve mechanical retention and chemical bonding to the dentinal walls. A physical barrier to fluids and nutrients is then formed [7]. They are widely indicated with the single cone (SC) technique [8].

However, thermoplasticized gutta-percha shows better canal irregularities in fillings than cold gutta-percha points and promotes the creation of a three-dimensional obturation [9]. Nevertheless, some studies reported that excessive heat might alter the sealers' properties [10], while others proved the opposite [11,12].

Recently, two new modified sealers HiFlow (Brasseler, Savannah, GA, SA) and Bio-C (Angelus, Londrína, PR, Brazil) have been proposed with warm vertical gutta-percha obturation techniques. According to the manufacturer, HiFlow exhibits a lower viscosity compared to standard BC Sealer when heated and is more radiopaque, making it optimal for warm vertical compaction (WVC). (**Stephen Buchanan**. Warm gutta-percha obturation with BC HiFlow™ Sealer. Endodontic practice US 2018).

To our knowledge, no study has yet evaluated the impact of the warm vertical compaction on the dentinal tubule penetration. The aim of this in vitro study was to evaluate the impact of heat application on the tubular penetration of two silicate-based sealers in comparison with the cold single cone technique using confocal laser scanning microscopy. The null hypothesis tested was that WVC does not enhance both sealers' penetration compared with the SC technique.

## 2. Materials and Methods

This study was approved by the Ethical Committee of the Saint Joseph University-Beirut (FMD 186, 2018).

### 2.1. Selection of Specimen

Forty-four human mandibular permanent single-rooted premolars were selected in this study. Criteria for the selection of the teeth were one straight canal, no sign of fracture/cracks, absence of internal and external resorption, and no obstruction or calcification within the canal. Two digital radiographs (buccolingual and mesiodistal) were taken to confirm the presence of one canal and the glidepath in each tooth.

### 2.2. Root Canal Treatment

The crowns were removed at 16 mm to standardize the length of all the canals. A standard access preparation was performed for each tooth. Patency was checked with a #10 K-file (Dentsply Maillefer, Ballaigues, Switzerland) until the tip was visible at the apices. Then, the working length (WL) was established by subtracting 0.5 mm from this measurement. The root canals were prepared up to F3 (0.3 mm, 0.09 taper) with the ProTaper System (Dentsply Maillefer, Ballaigues, Switzerland) according to the manufacturer's instructions.

During instrumentation, the root canals were copiously irrigated with 10 mL 5.25% NaOCl. After instrumentation, the canals were irrigated with 10 mL of 17% Ethylenediaminetetraacetic acid (EDTA), followed by 3 mL of 5.25% sodium hypochlorite (NaOCl) for 1 min, followed by a final flush with 10 mL of deionized water. Irrigating solutions were delivered using a 27-gauge side-vented needle (Max-I-Probe; Dentsply Maillefer, Ballaigues, Switzerland) and sonically activated for 1 min using the Endoactivator system (Dentsply Maillefer, Ballaigues, Switzerland) with a 25/04 tip. The tip was placed at −2 mm from the WL. Root canals were then dried with paper points. Teeth were randomly divided into 4 equally experimental groups (n = 10) and 2 control groups according to the type of sealer and the obturation techniques.

### 2.3. Root Canal Obturation

The HiFlow and Bio-C sealers were placed in a disposable syringe. They were both labeled during the mixing procedure with 0.1% Rhodamine B dye (Sigma-Aldrich, St. Louis, MO, USA) to assess fluorescence for the confocal microscopy.

Four groups were randomly divided as follows:

In group 1 (B/SC, n = 10), Bio-C sealer (Angelus, Londrína, PR, Brazil) was labeled with 0.1% Rhodamine B dye (Sigma-Aldrich, St. Louis, MO, USA) to assess fluorescence for the confocal microscopy. Bio-C sealer was delivered in the canals with a size 30 lentulo spiral (Dentsply Maillefer, Ballaigues, Switzerland). An F3 gutta-percha cone was then slightly coated with 20 µL of sealer mixture and slowly inserted into the WL. The cone was cut at the orifice with the heat carrier.

In group 2 (B/WVC, n = 10), the cone was placed as previously described (group 1) then packed down using System B Pluggers (0.06) (Sybron Endodontics, Orange, CA, USA) to 4 mm from the apex at 200 °C for 10 s. Canals were backfilled using an Obtura II (Obtura Spartan, Fenton, MO, USA).

In group 3 (H/SC, n = 10) and group 4 (H/WVC, n = 10), teeth were obturated with the same procedure but with the HiFlow (Brasseler USA®, Savannah, GA, USA) sealer using the SC and WVC techniques, respectively. A temporary filling material (Cavit, 3 M; ESPE, St. Paul, MN, USA) was placed coronally in all the specimens. Teeth were stored in a 37 °C incubator at 100% humidity for 2 weeks for complete setting. Negative control groups (n = 2) were filled with either HiFlow sealer or Bio-C without the fluorescent agent. Positive controls (n = 2) were left unobturated.

### 2.4. Sectioning of Roots and Preparation of Root Surfaces

Teeth were vertically embedded in an orthodontic resin block. They were sliced perpendicular to their long axis using slow speed diamond disks (25,000 rpm) under continuous water cooling at levels of 1 and 5 mm from the apex. Two slices of 2 mm thickness were obtained from each tooth. Apical and middle portions were polished with abrasive papers (500, 700, and 1200) to eliminate the debris from the cutting process. Sections were placed in an ultrasonic bath for 1 min at 45 °C and were mounted on glass slides.

### 2.5. Confocal Laser Analysis

Each section was examined under CLSM (10× magnification) (Zeiss LSM 710, Wetzlar, Germany). The emission wavelength was set at 561 nm. Digital images were analyzed with the software Image J (ImageJ software, NIH) to measure the maximum sealer penetration depths (µm) in the dentinal tubules at 4 circumferential points (12, 3, 6, and 9 o'clock). The tool "distance" was applied from the root canal surface to the deepest extent of the visible sealer. Measurements were performed by 1 observer and repeated 2 times to ensure reliability.

### 2.6. Statistical Analysis

The normality of the distribution was analyzed using the Kolmogorov–Smirnov test. The significance level was set at $p \leq 0.05$ and the confidence interval at 95%. The Kruskal–Wallis test was used within groups to compare differences between middle and apical portions. The nonparametric Mann–Whitney U test was used for pairwise comparison between the type of sealers and the filling techniques ($p < 0.05$). Data statistical analysis was conducted by using SPSS 16.0 software (Chicago, IL, USA).

## 3. Results

### 3.1. Comparison between Cuts at 1 mm and 5 mm from the Apex in Each Group

The Kruskal–Wallis test showed that there was a statistical difference between the four groups at 1 mm from the apex ($p = 0.0116$). The mean penetration was more variable between the groups. However, similar statistical results were observed at 5 mm ($p = 0.2026$). Moreover, the sealer penetrated deeper at the $-5$ mm level compared with the $-1$ mm level in the four experimental groups (results shown in Table 1).

**Table 1.** Mean penetration depth (μm) of two calcium silicate-based sealers.

| Level \ Group | Bio-C-SC | Bio-C-WVC | HiFlow-SC | HiFlow-WVC | Sig |
|---|---|---|---|---|---|
| 1 mm | 397.428 μm ± 77.46 | 447.076 μm ± 303.082 | 194.24 μm ± 227.369 | 672.82 μm ± 390.807 | 0.0116 |
| 5 mm | 1080.92 μm ± 575.228 | 1421.98 μm ± 509.75 | 1115.051 μm ± 619.506 | 1567.634 μm ± 666.873 | 0.2026 * |
| Sig | 0.0065 | 0.0007 | 0.0007 | 0.0052 | |

* Analysis of variance: no statistically significant difference among the mean maximum depth measurements.

### 3.2. Comparison between the Sealers (HiFlow/BioC) Regardless of the Technique Used

Both sealers showed no statistically significant difference for the maximum diffusion at 1 mm ($p = 0.7455$) and 5 mm ($p = 0.7251$).

### 3.3. Comparison between the Obturation Techniques (SC/WVC) Regardless of the Sealer Used

The WVC technique allowed for a better diffusion at 1 mm ($p = 0.011$) and at 5 mm from the apex ($p = 0.034$) than the SC (results shown in Table 2 and Figure 1).

**Table 2.** Penetration depth (μm) according to the obturation techniques at different levels (1 and 5 mm).

| Level \ Obturation Technique | Single Cone | Warm Vertical Compaction | Sig |
|---|---|---|---|
| 1 mm | 295.776 μm ± 252.568 | 559.488 μm ± 359.539 | 0.011 |
| 5 mm | 1097 μm ± 582.119 | 1494.457 μm ± 582.511 | 0.0349 |

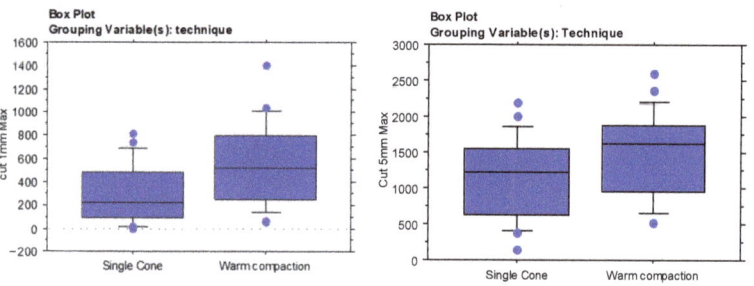

**Figure 1.** Box plot representation of the sealers penetration depth at 1 mm (left) and 5 mm (right) depending on the obturation techniques.

## 4. Discussion

Many microorganisms persist in ramifications and isthmuses despite proper chemomechanical preparation. Therefore, the penetration of a sealer is required for the elimination of residual bacteria and biofilms sheltering into these anatomies [13]. The sealer's diffusion in the tubules should be optimal to also obtain a hermetic seal and improve retention for a better long-term outcome [14]. Nevertheless, it is affected by various factors such as the physical and chemical properties of the sealer, the effectiveness of the removal of the smear layer, the anatomy of the root canal system, and the filling technique [15]. Moreover, the fine particles of the calcium silicate-based sealers (<1 μm) represent one of the major reasons why their deep diffusion is more likely to occur even with the SC technique, in addition to their basic pH which denatures the collagen fibers, their high flow rate, and their volume expansion of 0.2% with the setting results in tubular penetration [13,16].

It has been reported that the flushing effect and hydrodynamic agitation might affect the irrigation solutions' efficiency and the smear layer removal [17]. In fact, its adherence forms physical barriers and contamination in the dentinal tubules, blocking the penetration of the sealer [18]. Therefore, the irrigation protocol provided in this study was characterized by the use of EDTA and sonic activation with Endoactivator [19].

CLSM was used to assess the diffusion; measures were taken with a method similar to that used by Bitter et al. [20]. Different techniques were proposed in the literature, like the use of scanning electron microscopy (SEM), optical microscopy, transmission electron microscopes (TEM), and stereomicroscopy. CLSM was chosen over all other techniques as sections are visualized at different levels, creating a 3D image. Moreover, no dehydration or gold coatings were required for specimen preparation. The integrity of the dentin was later preserved [18]. This method, unlike SEM, offers a wide and detailed vision without artifacts [21,22]. Previous studies showed that leaching of the fluorescent Rhodamine B was not possible. The very limited quantity (0.1%) used did not alter the sealer's properties [21]. However, another agent, Fluo-3, was also used in a previous study by Jeong et al. An average penetration depth ranging between 200 and 400 μm was found [15], while others visualized a depth of up to approximately 1500 μm [21]. This difference was explained by the use of Rhodamine B, which was capable of leaching out and modifying the results [15]. In our study, no diffusion of this agent was noted. Rhodamine B could be suitable with the calcium silicate-based sealers. In addition, the complexity of the canal system might also interfere with the measurements. The oval shaped canals had a very challenging anatomy and should be taken into account in the selection of the specimen. The butterfly effect described by Russell was more likely to be seen in these configurations. Greater penetration was observed bucco-lingually than mesio-distally in some sections. This might explain the wide range of diffusion found with both sealers in our research as well as in various previous studies [15,21,23].

BC sealer is typically recommended with the single cone technique because heat might deteriorate its physical properties by decreasing the bond strength. The setting time and flow rate were reduced [24]. However, Heran et al. showed that calcium silicate-based sealers were not influenced by heat [25], whereas Fernandez et al. described filling more of the lateral canals with WVC [26]. Celikten et al. indicated that EndoSequence BC sealer had similar significant results in the number of voids and gaps, regardless of the three different obturation techniques applied [27].

The use of one tapered master cone matched better with the canal anatomy, which allowed similar obturation quality to WVC according to Alshehri et al. [28]. Some studies reported a predominance of one method over the other, while others advocated no significant difference between the techniques. No clear consensus has been reached indicating better tightness with one method over the other [21]. In fact, the major difference between the techniques is that endodontic sealer is mainly filled into the irregularities with the SC technique, whereas thermoplastified gutta-percha penetrates more completely in these areas with WVC [22].

Concerning the epoxy resin sealer AH Plus (Dentsply), it was reported that heat affects its properties [11,12,20]. Therefore, it was not exploited in these conditions in our study. Wang Y et al. found similar results with the iRoot SP using the two obturation techniques. They explained that heat had not shown an impact on the apical third [29]. McMichael et al. found similar tubule penetration of Endosequence BC with both single cone and warm vertical compaction at both levels [21]. However, the results in our study showed deeper penetration with WVC (Figure 2B,D). This difference might be related to the greater compressive forces applied coronally during obturation which would improve the sealer's penetration in the apical third (Figure 3). Maximum measurements were also observed in the middle portion for both sealers regardless of the filling technique ($p > 0.7$). The significant difference can be attributed to the increase in the tubules' density and diameter in the coronal direction. Moreover, the sclerotic dentin and the hardness of the smear layer in the apical third might create a physical barrier to the sealer's penetration [27].

The new modified tricalcium silicate sealers could still be promising even when thermoplastic techniques such as WVC are used, resulting in an improvement in the quality of the filling. Therefore, the best obturation technique for this material is still a matter of debate. However, despite the temperature of the devices being set at 200 °C, the true temperature generated by most heat carriers appears to be much lower [30].

Parameters such as physicochemical properties, cellular responses, and long-term clinical considerations should be investigated further.

Nevertheless, some authors showed that retreatment techniques were not able to fully remove BC sealers [14]. Further investigations are needed concerning their retreatment.

The null hypothesis of this study was rejected: the application of heat using WVC enhanced the calcium silicate-based sealer penetration in the dentinal tubules. No differences were observed comparing the HiFlow with the Bio-C sealer. Although the BC sealers are recommended with the SC technique, it might be interesting to reconsider the application of Schilder's principles with these newly introduced sealers.

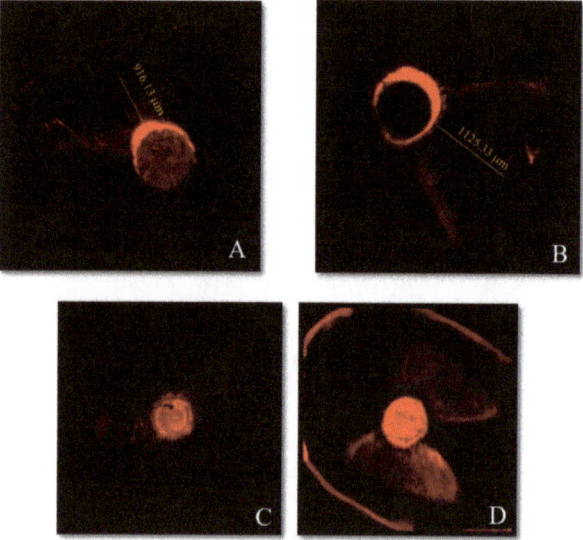

**Figure 2.** Representative confocal microscopic images of each sealer's depth penetration in the dentinal tubules at 1 mm from the apex: (**A**) HiFlow sealer with the single cone (SC) technique and (**B**) HiFlow sealer with warm vertical compaction (WVC). Moreover, at 5 mm from the apex: (**C**) HiFlow sealer with the SC and (**D**) HiFlow sealer with WVC.

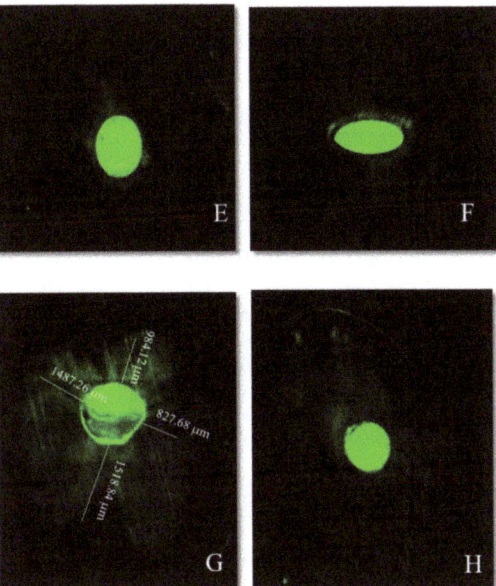

**Figure 3.** Representative confocal microscopic images of each sealer's depth penetration in the dentinal tubules at 1 mm from the apex: (**E**) Bio-C sealer with the SC technique and (**F**) Bio-C sealer with WVC. Moreover, at 5 mm from the apex: (**G**) Bio-C sealer with the SC and (**H**) Bio-C sealer with WVC.

**Author Contributions:** Conceptualization, D.E. and C.Z.; methodology, E.M.; software, E.M.; validation, D.E., I.K., A.N. and C.Z.; investigation, D.E.; resources, D.E., A.N. and C.Z.; writing—original draft preparation, D.E.; writing—review and editing, G.D.-D.; G.D.-D. contributed in the interpretation of data for the work and revised this work critically for important intellectual content; visualization, D.E.; supervision, E.M. and C.Z. All authors have read and agreed to the published version of the manuscript.

**Funding:** This research received no external funding.

**Institutional Review Board Statement:** The study was conducted according to the guidelines of the Declaration of Helsinki, and approved by the Institutional Review Board (or Ethics Committee) of Saint Joseph University (protocol code FMD186 and 15-7-2019).

**Informed Consent Statement:** Not applicable.

**Data Availability Statement:** The data presented in this study are available on request from the corresponding author.

**Acknowledgments:** The authors wish to thank Mario Zuolo for the precious corrections he added to this paper.

**Conflicts of Interest:** The authors declare no conflict of interest.

# References

1. Benezra, M.K.; Wismayer, P.S.; Camilleri, J. Interfacial Characteristics and Cytocompatibility of Hydraulic Sealer Cements. *J. Endod.* **2018**, *44*, 1007–1017. [CrossRef]
2. Trope, M.; Bunes, A.; Debelian, G. Root filling materials and techniques: Bioceramics a new hope? *Endod. Top.* **2015**, *32*, 86–96. [CrossRef]
3. De Deus, G.A.; Gurgel-Filho, E.D.; Maniglia-Ferreira, C.; Coulinho-Filho, T. The influence of filling technique on depth of tubule penetration by root canal sealer: A study using light microscopy and digital image processing. *Aust. Endod. J.* **2004**, *30*, 23–28. [CrossRef]

4. Giacomino, C.M.; Wealleans, J.A.; Kuhn, N.; Diogenes, A. Comparative Biocompatibility and Osteogenic Potential of Two Bioceramic Sealers. *J. Endod.* **2019**, *45*, 51–56. [CrossRef]
5. Jafari, F.; Jafari, S. Composition and physicochemical properties of calcium silicate based sealers: A review article. *J. Clin. Exp. Dent.* **2017**, *9*, e1249–e1255. [CrossRef]
6. Munitić, M.; Peričić, T.P.; Utrobičić, A.; Bago, I.; Puljak, L. Antimicrobial efficacy of commercially available endodontic bioceramic root canal sealers: A systematic review. *PLoS ONE* **2019**, *14*, e0223575. [CrossRef]
7. Almeida, L.H.S.; Moraes, R.R.; Morgental, R.D.; Pappen, F.G. Are Premixed Calcium Silicate-based Endodontic Sealers Comparable to Conventional Materials? A Systematic Review of in Vitro Studies. *J. Endod.* **2017**, *43*, 527–535. [CrossRef]
8. Al-Haddad, A.; Ab Aziz, Z.A.C. Bioceramic-Based Root Canal Sealers: A Review. *Int. J. Biomater.* **2016**, *2016*, 1–10. [CrossRef] [PubMed]
9. Schilder, H. Filling root canals in three dimensions. *J. Endod.* **2006**, *32*, 281–290. [CrossRef] [PubMed]
10. Camilleri, J. Sealers and warm gutta-percha obturation techniques. *J. Endod.* **2015**, *41*, 72–78. [CrossRef]
11. Viapiana, R.; Baluci, C.A.; Tanomaru-Filho, M.; Camilleri, J. Investigation of chemical changes in sealers during application of the warm vertical compaction technique. *Int. Endod. J.* **2014**, *48*, 16–27. [CrossRef] [PubMed]
12. Atmeh, A.R.; AlShwaimi, E. The Effect of Heating Time and Temperature on Epoxy Resin and Calcium Silicate-based Endodontic Sealers. *J. Endod.* **2017**, *43*, 2112–2118. [CrossRef] [PubMed]
13. Akcay, M.; Arslan, H.; Durmus, N.; Mese, M.; Capar, I.D. Dentinal tubule penetration of AH Plus, iRoot SP, MTA fillapex, and guttaflow bioseal root canal sealers after different final irrigation procedures: A confocal microscopic study. *Lasers Surg. Med.* **2016**, *48*, 70–76. [CrossRef] [PubMed]
14. Donnermeyer, D.; Bunne, C.; Schäfer, E.; Dammaschke, T. Retreatability of three calcium silicate-containing sealers and one epoxy resin-based root canal sealer with four different root canal instruments. *Clin. Oral Investig.* **2018**, *22*, 811–817. [CrossRef] [PubMed]
15. Jeong, J.W.; Degraft-Johnson, A.; Dorn, S.O.; Di Fiore, P.M. Dentinal Tubule Penetration of a Calcium Silicate-based Root Canal Sealer with Different Obturation Methods. *J. Endod.* **2017**, *43*, 633–637. [CrossRef]
16. Khaord, P.; Amin, A.; Shah, M.B.; Uthappa, R.; Raj, N.; Kachalia, T.; Kharod, H. Effectiveness of different irrigation techniques on smear layer removal in apical thirds of mesial root canals of permanent mandibular first molar: A scanning electron microscopic study. *J. Conserv. Dent.* **2015**, *18*, 321–326. [CrossRef]
17. Mancini, M.; Cerroni, L. Evaluation of Smear Layer Removal Using Different Irrigant Activation Methods (EndoActivator, EndoVac, PUI and LAI). An in Vitro Study. *Clin. Oral Investig.* **2018**, *22*, 993–999. [CrossRef]
18. Kuçi, A.; Alaçam, T.; Yavaş, Özer; Ergul-Ulger, Z.; Kayaoglu, G. Sealer penetration into dentinal tubules in the presence or absence of smear layer: A confocal laser scanning microscopic study. *J. Endod.* **2014**, *40*, 1627–1631. [CrossRef]
19. Virdee, S.S.; Seymour, D.W.; Farnell, D.; Bhamra, G.; Bhakta, S. Efficacy of irrigant activation techniques in removing intracanal smear layer and debris from mature permanent teeth: A systematic review and meta-analysis. *Int. Endod. J.* **2017**, *51*, 605–621. [CrossRef]
20. Bitter, K.; Paris, S.; Martus, P.; Schartner, R.; Kielbassa, A.M. A Confocal Laser Scanning Microscope investigation of different dental adhesives bonded to root canal dentine. *Int. Endod. J.* **2004**, *37*, 840–848. [CrossRef]
21. McMichael, G.E.; Primus, C.M.; Opperman, L.A. Dentinal Tubule Penetration of Tricalcium Silicate Sealers. *J. Endod.* **2016**, *42*, 632–636. [CrossRef] [PubMed]
22. Ortiz, F.G.; Jimeno, E.B. Analysis of the porosity of endodontic sealers through micro-computed tomography: A systematic review. *J. Conserv. Dent.* **2018**, *21*, 238–242. [CrossRef] [PubMed]
23. Piai, G.G.; Duarte, M.A.H.; Nascimento, A.L.D.; Da Rosa, R.A.; Nascimento, A.L.D.; Vivan, R. Penetrability of a new endodontic sealer: A confocal laser scanning microscopy evaluation. *Microsc. Res. Tech.* **2018**, *81*, 1246–1249. [CrossRef] [PubMed]
24. Qu, W.; Bai, W.; Liang, Y.-H.; Gao, X.-J. Influence of Warm Vertical Compaction Technique on Physical Properties of Root Canal Sealers. *J. Endod.* **2016**, *42*, 1829–1833. [CrossRef]
25. Heran, J.; Khalid, S.; Albaaj, F.; Tomson, P.L.; Camilleri, J. The single cone obturation technique with a modified warm filler. *J. Dent.* **2019**, *89*, 103181. [CrossRef]
26. Fernández, R.; Restrepo, J.S.; Aristizábal, D.C.; Alvarez, L.G. Evaluation of the filling ability of artificial lateral canals using calcium silicate-based and epoxy resin-based endodontic sealers and two gutta-percha filling techniques. *Int. Endod. J.* **2015**, *49*, 365–373. [CrossRef]
27. Celikten, B.; Uzuntas, C.F.; Orhan, A.I.; Tufenkci, P.; Misirli, M.; Demiralp, K.O.; Orhan, K. Micro-CT assessment of the sealing ability of three root canal filling techniques. *J. Oral Sci.* **2015**, *57*, 361–366. [CrossRef]
28. AlShehri, M.; Alamri, H.M.; AlShwaimi, E.; Kujan, O. Micro-computed tomographic assessment of quality of obturation in the apical third with continuous wave vertical compaction and single match taper sized cone obturation techniques. *Scanning* **2015**, *38*, 352–356. [CrossRef]
29. Wang, Y.; Liu, S.; Dong, Y.-M. In vitro study of dentinal tubule penetration and filling quality of bioceramic sealer. *PLoS ONE* **2018**, *13*, e0192248. [CrossRef]
30. Atmeh, A.R.; Hadis, M.; Camilleri, J. Real-time chemical analysis of root filling materials with heating: Guidelines for safe temperature levels. *Int. Endod. J.* **2020**, *53*, 698–708. [CrossRef]

# Analysis of the Morpho-Geometrical Changes of the Root Canal System Produced by TF Adaptive vs. BioRace: A Micro-Computed Tomography Study

Loai Alsofi [1,*], Muhannad Al Harbi [1,2], Martin Stauber [3] and Khaled Balto [1]

1. Department of Endodontics, Faculty of Dentistry, King Abdulaziz University, Jeddah 21589, Saudi Arabia; Mohannada@moh.gov.sa (M.H.); kbalto@kau.edu.sa (K.B.)
2. Ministry of Health, Al Thaghr Hospital, Al Thaghr, Jeddah 22361, Saudi Arabia
3. SCANCO Medical AG, 8306 Brüttisellen, Switzerland; martin.stauber@gratxray.com
* Correspondence: lalsofi@kau.edu.sa; Tel.: +966-55-531-8481

**Abstract:** We aimed to analyze the morpho-geometric changes of the root canal system created by two rotary systems (TF Adaptive and BioRace) using micro-CT technology. Two concepts of rotary file system kinematics, continuous rotation and adaptive kinematics, were used in root canal preparation. Twenty mandibular molars (n = 20) were selected with the following criteria: the teeth have mesial roots with a single and continuous isthmus connecting the mesiobuccal and mesiolingual canals (Vertucci's Type I configuration) and distal roots with independent canals. Teeth were scanned at a resolution of 14 μm. Canals were divided equally into two groups and then enlarged sequentially using the BioRace system and TF Adaptive system according to manufacturer protocol. Co-registered images, before and after preparation, were evaluated for morphometric measurements of canal surface area, volume, structure model index, thickness, straightening, and un-instrumented surface area. Before and after preparation, data were statistically analyzed using a paired sample $t$-test. After preparation, data were analyzed using an unpaired sample test. The preparation by both systems significantly changed canal surface area, volume, structure model index, and thickness in both systems. There were no significant differences between instrument types with respect to these parameters ($p > 0.05$). TF Adaptive was associated with less straightening (8% compared with 17% for BioRace in the mesial canal, $p > 0.05$). Both instrumentation systems produced canal preparations with adequate geometrical changes. BioRace straightened the mesial canals more than TF Adaptive.

**Keywords:** micro-computed tomography; nickel-titanium instruments; root canal preparation; endodontic drills; TF Adaptive; iRace

## 1. Introduction

Three-dimensional cleaning and shaping of the root canal system of the teeth is the key for three-dimensional obturation [1,2]. Several nickel–titanium (NiTi) instrument systems have been introduced on the market. These instruments along with the different irrigation solutions facilitate the biomechanical cleaning and shaping of the root canal system. NiTi rotary files may undergo fatigue without showing signs of deterioration on the flutes [3–5]. Most companies are trying to develop novel manufacturing technologies to overcome the inherent deficiencies. Such new technologies include M-wire, the newly introduced controlled memory, and thermal technology [6–10]. Alteration to the root canal anatomy, particularly in the apical third of the root canal space, is another key shortcoming of the current instrumentation systems [7,8]. This may create space inside the root canal, which may harbor bacteria and other microbes.

All NiTi rotary file systems available on the market are manufactured using the machine grinding technique, except two, which are twisted files (TF) and TF Adaptive systems (Kerr, Brea, CA, USA). The Twisted File Adaptive system (TF Adaptive) is used in combination with continuous rotation and reciprocation (Kerr, Brea, CA, USA). Reports indicate that reciprocating files result in a marked improvement in cyclic fatigue resistance [11]. The file operates in continuous rotation when minimal pressure is applied, and in reciprocal mode when it engages dentin and the load is increased. Manufacturers argue that this adaptive technology and twisted file design enhances flexibility and allows files to adjust to intracanal torsional stress.

The BioRace system (FKG Dentsaire SA, La Chaux-de-Fonds, Switzerland) is a simplified version of the original Race system (FKG Dentsaire SA). It has active cutting regions, which are electrochemically polished, and twisted areas with alternating cutting edges [12]. BioRace files are another promising option to improve clinical performance [13]. We aimed to evaluate and compare, in an ex vivo model, the shaping ability of adaptive reciprocation kinematics and continuous rotation instrumentation movement using TF Adaptive files and BioRace files, respectively, using micro-computed tomography (micro-CT).

The null hypothesis of the study was that there is no statistically significant difference in the morpho-geometric changes produced in root canals by BioRace and TF Adaptive system.

## 2. Materials and Methods

### 2.1. Experimental Teeth Selection

After local research ethics committee approval from King Abdulaziz University, Jeddah, Saudi Arabia (protocol no. 2016/145), one hundred extracted human mandibular first molars were obtained from a pool of teeth. Preapical radiographs were taken from buccolingual and mesiodistal views to ensure they had noncalcified canals. Teeth were stored in 0.1% thymol solution at 4 °C [14]. Inclusion criteria were: teeth with two mesial canals and one distal canal, teeth that had completely formed roots, had both mesial canals connected by a single and continuous isthmus (Vertucci type II configuration), and had a root curvature range of 15°–20° in both the mesiodistal and buccolingual directions. Exclusion criteria were carious teeth and teeth with root resorption or visible cracks. With these criteria, twenty human mandibular first molars were included in this study. Teeth were cleaned using Kavo ultrasonic peizo scaler (Kavo, Biberach an der Riss, Germany) and inspected under magnification (20×) using a dental operating microscope (Zeiss, Oberkochen, Germany)

### 2.2. Teeth Preparation

The twenty teeth were randomly divided into two groups (10 teeth in each group): group A (TF, n = 20 canals) and group B (BioRace, n = 20 canals). The teeth were mounted to a special-purpose sample holder. The tips of the roots were covered with utility wax to create a closed-end system and to prevent the intrusion of the rubber base material into the apical part of the canal. Standard access cavity preparation was performed using a diamond-coated bur [15]. Working length was determined using a size 15 K-file with the aid of periapical radiographs [16]. In group A, ten first mandibular molars were prepared using the TF Adaptive rotary system (Kerr, Brea, CA, USA) according to the manufacturer's instructions after establishing the glide path to full working length using a size 15 K-file. Teeth were prepared with TF Adaptive small canal system SM1 20/0.4, SM2 25/0.6, and SM3 35/0.4 to full working length using an elements motor (Kerr, Brea, CA, USA) at the installed recommended setting for the TF Adaptive in adaptive motion. Standard irrigation, as described above, was performed between each file. The rotary system files were used once per tooth. Each canal was dried with absorbent paper (35/4%; Dentsply Maillefer). Each file was carefully cleaned of debris after the preparation of each root canal using Korsolex Endo-Cleaner [17]. In group B, ten first mandibular molars were prepared using the BioRace rotary system (FKG, La Chaux-de-Fonds, Switzerland) according to the manufacturer's instructions after establishing the glide path to full working length using a size 15 K-file (Dentsply Maillefer, Ballaigues, Switzerland). Teeth were prepared with R1 15/0.6, R2 25/0.4, R3 30/0.4, and BioRace 35/0.4 to full working length using an elements motor (Kerr, Brea, CA, USA) with 600 rpm and 1.5 N/cm torque in continuous rotation [18].

Irrigation was performed using a 30 gauge side-vented needle (Ultradent, South Jordan, UT, USA) with a 5 mL syringe. The needle was inserted up to 1 mm shorter than the working length. The total amount of fluid for each canal was 5 mL of 5.25% NaOCl and 2 mL of 17% Ethylenediaminetetraacetic acid (EDTA) as a final flush after canal preparation. Teeth were irrigated with 1 mL of 5.25% NaOCl for each step of canal preparation as follows: irrigation with 1 mL of 5.25% NaOCl before instrumentation, between each instrument, and after instrumentation. A final flush was conducted with 2 mL of 17% EDTA [19].

Standard irrigation, as described above, was performed between each file. The rotary system files were used once per tooth. Each canal was dried with absorbent paper (35/4%; Dentsply Maillefer). Each file was carefully cleaned of debris after the preparation of each root canal using Korsolex Endo-Cleaner.

*2.3. Micro-CT Analysis*

The teeth were embedded in a special sample holder to ensure reproducible positioning for the repetitive measurements. The specimens were scanned with a μCT 100 (Scanco Medical AG, Brüttisellen, Switzerland) at an energy of 90 kVp, an intensity of 88 μA, and an integration time of 500 ms per projection. The data were reconstructed to an isotropic voxel size of 14 μm using a filtered back-projection algorithm. These settings were used for all base and follow-up measurements.

The outer contour of each tooth was generated automatically using a special-purpose algorithm. This outer contour was limited to a region that started at 50 slices above the slice where the root canals merged, and ended at the tip of the root. This outer contour was used for separating the background from the root canal, which was important for teeth where the root was cracked. Within this outer contour, the root canals could be extracted using global segmentation procedures.

Although the teeth were embedded, corresponding follow-up measurements did not fit perfectly. For this reason, a rigid registration algorithm was used to register the gray-level images. The main challenge with this procedure is that there are not many internal structures or features that allow for accurate registration. Therefore, the outer shape and gray-level intensities were the most significant features that could be used for the registration. With this registration, an accurate result could be achieved. Qualitative assessment was accomplished by the superimposition of constructed three-dimensional images showing the un-instrumented canal in green and the instrumented canal in red. Cross-section images perpendicular to the root canal were extracted and compared for each phase of the experiment. Volume and surface area of root canals were evaluated before and after instrumentation, and the changes were calculated as the difference between the pre- and post-instrumentation scores. The thickness was calculated along the canal using distance transformation techniques [20]. The structure model index (SMI) was calculated to determine the flatness of the root canal [21]. The centers of gravity of the canal were calculated slice-wise and connected by fitting a line, which was further used to calculate the curvature of the root canal [20]. Straightening is expressed as the difference between the post-instrumentation canal curvature (fitted line) and the initial curvature (in %). The un-instrumented surface area was calculated by evaluating the superimposed images through matching images of the surface area of the canal before and after preparation. A key assumption, in this case, was that surface voxels remained in the same places before and after preparation.

*2.4. Statistical Analysis*

The Shapiro–Wilk normality test was used to test all baseline measurements from mesial and distal roots. After instrumentation, we compared data from the baseline and data from after instrumentation measurements of the two file systems. Statistical analysis was performed using a paired sample *t*-test for normally distributed data (before and after instrumentation). An unpaired sample $t$-test was used for normally distributed data between nonparametric Mann–Whitney test for non-normally distributed data at a $p$-value of 0.05. Prism 8 software (Version 8, GraphPad Software, La Jolla, CA, USA) was used for analysis.

## 3. Results

All baseline parameters of mesial and distal roots showed normal distribution except for canal volume of both mesial and distal roots. Normally distributed data included structure model index (SMI), surface area, and the thickness of the canal. Table 1 shows µCT data before and after the preparation of the mesial canal for both TF Adaptive and BioRace systems. Table 2 shows µCT data before and after the preparation of the distal canal for both TF Adaptive and BioRace systems. The indices shown are as follows: volume, surface area, structural model index, average root canal thickness, and unprepared surface area. Both systems resulted in a significant change in root canal parameters when comparing before and after data in both mesial and distal canals.

**Table 1.** Morphometric indices before and after instrumentation of mesial canals.

| Parameters | | BioRace n = 20 Mean ± SD | $p$ ** | TF Adaptive n = 20 Mean ± SD | $p$ ** | $p$ * |
|---|---|---|---|---|---|---|
| Volume | Before (mm³) | 4.18 ± 1.48 | | 5.12 ± 2.62 | | 0.338 |
| | After (mm³) | 5.84 ± 1.13 | | 6.67 ± 2.57 | | 0.365 |
| | Increase (Δ%) | 1.67 ± 0.74 | <0.001 ** | 1.56 ± 1.07 | 0.001 ** | 0.969 |
| Surface Area | Before (mm²) | 42.37 ± 12.56 | | 44.72 ± 17.26 | | 0.732 |
| | After (mm²) | 46.99 ± 10.69 | | 49.43 ± 17.50 | | 0.711 |
| | Increase (Δ%) | 4.62 ± 6.07 | 0.039 ** | 4.71 ± 3.97 | 0.005 ** | 0.789 |
| Structural Model Index (SMI) | Before | 1.80 ± 1.07 | | 1.95 ± 0.91 | | 0.739 |
| | After | 2.51 ± 1.24 | | 2.10 ± 0.78 | | 0.385 |
| | Increase (Δ%) | 0.71 ± 0.88 | 0.030 ** | 0.15 ± 0.52 | 0.384 | 0.195 |
| Thickness | Before (mm) | 0.321 ± 0.14 | | 0.375 ± 0.14 | | 0.394 |
| | After (mm) | 0.53 ± 0.09 | | 0.53 ± 0.07 | | 0.915 |
| | Increase (Δ%) | 0.21 ± 0.099 | <0.001 ** | 0.15 ± 0.09 | 0.001 ** | 0.195 |
| Unprepared Area | Static Voxels | 80,468.20 ± 35 | | 67,006.70 ± 22 | | 0.323 |
| | After (%) | 42 ± 15% | | 36 ± 14% | | 0.405 |

* $p$-value for significance between TF Adaptive and BioRace. ** $p$-value for significance between before and after instrumentation data for the same instrument.

In mesial canals, 36–42% of the root canal surface was unprepared. The BioRace group showed slightly higher untreated voxels than the TF group. This indicated that the TF group touched more surface area in the mesial canals (Table 1). In the distal canal, the after preparation un-instrumented canal surface area ranged from 46–52%. The TF group showed slightly more untreated voxels in the distal canal, indicating that BioRace group touched more surface area in the distal canal. However, differences were not statistically significant between the groups, nor in the mesial or the distal canals (Table 2).

Figure 1a shows 3D-constructed images of the root canal system prepared using TF files before (left) and after (middle) instrumentation, as well as a superimposed image (right) from the mesial view. Figure 1b shows the 3D-constructed images of the root canal system prepared using BioRace system before (left) and after (middle) instrumentation, as well as a superimposed image (right) from the mesial view.

Table 2. Morphometric indices before and after instrumentation of distal canals.

| | Parameters | BioRace n = 20 Mean ± SD | p ** | TF Adaptive n = 20 Mean ± SD | p ** | p * |
|---|---|---|---|---|---|---|
| Volume | Before (mm$^3$) | 5.85 ± 1.86 | | 7.58 ± 4.59 | | 0.283 |
| | After (mm$^3$) | 7.25 ± 1.97 | | 8.22 ± 4.46 | | 0.534 |
| | Increase (Δ%) | 1.40 ± 0.88 | 0.001 ** | 0.64 ± 0.66 | 0.014 ** | 0.043 |
| Surface Area | Before (mm$^2$) | 48.71 ± 14.99 | | 47.55 ± 25.22 | | 0.902 |
| | After (mm$^2$) | 51.86 ± 14.78 | | 49.93 ± 29.59 | | 0.856 |
| | Increase (Δ%) | 3.14 ± 4.67 | 0.062 | 2.38 ± 5.92 | 0.236 | 0.751 |
| SMI | Before | 1.04 ± 1.32 | | 1.28 ± 0.87 | | 0.638 |
| | After | 1.50 ± 1.21 | | 1.46 ± 1.14 | | 0.942 |
| | Increase (Δ%) | 0.46 ± 0.93 | 0.154 | 0.18 ± 1.04 | 0.595 | 0.536 |
| Thickness | Before (mm) | 0.38 ± 0.16 | | 0.47 ± 0.12 | | 0.193 |
| | After (mm) | 0.52 ± 0.10 | | 0.57 ± 0.11 | | 0.288 |
| | Increase (Δ%) | 0.14 ± 0.09 | 0.001 ** | 0.10 ± 0.07 | 0.001 ** | 0.358 |
| Unprepared Area | Static Voxels | 86,191.50 ± 42,415.72 | | 100,673.80 ± 40,002.76 | | 0.442 |
| | After (%) | 46 ± 22 | | 52 ± 17 | | 0.551 |

\* *p*-value for significance between TF Adaptive and BioRace. \*\* *p*-value for significance between before and after instrumentation data for the same.

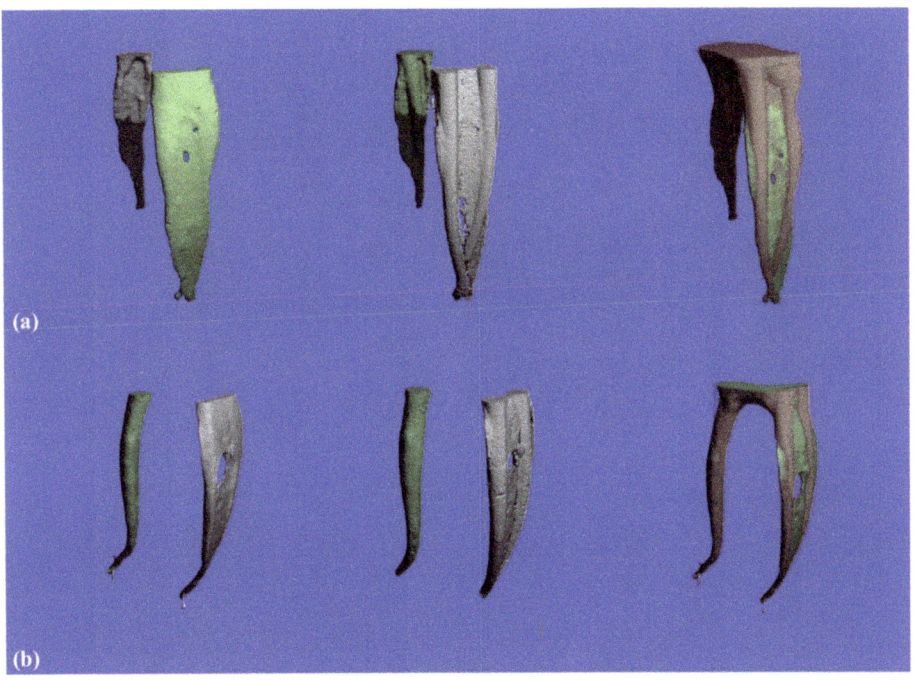

**Figure 1.** (**a**) 3D-constructed images from the TF Adaptive group of root canal system before (left) and after (middle) instrumentation and superimposed image (right) from the mesial. (**b**) 3D constructed images from BioRace group of root canal system before (left) and after (middle) instrumentation and superimposed image (right) from the mesial. Green indicates un-instrumented areas while red indicates instrumented areas.

Figure 2a shows cross-section images from different levels: 700 μm (top), 950 μm (middle), and 1200 μm (bottom) obtained from micro-CT image before (images on the left) and after (images on the right) root canal preparation using TF system. Figure 2b shows cross-section images from different level slices 700 μm (top), 950 μm (middle), and 1200 μm (bottom) obtained from micro-CT image before (images on the left) and after (images on the right) root canal preparation using BioRace system preparation. The relative degrees of canal straightening in BioRace and TF Adaptive groups were 17.56% ± 10.7% and 8.87% ± 6.84% in mesial canals, respectively, with no significant differences between instrument type ($p > 0.5$). In the distal canal, there was no significant difference in canal straightening for BioRace and TF Adaptive groups, 12.1% ± 12.9%, and 9.6% ± 5.6% respectively.

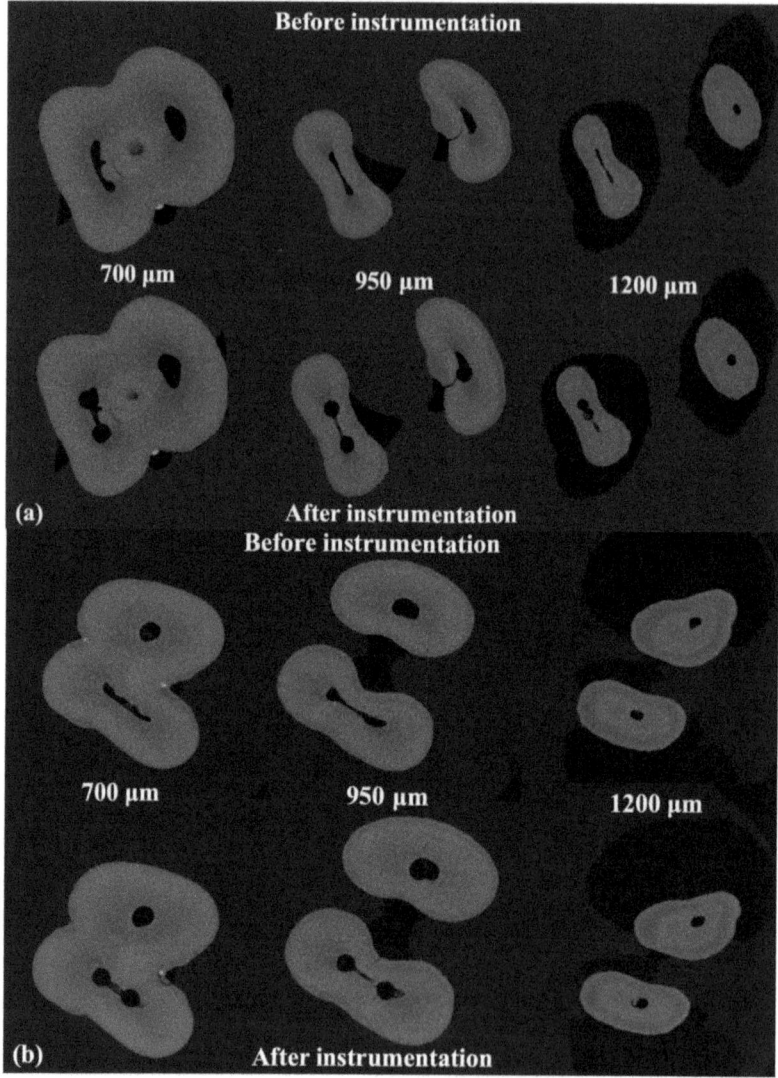

**Figure 2.** (a) Cross-section images from different level slices 700 μm (top), 950 μm (middle), and 1200 μm (bottom) obtained from micro-CT image before (images on the left) and after (images on the right) root canal preparation using TF system. (b) Cross-section images from deferent level slices 700 μm (top), 950 μm (middle), and 1200 μm (bottom) obtained from micro-CT image before (images on the left) and after (images on the right) root canal preparation using BioRace system.

## 4. Discussion

The main objective of root canal preparation is to create a tapered shape from apical to coronal areas while maintaining the original shape and keeping the apical diameter as small as possible [22]. This procedure may result in several preparation errors, such as ledge formation, perforation, canal transportation, file separation, elbow, apical zip, and canal blockage [23]. BioRace and TF Adaptive systems were designed to improve the canal shape while reducing unwanted procedural side effects.

When comparing the morpho-geometric changes after root canal preparation, it is important to have apical preparation diameters and similar tapers [24]. In this study, we compared the effects of two root canal instrumentation systems on the morpho-geometric changes. We chose BioRace and TF Adaptive systems because of their similarity in cross-section and instrument design. The only differences between these two devices are the kinematics and manufacturing process, which could be one of the limitations of this study. A recent study by Alghamdi et al. compared the effect of thermomechanical treatment of two rotary systems with similar design on the morpho-geometric morphology of prepared root canals [25].

In this study, the morpho-geometric changes were quantitatively analyzed using a set of measures such as the surface area, volume, thickness, and SMI. Furthermore, the mean values of the entire length of the canal's three-dimensional geometry were calculated [20]. We found that changes in canal geometry after instrumentation depend more on the canal type rather than the technique. This adds another limitation to the study, which is the variability in teeth anatomy between experimental groups.

In the mesial canals, instrumentation changed the geometry of the root canals. With the BioRace system, significant changes in volume and SMI were found. The significant change in volume could be explained by BioRace files working in continuous rotation only and thus lack the adaptive counterclockwise motion. This is especially pronounced in narrow canals such as the mesial canals in lower molars. The changes in SMI with BioRace indicated that it tends to change the general geometry of the root canal by transforming the original flat canals to conical ones. This indicated that the BioRace system left larger and more rounded canals after preparation than TF Adaptive in the mesial canal.

In the distal canals, the surface area and SMI were slightly increased, without being statistically significant, with both systems. This indicated that surface area and canal roundness in the distal canals were less affected than in mesial canals. This may be explained by anatomical variations and the size of the canal, which is much larger compared to mesial canals. Therefore, the instrumentation method has less influence on the resulting canal shape.

The mean untouched canal walls ranged from 36–42%. Both systems were unable to clean the root canal completely, which agrees with previous studies [8,21,26,27]. A comparable study by Velozo et al. showed that XP-Endo Shaper and ProTaper Next have similar canal-shaping ability when used in oval canals in mandibular incisors. All preparation parameters (volume, surface area, structure model index, and untouched walls) were significantly increased with no statistically significant difference between the two systems [28]. However, in our study, the tissue volume removed from the canals was higher than in other reports with similar methodology (5–30%) [29–31]. This may be due to the complex anatomy of the selected teeth, which may have a greater effect than the instrumentation techniques [20]. However, no significant difference was found between the two systems. If the amount of dentin removed was <34 µm, it would not have been registered [20] in this study; however, removing <34 µm of dentin was not sufficient because microorganisms can penetrate up to 150 µm inside the dentinal tubules [32].

NiTi rotary instruments tend to maintain the original canal curvature, even in extremely curved canals [33,34]. In this study, canal curvature was evaluated by fitting a line through the centers of gravity of each slice along the z-axis. This line was calculated for the un-instrumented and instrumented canals to calculate the straightening. In agreement with previous studies [35–37], we found that TF Adaptive maintained the original canal curvature better than BioRace in the mesial canal. This may be due to its alloy martensitic nature and unique adaptive motion. As the distal canals are much wider, they have less resistance; thus, the adaptive motion has little effect. Therefore, we found no difference between the two techniques in distal canals. However, further studies are needed to better evaluate the effect of adaptive motion on the straightening of the canal.

Excessive removal of dentin may lead to root fracture [37–39]. However, if the instrument is well-centered, more dentin can be preserved and the stability of the roots can be maintained [1]. In our study, the dentin was much better preserved than in studies performed with conventional instruments. This may be explained by the similar design of the two systems. The effect of the heat treatment of the NiTi in the TF group did not produce a superior result compared to BioRace in terms of remaining thickness, which is a conventional NiTi. It is expected that heat-treated NiTi systems would produce superior results to conventional NiTi systems with a similar design. This can be attributed to their plastic deformation, which can improve the cutting efficiency of the cutting edges during instrumentation, as mentioned in previous studies [31,40]. The limitations of our study include the different design features between both systems and the selection of the teeth based on clinical criteria and conventional radiographs rather than micro-CT evaluation.

## 5. Conclusions

Both rotary systems produced canal preparations with adequate geometrical changes. The BioRace system tended to produce more changes in canal geometry, volume, and more straightening, whereas the TF Adaptive system did not induce significant changes to the original canal curvature and geometry as much as BioRace. Neither of the two systems could touch all the canal walls.

**Author Contributions:** Conceptualization, L.A. and K.B.; methodology, M.H.; software, M.S.; validation, M.H., K.B., and M.S.; formal analysis, M.H.; investigation, M.S.; resources, K.B.; data curation, M.H.; writing—original draft preparation, L.A.; writing—review and editing, L.A.; visualization, K.B.; supervision, K.B.; project administration, K.B.; funding acquisition, M.H. All authors have read and agreed to the published version of the manuscript.

**Funding:** This research was funded by King Abdulaziz City for Science and Technology (KACST) grant number 285-36.

**Institutional Review Board Statement:** Ethical review and approval were waived for this study, due to the fact that the stury is in accordance with the guidelines of the Ethical Review Committee, Faculty of Dentistry, King Abdulaziz University, Jeddah 21589, Saudi Arabia.

**Informed Consent Statement:** Patient consent was waived because the study was done on extracted teeth.

**Data Availability Statement:** The data presented in this study are available on request from the corresponding author. The data are not publicly available due to intellectual reasons.

**Conflicts of Interest:** The authors declare no conflict of interest.

## References

1. Hulsmann, M.; Peters, O.A.; Dummer, P.M. Mechanical preparation of root canals: Shaping goals, techniques and means. *Endod. Top.* **2005**, *10*, 30–76. [CrossRef]
2. Schilder, H. Cleaning and shaping the root canal. *Dent. Clin. N. Am.* **1974**, *18*, 269–296. [PubMed]
3. Aydin, C.; Inan, U.; Tunca, Y.M. Comparison of cyclic fatigue resistance of used and new RaCe instruments. *Oral Surg. Oral Med. Oral Pathol. Oral Radiol. Endod.* **2010**, *109*, e131–e134. [CrossRef] [PubMed]
4. Aydin, C.; Inan, U.; Yasar, S.; Bulucu, B.; Tunca, Y.M. Comparison of shaping ability of RaCe and Hero Shaper instruments in simulated curved canals. *Oral Surg. Oral Med. Oral Pathol. Oral Radiol. Endod.* **2008**, *105*, e92–e97. [CrossRef] [PubMed]
5. Sattapan, B.; Nervo, G.J.; Palamara, J.E.; Messer, H.H. Defects in rotary nickel-titanium files after clinical use. *J. Endod.* **2000**, *26*, 161–165. [CrossRef] [PubMed]
6. Bidar, M.; Moradi, S.; Forghani, M.; Bidad, S.; Azghadi, M.; Rezvani, S.; Khoynezhad, S. Microscopic evaluation of cleaning efficiency of three different nickel-titanium rotary instruments. *Iran. Endod. J.* **2010**, *5*, 174–178.

7. Capar, I.D.; Arslan, H.; Akcay, M.; Ertas, H. An in vitro comparison of apically extruded debris and instrumentation times with ProTaper Universal, ProTaper Next, Twisted File Adaptive, and HyFlex instruments. *J. Endod.* **2014**, *40*, 1638–1641. [CrossRef]
8. Capar, I.D.; Ertas, H.; Ok, E.; Arslan, H.; Ertas, E.T. Comparative study of different novel nickel-titanium rotary systems for root canal preparation in severely curved root canals. *J. Endod.* **2014**, *40*, 852–856. [CrossRef]
9. Shen, Y.; Zhou, H.M.; Zheng, Y.F.; Campbell, L.; Peng, B.; Haapasalo, M. Metallurgical characterization of controlled memory wire nickel-titanium rotary instruments. *J. Endod.* **2011**, *37*, 1566–1571. [CrossRef]
10. Alapati, S.B.; Brantley, W.A.; Iijima, M.; Clark, W.A.; Kovarik, L.; Buie, C.; Liu, J.; Ben Johnson, W. Metallurgical characterization of a new nickel-titanium wire for rotary endodontic instruments. *J. Endod.* **2009**, *35*, 1589–1593. [CrossRef]
11. Jin, S.Y.; Lee, W.; Kang, M.K.; Hur, B.; Kim, H.C. Single file reciprocating technique using conventional nickel-titanium rotary endodontic files. *Scanning* **2013**, *35*, 349–354. [CrossRef] [PubMed]
12. Saber, S.E.; Nagy, M.M.; Schäfer, E. Comparative evaluation of the shaping ability of ProTaper Next, iRaCe and Hyflex CM rotary NiTi files in severely curved root canals. *Int. Endod. J.* **2015**, *48*, 131–136. [CrossRef] [PubMed]
13. Vadhana, S.; SaravanaKarthikeyan, B.; Nandini, S.; Velmurugan, N. Cyclic fatigue resistance of RaCe and Mtwo rotary files in continuous rotation and reciprocating motion. *J. Endod.* **2014**, *40*, 995–999. [CrossRef] [PubMed]
14. Strawn, S.E.; White, J.M.; Marshall, G.W.; Gee, L.; Goodis, H.E.; Marshall, S.J. Spectroscopic changes in human dentine exposed to various storage solutions–short term. *J. Dent.* **1996**, *24*, 417–423. [CrossRef]
15. Yamamura, B.; Cox, T.C.; Heddaya, B.; Flake, N.M.; Johnson, J.D.; Paranjpe, A. Comparing canal transportation and centering ability of endosequence and vortex rotary files by using micro-computed tomography. *J. Endod.* **2012**, *38*, 1121–1125. [CrossRef]
16. Turkistani, A.K.; Gomaa, M.M.; Shafei, L.A.; Alsofi, L.; Majeed, A.; AlShwaimi, E. Shaping Ability of HyFlex EDM and ProTaper Next Rotary Instruments in Curved Root Canals: A Micro-CT Study. *J. Contemp. Dent. Pract.* **2019**, *20*, 680–685. [CrossRef]
17. Gambarini, G.; Testarelli, L.; De Luca, M.; Milana, V.; Plotino, G.; Grande, N.M.; Rubini, A.G.; Al Sudani, D.; Sannino, G. The influence of three different instrumentation techniques on the incidence of postoperative pain after endodontic treatment. *Ann. Stomatol. (Roma)* **2013**, *4*, 152–155. [CrossRef]
18. Bonaccorso, A.; Cantatore, G.; Condorelli, G.G.; Schafer, E.; Tripi, T.R. Shaping ability of four nickel-titanium rotary instruments in simulated S-shaped canals. *J. Endod.* **2009**, *35*, 883–886. [CrossRef]
19. Paque, F.; Zehnder, M.; De-Deus, G. Microtomography-based comparison of reciprocating single-file F2 ProTaper technique versus rotary full sequence. *J. Endod.* **2011**, *37*, 1394–1397. [CrossRef]
20. Peters, O.A.; Laib, A.; Göhring, T.N.; Barbakow, F. Changes in root canal geometry after preparation assessed by high-resolution computed tomography. *J. Endod.* **2001**, *27*, 1–6. [CrossRef]
21. Peters, O.A.; Schonenberger, K.; Laib, A. Effects of four Ni-Ti preparation techniques on root canal geometry assessed by micro computed tomography. *Int. Endod. J.* **2001**, *34*, 221–230. [CrossRef] [PubMed]
22. Thompson, S.A.; Dummer, P.M. Shaping ability of Hero 642 rotary nickel-titanium instruments in simulated root canals: Part 2. *Int. Endod. J.* **2000**, *33*, 255–261. [CrossRef] [PubMed]
23. Al-Omari, M.A.; Dummer, P.M. Canal blockage and debris extrusion with eight preparation techniques. *J. Endod.* **1995**, *21*, 154–158. [CrossRef]
24. Bergmans, L.; Van Cleynenbreugel, J.; Beullens, M.; Wevers, M.; Van Meerbeek, B.; Lambrechts, P. Progressive versus constant tapered shaft design using NiTi rotary instruments. *Int. Endod. J.* **2003**, *36*, 288–295. [CrossRef]
25. Alghamdi, A.; Alsofi, L.; Balto, K. Effects of a Novel NiTi Thermomechanical Treatment on the Geometric Features of the Prepared Root Canal System. *Materials* **2020**, *13*, 5546. [CrossRef]
26. Gergi, R.; Osta, N.; Bourbouze, G.; Zgheib, C.; Arbab-Chirani, R.; Naaman, A. Effects of three nickel titanium instrument systems on root canal geometry assessed by micro-computed tomography. *Int. Endod. J.* **2015**, *48*, 162–170. [CrossRef]
27. Zhao, D.; Shen, Y.; Peng, B.; Haapasalo, M. Root canal preparation of mandibular molars with 3 nickel-titanium rotary instruments: A micro-computed tomographic study. *J. Endod.* **2014**, *40*, 1860–1864. [CrossRef]
28. Velozo, C.; Silva, S.; Almeida, A.; Romeiro, K.; Vieira, B.; Dantas, H.; Sousa, F.; De Albuquerque, D.S. Shaping ability of XP-endo Shaper and ProTaper Next in long oval-shaped canals: A micro-computed tomography study. *Int. Endod. J.* **2020**, *53*, 998–1006. [CrossRef]
29. Peters, O.A.; Boessler, C.; Paqué, F. Root canal preparation with a novel nickel-titanium instrument evaluated with micro-computed tomography: Canal surface preparation over time. *J. Endod.* **2010**, *36*, 1068–1072. [CrossRef]
30. Paque, F.; Balmer, M.; Attin, T.; Peters, O.A. Preparation of oval-shaped root canals in mandibular molars using nickel-titanium rotary instruments: A micro-computed tomography study. *J. Endod.* **2010**, *36*, 703–707. [CrossRef]
31. Gagliardi, J.; Versiani, M.A.; de Sousa-Neto, M.D.; Plazas-Garzon, A.; Basrani, B. Evaluation of the Shaping Characteristics of ProTaper Gold, ProTaper NEXT, and ProTaper Universal in Curved Canals. *J. Endod.* **2015**, *41*, 1718–1724. [CrossRef] [PubMed]
32. Sen, B.H.; Piskin, B.; Demirci, T. Observation of bacteria and fungi in infected root canals and dentinal tubules by SEM. *Endod. Dent. Traumatol.* **1995**, *11*, 6–9. [CrossRef] [PubMed]
33. Hülsmann, M.; Gressmann, G.; Schäfers, F. A comparative study of root canal preparation using FlexMaster and HERO 642 rotary Ni-Ti instruments. *Int. Endod. J.* **2003**, *36*, 358–366. [CrossRef] [PubMed]
34. Versümer, J.; Hülsmann, M.; Schäfers, F. A comparative study of root canal preparation using Profile .04 and Lightspeed rotary Ni-Ti instruments. *Int. Endod. J.* **2002**, *35*, 37–46. [CrossRef] [PubMed]

35. Aminsobhani, M.; Razmi, H.; Nozari, S. Ex Vivo Comparison of Mtwo and RaCe Rotary File Systems in Root Canal Deviation: One File Only versus the Conventional Method. *J. Dent. (Tehran)* **2015**, *12*, 469–477.
36. Qiu, N.; Wang, C.Y.; Liu, Y.F.; Yu, X.Q.; Xue, M. Comparison of the shaping ability of three Ni-Ti rotary instruments in the preparation of simulated curved root canals. *Shanghai Kou Qiang Yi Xue* **2016**, *25*, 191–194. [PubMed]
37. Ordinola-Zapata, R.; Bramante, C.M.; Duarte, M.A.; Cavenago, B.C.; Jaramillo, D.; Versiani, M.A. Shaping ability of reciproc and TF adaptive systems in severely curved canals of rapid microCT-based prototyping molar replicas. *J. Appl. Oral Sci.* **2014**, *22*, 509–515. [CrossRef]
38. Kishen, A. Mechanisms and risk factors for fracture predilection in endodontically treated teeth. *Endod. Top.* **2006**, *13*, 57–83. [CrossRef]
39. Tang, W.; Wu, Y.; Smales, R.J. Identifying and reducing risks for potential fractures in endodontically treated teeth. *J. Endod.* **2010**, *36*, 609–617. [CrossRef]
40. Shen, Y.; Coil, J.M.; Zhou, H.; Zheng, Y.; Haapasalo, M. HyFlex nickel-titanium rotary instruments after clinical use: Metallurgical properties. *Int. Endod. J.* **2013**, *46*, 720–729. [CrossRef]

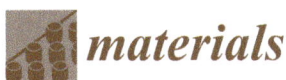 

*Article*

# Quantitative and Qualitative Assessment of Fluorescence in Aesthetic Direct Restorations

Zsuzsanna Bardocz-Veres [1], Melinda Székely [1,*], Pál Salamon [2,3], Előd Bala [1], Előd Bereczki [1] and Bernadette Kerekes-Máthé [1]

[1] Faculty of Dental Medicine, George Emil Palade University of Medicine, Pharmacy, Science, and Technology of Târgu Mureș, 38 Gh. Marinescu Str., 540139 Târgu Mureș, Romania; zsuzsanna.bardocz-veres@umfst.ro (Z.B.-V.); ballaelod59@gmail.com (E.B.); elodberecki@gmail.com (E.B.); bernadette.kerekes-mathe@umfst.ro (B.K.-M.)

[2] Department of Bioengineering, Faculty of Economics, Socio-Human Sciences and Engineering, Sapientia Hungarian University of Transylvania [EMTE], Libertatii sq. 1, 530104 Miercurea Ciuc, Romania; salamonpal@uni.sapientia.ro

[3] Molecular Diagnostics Laboratory, Emergency County Hospital of Miercurea Ciuc, Dr. Denes Laszlo 2, 530173 Miercurea Ciuc, Romania

\* Correspondence: melinda.szekely@umfst.ro; Tel.: +40-744-878-610

**Abstract:** Currently available direct restoration materials have been developed to have improved optical properties to interact with light in the same manner as the natural tooth. The objective of this study was to investigate the fluorescence of different enamel resin composites. In the present study, nine brands of enamel composites were tested in vitro, some of which are cited by manufacturers as having color adjustment potential. Fluorescence spectra of the composite specimens and the human natural enamel were measured with a fluorescence spectrophotometer immediately after preparation and after 6 months. Qualitative data of the specimens were also collected. Statistical analyses were conducted by Kruskal–Wallis and Mann–Whitney U nonparametric tests ($p < 0.05$). Almost all tested resin composites presented a significant decrease in the fluorescence values after a period of 6 months. There was no significant decrease in fluorescence in the case of Harmonize™ resin composite samples, which presented the lowest initial fluorescence values. The highest value in the reduction of the initial fluorescence intensity after 6 months (22.95%) was observed for the Charisma® specimens. Composites with a color adjustment did not perform significantly better than other composites in terms of reduction in fluorescence intensity.

**Keywords:** dental materials; fluorescence properties; restorative materials; resin-based composite; enamel

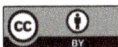

## 1. Introduction

Modern composites can reproduce the beauty of the appearance of a natural tooth, a potential reason for widespread use in the direct restorations of the anterior region. Currently available enamel direct composite materials differ not only in color but also in fundamental optical properties, such as translucency, opalescence, and fluorescence. These optical properties form the basis for clinical shade-matching.

Light can be broken into three primary colors: red, green, and blue, and in their merging point, they produce three more colors, evidenced in prism light. Our brain perceives the reflected waves as color. The color that we perceive is the sum of all the colors reflected by the object. Color perception is regulated by absorption and reflection mechanisms. The human eye can perceive wavelengths included in a range between 380 and 760 nm. Light absorption and reflection phenomena work at the expense of the object's translucency and opacity. Transparent and translucent objects allow light to pass partially or completely, while opaque objects block the passage of light [1].

The enamel is considered a crystalline tissue that, due to the arrangement of the prisms, translucency, and opalescence, confers the ability to transmit light to the underlying dentin, which features several nuances and three-dimensional aspects of color. The enamel is primarily responsible for regulating the tooth brightness and is characterized by a high degree of translucency and unique light effects. Enamel is composed mainly of hydroxyapatite and a lesser percentage of organic matter and water. The crystalline structure of the enamel prism allows light to pass with little restraint, while the organic interprismatic substance shows high opacity. The composition of the enamel enables a unique complex of reflection, transmission, and absorption of light. The interaction between the enamel and dentin makes the tooth an object that uniquely plays with light. Compared with other dental tissues, the enamel structure has a highly translucent appearance and a high degree of opacity. Even though no tooth structure is transparent, enamel allows light to pass through, providing translucent and opalescent effects [2,3].

Fluorescence is defined as the optical property of a substance that, while exposed to the exciting irradiation, absorbs the light and consequently emits the light at a longer wavelength (Figure 1). Fluorescence, as an optical property, can determine the aesthetic quality, success, or failure of restorative treatment. Unfortunately, the fluorescence intensity of dental tissues and restorative materials cannot be certified visually, the phenomenon is evident under fluorescent light but still stands out significantly, although less obviously under natural light. The use of fluorescent materials has marked a revolution in aesthetic dentistry, therefore, today's restorative materials that lack fluorescence are not considered to be optimal materials. The most important feature of the fluorescence is the light emission from inside, e.g., endodontic treatment and aging result in a decrease in the fluorescence because of protein loss, tissue mineralization, and pigmentation [4].

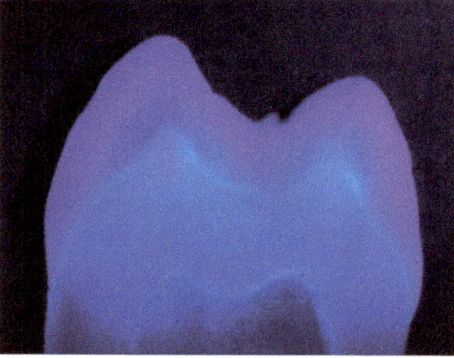

**Figure 1.** Fluorescence of a premolar slice (in 385 nm UV light). The digital equipment used was a DSLR camera (Nikon D3100, Nikon Corporation, Tokyo, Japan) equipped with a macro objective (Tamron 90 mm), ISO 200, f/22, exposure time: 1/200 s.

Fluorescence belongs to the family of photoluminescence processes, in which case, the molecules can emit light through electronically excited states. Photoluminescence is defined as the ability of bodies to emit certain types of light when subjected to invisible ultraviolet rays. It can be divided into two bodies: phosphorescent (bodies that have the ability to continue to emit visible light even after the removal of the ultraviolet rays) and fluorescents (bodies that emit visible light only during exposure to ultraviolet rays).

The first studies related to fluorescence in natural teeth defined that the teeth presented white–blue fluorescent properties when exposed to low-intensity radiation of the ultraviolet rays. This characteristic makes the natural teeth whiter and brighter in daylight, giving them an aspect of vitality and naturalness.

Fluorescence is a phenomenon capable of absorbing light energy of ultraviolet origin and re-emitting it in the visible light spectrum in the form of blue–violet light. This means that the absorption of electromagnetic waves invisible to the human eye is converted by the body irradiated with ultraviolet light, which re-emits it as visible energy [5].

Restorative materials that stimulate the natural tooth color have different particle size distribution and optical characteristics: they absorb some rays while transmitting and reflecting others. The synergy among them creates the colors perceived by the eye. Composite resins and dental ceramics are materials that absorb a relatively large amount of light [6].

The enamel and dentin interrelation in the natural tooth determines their color through the processes of reflection and refraction of light. This means that restorative materials need to have similar optical properties to the dental structure, making the restorations almost undetectable. The dentin and the enamel differ in fluorescence (Figure 2).

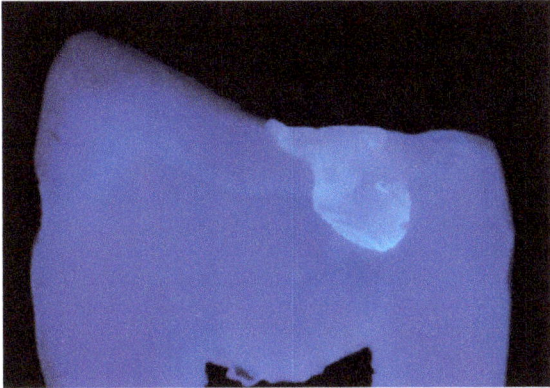

**Figure 2.** Image of a cross-section premolar slice in UV light (385 nm), revealing the differences in fluorescence between dental tissues and a restoration with Charisma®. The digital equipment used was a DSLR camera (Nikon D3100) equipped with a macro objective (Tamron 90 mm), ISO 200, f/22, exposure time: 1/200 s.

Manufacturers have included special agents from metals like europium, terbium, ytterbium, and cerium to reproduce the phenomena of fluorescence. Clinically, fluorescence contributes to the aspect of the vitality of the restoration and helps to obtain the correct luminosity. Different composites have different degrees of fluorescence, depending on the manufacturer's approach or the optical properties of the material. The lighter the chroma, the more fluorescent the material becomes. However, the fluorescence of the composites still does not completely mimic that of natural teeth [7,8].

Several studies have dealt with the opalescence and fluorescence properties of resin composites. Since UV light causes fluorescent emission in dental resin composites, this may influence the opalescence property and translucency of materials. Therefore, inclusion or exclusion of the UV component of illumination may have an influence on the translucency and masking effect [9].

The objective of the present study was to evaluate, in vitro, the fluorescence intensity of resin composites, focusing on the direct restoration of the enamel. The null hypotheses tested were that the fluorescence intensity of composite samples: (i) does not differ significantly from the enamel samples and (ii) does not reduce over time.

## 2. Materials and Methods

A total number of 9 different brands of restorative materials used for the direct restoration of enamel were analyzed. The materials included in the study are presented in Table 1.

Table 1. Materials included in the study.

| Materials | Composition | Manufacturer | Shade |
|---|---|---|---|
| Omnichroma | UDMA, TEGDMA, uniform-sized supra-nano spherical filler (260 nm spherical $SiO_2$-$ZrO_2$), composite filler ($SiO_2$-$ZrO_2$) | Tokoyama Dental, Tokyo, Japan | One shade (Special) |
| Harmonize™ | Bis-GMA, Bis-EMA, TEGDMA, spherical silica, and zirconia particles 5 to 400 nm formed from a molecular suspension in ART, barium glass | Kerr Dental, Orange, CA, USA | A2 |
| Filtek™ Z250 | Bis-GMA, UDMA, and Bis-EMA; 66% of filler: Zirconium/Silica | 3M ESPE Dental Products, St. Paul, MN, USA | A2 |
| Gaenial Anterior | UDMA, dimethacrylate co-monomers. Filler: silica, strontium, lanthanoid fluoride (16–17 µm), silica (>100 nm) fumed silica | GC Corporation, Tokyo, Japan | A2 |
| Enamel Plus Function HRI | Bis-GMA, UDMA, butanediol dimethacrylate Nano-hybrid composite content of filler (80% weight) | Micerium, Avegno, Italy | EF3 (Special) |
| Essentia | UDMA, Bis-MEPP, Bis-EMA, Bis-GMA, TEGDMA, Filler: pre polymerized fillers, barium glass, fumed silica | GC Corporation, Tokyo, Japan | LE (Special) |
| Charisma | Bis-GMA, TEGMA, Ba-Al-F glass fillers, pre-polymerized filler, pyrogenic silica, initiator | Heraeus Kulzer, Hannau, Germany | A2 |
| Luna | UDMA/Bis-EMA/TEGDMA, (61%) SAS, AS0.02-2 µm, 200–400 nm | SDI GmbH, Cologne, Germany | A2 |
| Brilliant Flow | Bis-GMA, Bis-EMA, TEGDMA, barium glass, silanized silica (0.6 µm), 42%vol | Coltene-Whaledent, Altstatten, Switzerland | A2/B2 |

In the first part of the study, six specimens from each of the nine brands of the composite were prepared according to the manufacturers' instructions. The sample size was calculated using a sample size calculator (SSCALC, at a confidence level of 95%, the value of the confidence interval was 10). Discs of 5 mm in diameter and 2 mm in thickness were made using a silicone mold (Elite HD Putty Soft, Zhermack, SpA, Badia Polesine (RO), Italy). A total number of 54 specimens were prepared. The resin was inserted in a single increment for each specimen, followed by the positioning of a polyester sheet and a glass plate on the surface. A force of 20 N was applied to eliminate the excess material. The curing of the specimens was realized using a hand light-curing unit (Noblesse Wireless LED, Max Dental Co, Seokcheon-ro, Ojeong-gu, Bucheon-si, Gyeonggi-do, Korea) for 20 s from one side of the mold, with an intensity setting of 1000 mW/cm$^2$. As a control group, we prepared eight natural enamel slices of 5 mm × 2 mm each from upper premolars extracted for orthodontic reasons. Enamel specimens were obtained by slicing the tooth with a high-speed diamond disc under water cooling. The dimension of the specimens was verified using a digital micrometer caliper (Powerfix, OWIM, Neckarsulm, Germany). As a polishing protocol, 600 grit sandpaper was applied for every specimen. The specimens were stored in plastic containers with artificial saliva to avoid desiccation which could bias the measured parameters. Just before the measurements, specimens were removed from the containers and blot-dried.

For the quantitative measurements, a fluorescence spectrophotometer was used (Cary Eclipse, Fluorescence Spectrophotometer, Agilent Technologies, Santa Clara, CA, USA). The samples were introduced in Quartz Microplate (Hellma Analytics, material: Quartz Glass, wells diameter: 6.6 mm, dimensions: 14.5 mm × 127 mm × 85.5 mm). A fluorescence emission spectrum was recorded at an excitation wavelength of 395 nm; the emission measurement range was 400–600 nm. The data were analyzed by the SpectraGryph 1.2 spectroscopy software. To assess the fluorescence intensity changes over time of the composite resin specimens, the same measurements were repeated after 6 months.

In the second part of the study, we collected qualitative data on the materials' fluorescence. Disc specimens of 12 mm in diameter and 1 mm in thickness were made using a custom-made silicone mold. Light curing was performed with the same protocol as described above. After curing, specimens were removed from the mold. Two specimens were made for each brand (a total number of 18 specimens) and all were made by the same operator (EB) at the same room temperature and humidity.

The qualitative evaluation of the fluorescence intensity was assessed by a qualitative visual method [10] by two of the authors (ZSBV and BKM). Therefore, the samples were introduced in a custom-made black box and illuminated by a UV light source at the intensity of 385 nm. All the specimens and the natural enamel samples were photographed using a DSLR camera (Nikon D3100) with a macro lens (Tamron 90 mm Macro lens) from the same distance and standardized adjustments (ISO 200, f/22, exposure time: 1/200 s). For the analysis, a blind-type experiment was utilized, in which the evaluator was unaware of the trademark of the composite resin that was being evaluated. The order of disposition of the specimens was predetermined. Each evaluator received a form to be filled in with the responses they observed and they were instructed to evaluate the degree of fluorescence by a numerical value: 0 = low fluorescence, 1 = medium fluorescence, 2 = high fluorescence.

The collected data were statistically analyzed using Microsoft Excel spreadsheets, Kruskal-Wallis and Mann-Whitney U nonparametric tests (GraphPadPrism), using $p$ values < 0.05.

## 3. Results

The lowest fluorescence intensity values were measured in the case of Harmonize™ (Kerr Dental) composite specimens (Table 2). The measured values in this group were significantly lower than the values of the enamel samples group ($p = 0.005$) and all the other composite groups ($p = 0.01$). All the other composite groups showed significantly higher values than natural enamel ($p = 0.01$). Fluorescence intensity data are given in Figures 3 and 4. The reduction of the values after 6 months and statistical significance are shown in Table 2.

**Table 2.** Reduction of the fluorescence intensity values after the second measurement for each material and the enamel specimens; $p$ values are based on Mann–Whitney nonparametric tests.

| Materials | Reduction after 6 Months, in Percentage | $p$-Value |
| --- | --- | --- |
| Omnichroma | 16.08% | 0.01 * |
| Harmonize™ | 5.22% | 0.149 |
| Filtek™ Z250 | 18.66% | 0.01 * |
| Gaenial Anterior | 13.05% | 0.01 * |
| Enamel Plus Function HRI | 11.39% | 0.01 * |
| Essentia | 20.91% | 0.006 * |
| Charisma | 22.95% | 0.01 * |
| Luna | 10.64% | 0.07 |
| Brilliant Flow | 13.33% | 0.03 * |
| Natural Enamel | 2.48% | 0.16 |

* Significant differences.

The qualitative assessment showed that only one of the composite materials belongs to the low fluorescence group, another composite belongs to the medium fluorescence, including all the brands with special shades (Table 3; Figure 5).

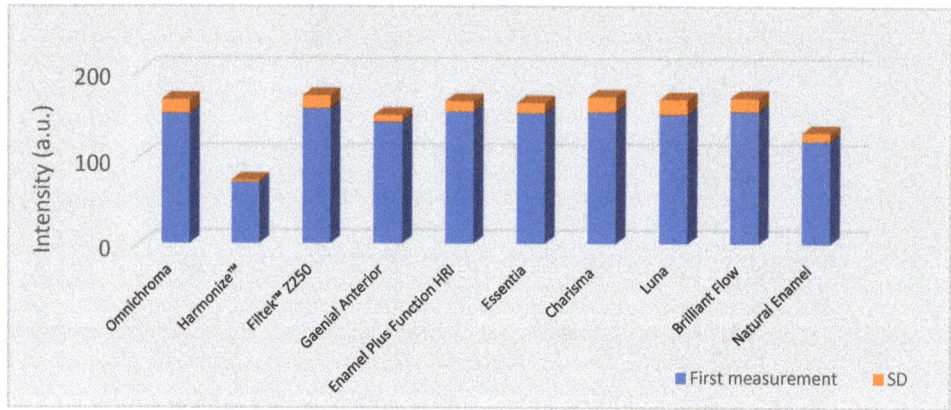

**Figure 3.** Column graph of the fluorescence intensity values (in arbitrary units) from the first measurement, representing the mean and standard deviation (SD) of each type of composite and the enamel.

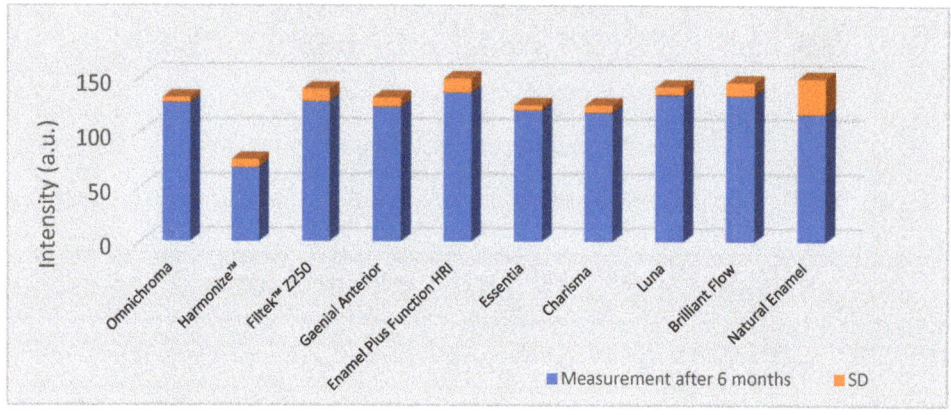

**Figure 4.** Column graph of the fluorescence intensity values (in arbitrary units) measured after 6 months, representing the mean and standard deviation (SD) of each type of composite and the enamel.

**Table 3.** The final values provided by the evaluators according to the defined fluorescence groups.

| Specimen | Dominant Fluorescence Group |
| --- | --- |
| Harmonize™ | 0 |
| Gaenial Anterior | 1 |
| Filtek™ Z250 | 2 |
| Omnichroma | 2 |
| Enamel Plus Function HRI | 2 |
| Essentia | 2 |
| Charisma | 2 |
| Luna | 2 |
| Brilliant Flow | 2 |

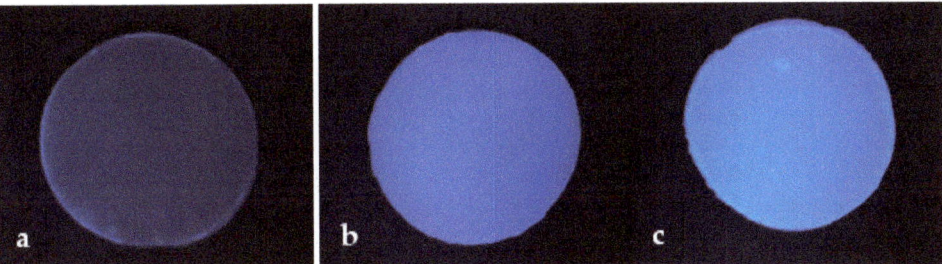

**Figure 5.** Samples under an ultraviolet light source showing the different fluorescence levels of the materials. Samples with different values: (**a**) low fluorescence (value 0); (**b**) medium fluorescence (value 1); (**c**) high fluorescence (value 2).

## 4. Discussion

Although we found multiple studies analyzing the fluorescence properties of the dental materials, no previous publication focused just on the enamel resin composites. The fluorescence of a resin composite is essential to reproduce the optical properties of dental hard tissues. Not all manufacturers consider this aspect important. Besides this, the precise composition of these materials is proprietary information, therefore, it is particularly hard to define which component is responsible for the fluorescent effect. In the international scientific literature, we found only comparative studies between different material brands or studies that compare natural teeth with restorative materials [4,5,10,11].

Garrido et al. reported increased fluorescence intensity as a function of time in the case of Filtek Z350 XT (3M ESPE). They considered that light absorption increases with aging, which leads to a slight increase in fluorescence emission over time, and this could be related to the organic components of this resin. In our study Filtek Z250, from the same manufacturer, showed a decrease in the fluorescence intensity after 6 months. A possible explanation could be the degradation of the organic complexes over time and with respect to the fact that rare earth metals have a low light absorption [12]. Although, in the present study, the fluorescence of Filtek Z250 was higher than that of other composites because Z250 has a smaller content of light scattering particles. These differences can be due to the nano behavior of Z250 and the presence of special particles in their composition. The difference in fluorescence of the composites tested in our study seems to be attributed to the difference in their composition and size of fillers.

All studies showed that composite resins that present fluorescent properties comparable to the enamels' have a mixture of several agents in their composition to achieve this characteristic. The organic and inorganic components, the type and the particle size of these, and any irregularity of the particles, can decrease light absorption and reflection. Resin composite has a high degree of translucency and value, absorbing, dispersing, and reflecting light in a similar way to dental structures. To understand that the final fluorescence is not equal to the sum of the fluorescence of each luminescent agent used in the material, manufacturers include fluorescent additives such as europium, cerium, and ytterbium, to improve the aesthetics of composite resins under all lighting conditions [13].

Previous studies have reported a gradual loss of the fluorescence properties of resin composites after aging, have included small sample sizes. With little differences between the brands, in all the nine resin composite specimens, a reduction in the fluorescence intensity was observed, however statistically significant differences could not be revealed in all cases. The fluorescence intensity of the specimens dropped to approximately 15% of the initial values after 6 months. Therefore, more awareness of the fluorescence properties of resin-based composites is needed [14].

Meller et al. examined composite samples of different brands and types, and they concluded that the fluorescence of different shades of the same brand is variable. They reported descriptive results and showed the different maximum intensity of fluorescence, which indicates the absence of standard fluorescent properties among different shades, even from the same brand [15].

The fluorescence of material reaches its optimal level at a certain concentration due to the interaction of light and fluorescent particles. Basically, after exceeding the optimal threshold, the fluorosed light is absorbed by other particles and decreases the efficiency of fluorescence (quenching effect). This phenomenon occurs when the thickness increases. In our study, the density of fluorescent particles in 1 mm thickness was too low to show the quenching effect. Thus, although thickness affects the fluorescence, this effect has an ascending trend to some extent and then descends due to the quenching effect [16].

Based on the fact that to generate distinct shades of composites, manufacturers add different amounts of chemicals like pigments, initiators, inhibitors, and activators, which influence the fluorescence phenomenon, Conceição et al. presented in their study a simple method to determine differences in fluorescence and reflectance. The Fluorescence and Reflectance Scale allow the examiner to identify a specific brand or restrict the possibilities down to two brands. This information about the fluorescence value of a dental restoration could help forensic experts in cases of identification, especially when antemortem data is limited [17].

Considering that each manufacturer uses specific compounds and combine these chemicals in different proportions, the fluorescence and reflectance phenomenon is unique for each manufacturer or brand.

In their study, Park et al. incorporated an organic fluorescent agent in varying concentrations in a resin matrix and measured the fluorescence intensity. Other manufacturers tried rare earth hybrid ions to polymerize into the resin matrix and as agents to achieve fluorescent composites [18].

Jablonski et al. showed a total reduction of 54.2% of the initial fluorescence intensity of Charisma®, however, the present study revealed a reduction of 22.95% of the initial fluorescence intensity after a half year by Jablonski et al. (23.5%). The differences between the study by Jablonski et al. and the present study probably result from the fact that in their study, two-color shades were evaluated, and in this study, only shade A2 was evaluated. We need to mention the fact that the specimens in their study were exposed to extreme conditions to simulate the aging process, while in our study, no aging conditions were used [19].

Stoleriu et al. analyzed the fluorescence properties of two composite resins; both materials presented low fluorescence, the results being in accordance with the present study. We would like to point out that in their study, both dentin and enamel shades were evaluated, and the results showed a higher emission of the fluorescence in dentine shades compared to the enamel shades [20].

Researchers conceptualized dental fluorescence around a wavelength between 430–450 nm, and they showed that surface characteristics of test specimens could cause changes in the optical properties of materials, either by the form of storage or even by the time taken for analysis [9]. Other studies showed that the different forms of storage of test specimens and different polishing protocols do not cause significant changes in the intensity of the fluorescence of the test specimens [11]. In the present study, specimens were stored in physiological serum, as we considered them more stable than artificial saliva.

The human eye is exposed to the range of light that forms the electromagnetic spectrum, which can decompose at various wavelengths, but only a small spectrum, the visible light spectrum initiates the process of color perception. However, the light source has numerous emission forms that differ in wavelength, so the perception of colors can suffer changes according to the amount of light that falls upon the object [21,22]. This could be one of the possible variables in the present study. Visual analysis of the images obtained under UV light showed extreme differences in the fluorescent contrast of the specimens, however, most of the specimens showed high fluorescence intensity. The evaluation of the data obtained was made by relating the results of the statistical analysis and the qualitative interpretation of the images obtained under UV light. In the case of Harmonize composite samples, very low initial fluorescence intensity values were assessed. Thus, the decrease in this sample group was not significant, while other materials, which had high initial values, were showing significant decreases.

## 5. Conclusions

Enamel composite resins' fluorescence intensity may differ significantly from the natural enamel's fluorescence intensity, presenting significantly lower or higher values than the natural enamel. Within the limitations of the present study, we can state that all the tested resin composites presented a decrease in fluorescence values after 6 months. The null hypotheses of the present study were rejected.

The results could be used as a reference value in the development of aesthetic restorative enamel composites. Although the first experimental data are encouraging, it would be recommended to carry out a controlled study with a larger number of shades, more brands of resin composites, and furthermore, in vivo studies, to verify possible changes in fluorescence of the materials in the oral environment.

**Author Contributions:** Conceptualization, Z.B.-V., M.S., E.B. (Előd Bala), E.B. (Előd Bereczki), and B.K.-M.; formal analysis, P.S. and E.B. (Előd Bereczki); investigation, E.B. (Előd Bala); methodology, Z.B.-V., P.S., E.B. (Előd Bala), E.B. (Előd Bereczki), and B.K.-M.; supervision, M.S.; validation, P.S.; writing-original draft, Z.B.-V.; writing-review and editing, M.S. and B.K.-M. All authors have read and agreed to the published version of the manuscript.

**Funding:** This paper was published under the framework of Internal Competition of Research Grants of George Emil Palade University of Medicine, Pharmacy, Science, and Technology of Târgu Mureș, Romania, grant number 15609/14/29.12.2017.

**Institutional Review Board Statement:** Not applicable.

**Informed Consent Statement:** Not applicable.

**Data Availability Statement:** Data supporting results can be found at the first author.

**Conflicts of Interest:** The authors declare no conflict of interest.

## References

1. Boyde, A. Microstructure of enamel. *Ciba Found. Symp.* **1997**, *205*, 18–27. [PubMed]
2. Vaarkamp, J.; ten Bosch, J.J.; Verdonschot, E.H. Propagation of light through human dental enamel and dentine. *Caries Res.* **1995**, *29*, 8–13. [CrossRef] [PubMed]
3. Mihu, C.M.; Dudea, D.; Melincovici, C.; Bocsa, B. Tooth Enamel, the Result of the Relationship between Matrix Proteins and Hydroxyapatite Crystals. *Appl. Med. Inform.* **2008**, *23*, 68–72.
4. Meller, C.; Klein, C. Fluorescence properties of commercial composite resin restorative materials in dentistry. *Dent. Mater. J.* **2012**, *31*, 916–923. [CrossRef] [PubMed]
5. Busato, P.M.R.; Saggin, P.G.; Camilotti, V.; Mendonça, M.J.; Busato, M.C.A. Evaluation of the fluorescence of enamel and dentin composite resins from different commercial sources. *Polímeros* **2015**, *25*, 200–204. [CrossRef]
6. Elgendy, H.; Maia, R.R.; Skiff, F.; Denehy, G.; Qian, F. Comparison of light propagation in dental tissues and nano-filled resin-based composite. *Clin. Oral. Investig.* **2019**, *23*, 423–433. [CrossRef] [PubMed]
7. Beolchi, R.S.; Mehta, D.; Pelissier, B.; Gênova, L.A.; Freitas, A.Z.; Bhandi, S.H. Influence of Filler Composition on the Refractive Index of Four Different Enamel Shades of Composite Resins. *J. Contemp. Dent. Pract.* **2021**, *22*, 557–561.
8. Uo, M.; Okamoto, M.; Watari, F.; Tani, K.; Morita, M.; Shintani, A. Rare earth oxide-containing fluorescent glass filler for composite resin. *Dent. Mater. J.* **2005**, *24*, 49–52. [CrossRef]
9. Lee, Y.K.; Lu, H.; Powers, J.M. Changes in opalescence and fluorescence properties of resin composites after accelerated aging. *Dent. Mater.* **2006**, *22*, 653–660. [CrossRef]
10. Lopes, G.M.; Prado, T.P.; Camilotti, V.; Bernardon, P.; Mendonça, M.J.; Ueda, J.K. In Vitro and in vivo evaluation of resin composites fluorescence. *J. Mech. Behav. Biomed. Mater.* **2021**, *114*, 104223. [CrossRef]
11. Volpato, C.A.M.; Pereira, M.R.C.; Silva, F.S. Fluorescence of natural teeth and restorative materials, methods for analysis and quantification: A literature review. *J. Esthet. Restor. Dent.* **2018**, *30*, 397–407. [CrossRef] [PubMed]
12. Garrido, T.M.; Hirata, R.; Sato, F.; Neto, A.M. In vitro evaluation of composite resin fluorescence after natural aging. *J. Clin. Exp. Dent.* **2020**, *12*, e461–e467. [CrossRef] [PubMed]
13. Klein, C.; Connert, T.; von Ohle, C.; Meller, C. How well can today's tooth-colored dental restorative materials reproduce the autofluorescence of human teeth?—Ambition and reality! *J. Esthet. Restor. Dent.* **2021**, *33*, 720–738. [CrossRef]

14. Klein, C.; Wolff, D.; Ohle, C.V.; Meller, C. The fluorescence of resin-based composites: An analysis after ten years of aging. *Dent. Mater. J.* **2021**, *40*, 94–100. [CrossRef] [PubMed]
15. Meller, C.; Klein, C. Fluorescence of composite resins: A comparison among properties of commercial shades. *Dent. Mater. J.* **2015**, *34*, 754–765. [CrossRef]
16. Tabatabaei, M.H.; Nahavandi, A.M.; Khorshidi, S.; Hashemikamangar, S.S. Fluorescence and Opalescence of Two Dental Composite Resins. *Eur. J. Dent.* **2019**, *13*, 527–534. [CrossRef]
17. Conceição, L.D.; Masotti, A.S.; Forgie, A.H.; Leite, F.R.M. New fluorescence and reflectance analyses to aid dental material detection in human identification. *Forensic. Sci. Int.* **2019**, *305*, 110032. [CrossRef]
18. Park, M.Y.; Lee, Y.K.; Lim, B.S. Influence of fluorescent whitening agent on the fluorescent emission of resin composites. *Dent. Mater.* **2007**, *23*, 731–735. [CrossRef]
19. Jablonski, T.; Takahashi, M.K.; Brum, R.T.; Rached, R.N.; Souza, E.M. Comparative study of the fluorescence intensity of dental composites and human teeth submitted to artificial aging. *Gen. Dent.* **2014**, *62*, 37–41.
20. Stoleriu, S.; Iovan, G.; Ghiorghe, A.; Pancu, G.; Topoliceanu, C.; Nica, I.; Andrian, S. Comparative study regarding the fluorescence of different types of composite resins. *Rom. J. Oral Rehabil.* **2015**, *7*, 45–49.
21. Brokos, I.; Stavridakis, M.; Lagouvardos, P.; Krejci, I. Fluorescence intensities of composite resins on photo images. *Odontology* **2021**, *109*, 615–624. [CrossRef] [PubMed]
22. Lefever, D.; Mayoral, J.R.; Mercade, M.; Basilio, J.; Roig, M. Optical integration and fluorescence: A comparison among restorative materials with spectrophotometric analysis. *Quintessence Int.* **2010**, *41*, 837–844. [PubMed]

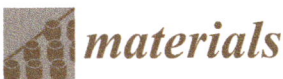 

*Article*

# Base Materials' Influence on Fracture Resistance of Molars with MOD Cavities

Gabriela Ciavoi [1,†], Ruxandra Mărgărit [2,†], Liana Todor [1,*], Dana Bodnar [2], Magdalena Natalia Dina [3], Daniela Ioana Tărlungeanu [4,*], Denisa Cojocaru [5], Cătălina Farcașiu [6,†] and Oana Cella Andrei [4]

1. Department of Dental Medicine, Faculty of Medicine and Pharmacy, University of Oradea, 10 1st December Square, 410068 Oradea, Romania; gciavoi@uoradea.ro
2. Department of Restorative Odontotherapy, Faculty of Dentistry, Carol Davila University of Medicine and Pharmacy, 37 Dionisie Lupu Str., 020021 Bucharest, Romania; ruxandra.margarit@gmail.com (R.M.); dana21bodnar@gmail.com (D.B.)
3. Department of Dental Techniques, Faculty of Midwifery and Nursing, Carol Davila University of Medicine and Pharmacy, 37 Dionisie Lupu Str., 020021 Bucharest, Romania; office@shinegrup.ro
4. Department of Removable Prosthodontics, Faculty of Dentistry, Carol Davila University of Medicine and Pharmacy, 37 Dionisie Lupu Str., 020021 Bucharest, Romania; cella.andrei@gmail.com
5. Independent Researcher, 020021 Bucharest, Romania; denisa.cojocaru96@yahoo.com
6. Faculty of Dentistry, Department of Pedodontics, Carol Davila University of Medicine and Pharmacy, 37 Dionisie Lupu Str., 020021 Bucharest, Romania; catalina.farcasiu@yahoo.com
* Correspondence: liana.todor@gmail.com (L.T.); ioanatarlungeanu@gmail.com (D.I.T.)
† These authors contributed equally to this work.

**Abstract:** The aim of this study was to compare fracture resistance of teeth presenting medium-sized mesial-occlusal-distal (MOD) cavities using different base materials. Thirty-six extracted molars were immersed for 48 h in saline solution (0.1% thymol at 4 °C) and divided into six groups. In group A, the molars were untouched, and in group B, cavities were prepared, but not filled. In group C, we used zinc polycarboxylate cement, in group D—conventional glass ionomer cement, in group E—resin modified glass ionomer cement, and in group F—flow composite. Fracture resistance was tested using a universal loading machine (Lloyd Instruments) with a maximum force of 5 kN and a crosshead speed of 1.0 mm/min; we used NEXYGEN Data Analysis Software and ANOVA Method ($p < 0.05$). The smallest load that determined the sample failure was 2780 N for Group A, 865 N for Group B, 1210 N for Group C, 1340 N for Group D, 1630 N for Group E and 1742 N for Group F. The highest loads were 3050 N (A), 1040 N (B), 1430 N (C), 1500 N (D), 1790 N (E), and 3320 N (F), the mean values being 2902 ± 114 N (A), 972 ± 65 N (B), 1339 ± 84 N (C), 1415 ± 67 N (D), 1712 ± 62 N (E), and 2334 ± 662 N (F). A $p = 0.000195$ shows a statistically significant difference between groups C, D, E and F. For medium sized mesial-occlusal-distal (MOD) cavities, the best base material regarding fracture resistance was flow composite, followed by glass ionomer modified with resin, conventional glass ionomer cement and zinc polycarboxylate cement. It can be concluded that light-cured base materials are a better option for the analyzed use case, one of the possible reasons being their compatibility with the final restoration material, also light-cured.

**Keywords:** mesial-occlusal-distal (MOD) cavities; fracture resistance; base materials

**Citation:** Ciavoi, G.; Mărgărit, R.; Todor, L.; Bodnar, D.; Dina, M.N.; Tărlungeanu, D.I.; Cojocaru, D.; Farcașiu, C.; Andrei, O.C. Base Materials' Influence on Fracture Resistance of Molars with MOD Cavities. *Materials* 2021, *14*, 5242. https://doi.org/10.3390/ma14185242

Academic Editor: Andrea Spagnoli

Received: 14 July 2021
Accepted: 9 September 2021
Published: 12 September 2021

**Publisher's Note:** MDPI stays neutral with regard to jurisdictional claims in published maps and institutional affiliations.

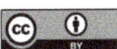

**Copyright:** © 2021 by the authors. Licensee MDPI, Basel, Switzerland. This article is an open access article distributed under the terms and conditions of the Creative Commons Attribution (CC BY) license (https://creativecommons.org/licenses/by/4.0/).

## 1. Introduction

Fractures of posterior teeth with mesial-occlusal-distal (MOD) cavities restored with different materials can occur in mastication more frequently than those of healthy ones, proportionally with the quantity of hard dental tissues loss [1–3]. As restoration materials, those that adhere most to the dentin are the most recommended [4], considering that using them increases the resistance of the restored tooth [5,6]. A material used as a base for replacing lost dentine in a medium-sized cavity ensures a uniformly distributed load and tension across the filled tooth [7], especially in MOD cavities [8,9]. Among the most used base materials are glass ionomer cements, zinc polycarboxylate cements, zinc phosphate cements and resins. Nowadays, composite resins are preferred for restoring MOD cavities [10], offering good esthetics for an acceptable price [11,12]. Some authors mostly recommend replacing dentin with a glass ionomer cement or a flow composite as a base material [13,14]. Glass ionomer cements adhere to dental structures because they develop an ion-enriched interfacial zone with dentine [15]; they present a minimum contraction setting and less marginal infiltration than most composite resins [16]. Their mechanical properties are moderate [17], but their cariostatic effect and adhesion to dentin recommend them as base materials. Zinc polycarboxylate cements present mechanical and adhesive properties similar to glass ionomer cements [18]. Better, such properties are gained by glass ionomer cements enriched with resins. Flow composites used as base materials present the advantage of good adherence to the composite restoration material. They can be applied in layers of up to 4 mm and they adapt perfectly to the form of the prepared cavity. Studies reported that using flow composites as base materials determined a decrease of tensions in the restored tooth in class II cavities [19,20]; the recommended final restoration material for such a base is a special composite resin for posterior teeth [21]. The aim of this study was to compare the fracture resistance of teeth presenting medium sized mesial-occlusal-distal (MOD) cavities filled with the same composite resin, but having different base materials, in order to find out which base material is best to use for the long-term resistance of tooth in mastication. Medium sized mesial-occlusal-distal cavities are those affecting both the enamel and the dentin, in consequence needing two layers of filling material, but far enough from the pulp so they do not require pulp capping. The interactions of the materials used in the experiment with the dental structures, elasticity modulus and compression strength values are presented in Table 1.

**Table 1.** Data regarding adhesion to the dental structures, elasticity modulus and compression strength.

| Material | Adhesion | Modulus of Elasticity | Compression Strength |
|---|---|---|---|
| Adhesor carbofine (Spofa Dental) | Natural adhesion to the hard dental tissues | 4.4 GPa | 47 MPa |
| Fuji IX (GC) | Intrinsic adhesion to dentine and enamel, without the need for etching and bonding | 8.3 GPa | 220 MPa |
| Fuji II LC (GC) | Strong adhesion, excellent bond strength to teeth even in presence of saliva | 5.33 GPa | 245 MPa |
| Charisma flow (Heraeus Kulzer) | Adhesive for any bonding technique | 14.3 GPa | 325 MPa |
| Charisma (Heraeus Kulzer) | Adhesive for any bonding technique | 8 GPa | 325 MPa |

## 2. Materials and Methods

### 2.1. Preparation of Teeth

We used 36 molars, extracted for orthodontic purposes, with no previous cavities or fillings, that were collected from 4 private clinics and divided into six groups (Group A–F) of six teeth each (Figure 1a). They were cleaned by removing the remnant soft tissues and immersed for 48 h in saline solution containing 0.1% thymol at 4 °C, until the cavities were prepared, in order to avoid dehydration.

### 2.2. Preparation of Test Specimens

In the first of the six groups, the control group, the molars were kept untouched (Group A) (Figure 1b). In the teeth from the remaining five groups, mesial-occlusal-distal (MOD) medium sized cavities were prepared using the same burs at high speed, 30 identical round burs ISO 001/014 with a diameter of 1.4 mm and 30 identical cylindrical burs ISO 111/012 with a diameter of 1.2 mm, two new burs for each prepared molar; the cavities' dimensions of 3.5 mm in width and 4.5 mm in height were verified using a digital caliper with an accuracy of 0.01 mm (Mitutoyo, Japan), cleaned and dried. In the second group, the medium-sized cavities were prepared, but were not filled at all, simulating a possible loss of the filling (Group B) (Figure 1c). In the other four groups, all final restorations were made with the same restoration material, using a universal composite (Charisma), but with four different types of base materials: Zinc polycarboxylate cement (zinc oxide with poly-acrylic acid-metallic oxide—ZPC) for Group C, conventional glass ionomer cement (silicate glass powder and polyacrylic acid—GIC) for Group D, resin modified glass ionomer cement (hybrid materials of traditional glass ionomer cement with a small addition of light-curing resin—RMGIC) for Group E, and flow composite (flowable resin-based composites that are conventional composites with the filler loading reduced to 37–53% in volume—FC) for Group F (Table 2). The chemical composition of the materials used for the experiment is presented in Table 2. All fillings were done according to the manufacturer's recommendations; the setting time was respected for all the materials used: 5–8 min for Adhesor carbofine, 6 min for Fuji IX and 20 s for the two light-cured materials.

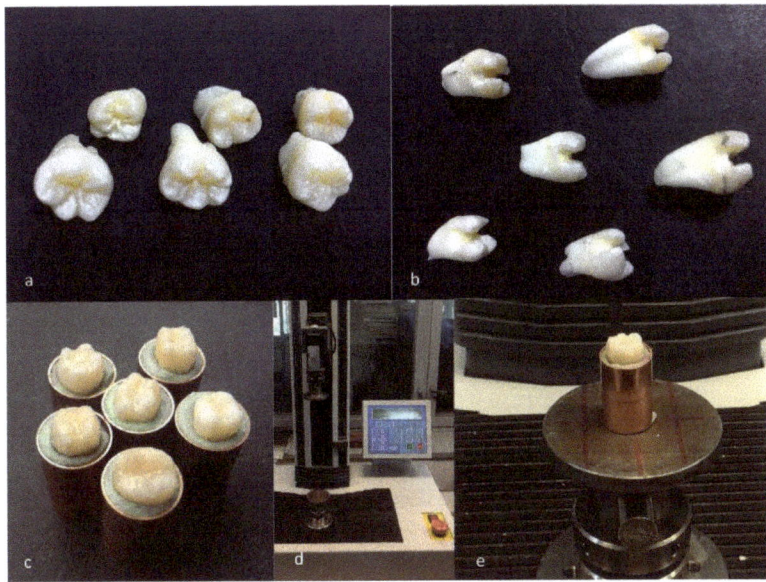

**Figure 1.** (a) Group of six molars unprepared; (b) group of six molars with MOD cavities; (c) group of samples prepared for testing; (d) universal loading machine; and (e) specimen before testing.

**Table 2.** The materials used for teeth restoration.

| Material | Purpose | Type | Chemical Composition |
|---|---|---|---|
| Adhesor carbofine (Spofa Dental) | Base | ZPC—zinc polycarboxylate cement | Zinc oxide, magnesium oxide, aluminum oxide, boric acid, acrylic acid, maleic anhydride, distilled water |
| Fuji IX (GC) | Base | GIC—glass ionomer cement | Alumino-silicate glass 95%, polyacrylic acid powder 5% |
| Fuji II LC (GC) | Base | RMGIC- Light-cured Resin Reinforced Glass Ionomer cement | Fluoro-alumino-silicate glass, polyacrylic acid 30–35%, distilled water 20–30%, 2HEMA 25–30%, initiator, urethan dymethylacrylate, camphorquinone multifunctional methacrylate monomers |
| Charisma flow (Heraeus Kulzer) | Base | FC-Flowable resin-micro-hybrid flowable composite, Light-cured | (EBADMA/TEGDMA); contains approximately 62% by weight or 38% by volume inorganic fillers such as Ba-Al-F silicate glass and $SiO_2$. The filler particle size is between 0.005 µm and 5 µm. |
| Charisma (Heraeus Kulzer) | Final restoration | Universal hybrid composite with microparticles, Light-cured | BIS-GMA matrix; contains 64% filler by volume: barium aluminum fluoride glass (0.02–2 microns); colloidal silica −0.01–0.07 µm. |

For this experiment, the roots of the teeth were introduced in 36 identical cylindrical-shaped containers filled with a putty silicone material, in order to resiliently support them during the experiment and to mimic the oral cavity conditions (Figure 1c).

## 2.3. Fracture Resistance Test

Fracture resistance was tested using a universal loading machine (Lloyd Instruments, Segensworth, Fareham, UK) (Figure 1d); samples were subjected to vertical compression, with a maximum force of 5 kN and a crosshead speed of 1.0 mm/min until the fracture of the tooth; the results were recorded with NEXYGEN Plus 3 Data Analysis Software. A representative specimen is shown in Figure 1e. The graphics show data regarding the maximum fracture force values till the fracture of the most resistant specimen of each group.

## 2.4. Statistical Analysis

Statistical analysis of obtained experimental values was performed using Microsoft Excel and ANOVA Method. For the variability of measured forces, mean values and standard deviations were analyzed. The level of significance was set at $p < 0.05$.

## 3. Results

For each group, the test results for each molar, the mean fracture force, median and the standard deviation are expressed in Table 3. The graphs with the maximum value of the force in which the most resistant sample from each group failed is represented in Figures 2–7. Group A, the control group, was stronger than all other groups, with a mean value of 2902 ± 114 N. Group B was weaker than all other groups, with a mean value of 972 ± 65 N. Group C and D were rather similar in terms of fracture resistance, with mean values of 1339 ± 84 N and 1415 ± 67 N. A more relevant difference was found between groups E and F, with mean values of 1712 ± 62 N and 2334 ± 662 N. In order to better compare the results for the four base materials that were used, the overlaid graphs of groups C–F are represented in Figure 8.

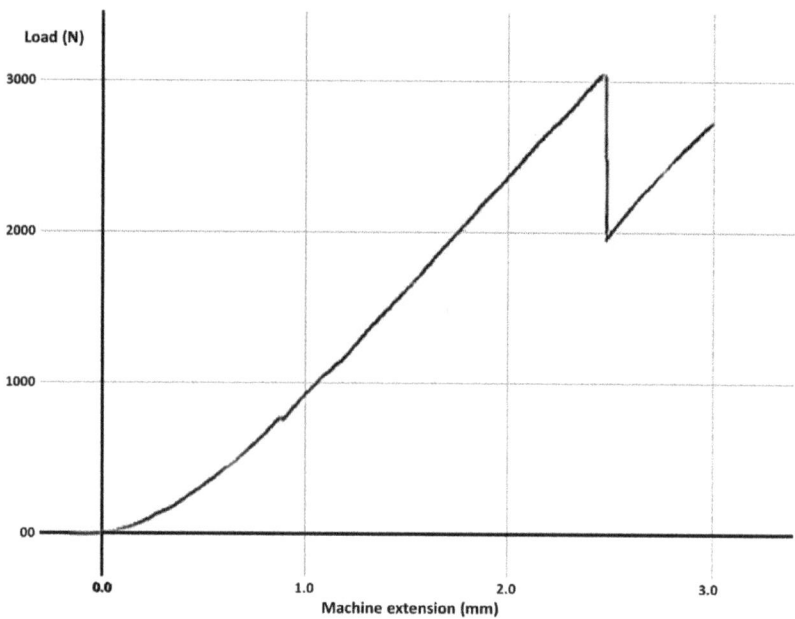

Figure 2. The maximum value of the force at which the most resistant molar from Group A failed.

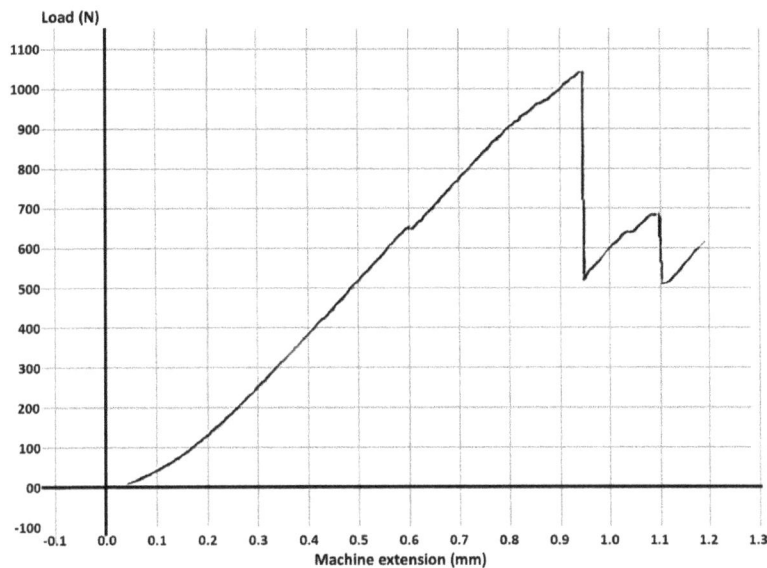

**Figure 3.** The maximum value of the force at which the most resistant molar from Group B failed.

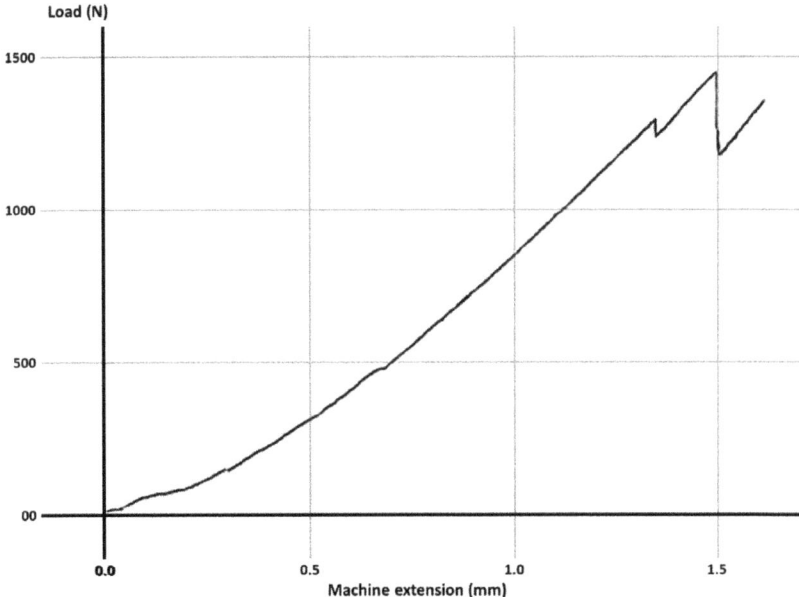

**Figure 4.** The maximum value of the force at which the most resistant molar from Group C failed.

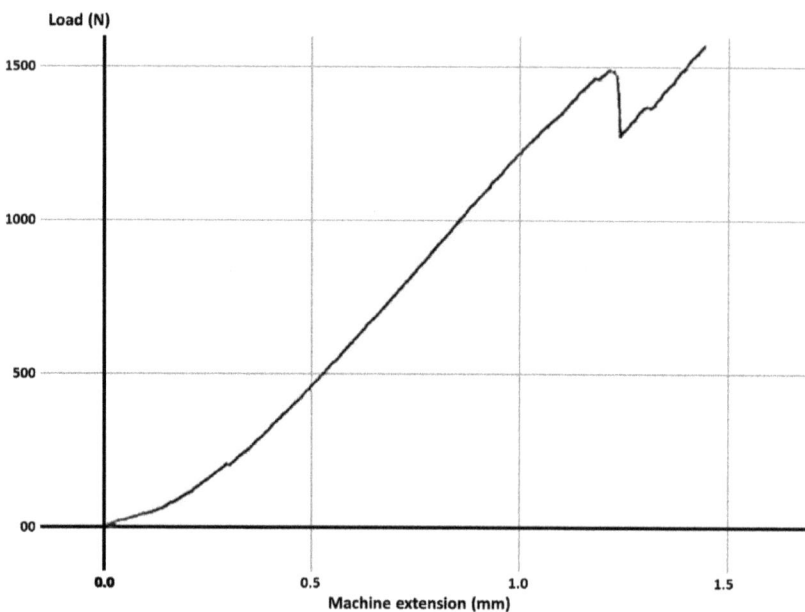

**Figure 5.** The maximum value of the force at which the most resistant molar from Group D failed.

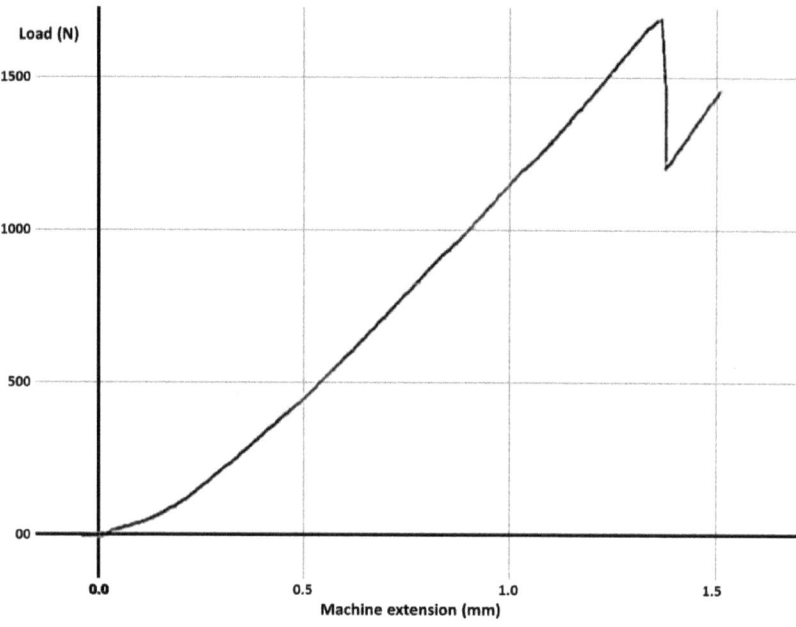

**Figure 6.** The maximum value of the force at which the most resistant molar from Group E failed.

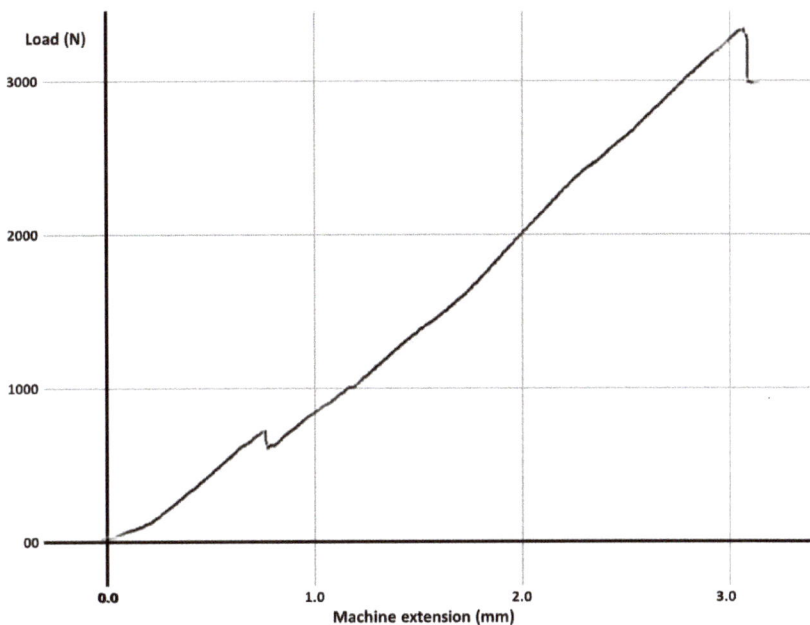

**Figure 7.** The maximum value of the force at which the most resistant molar from Group F failed.

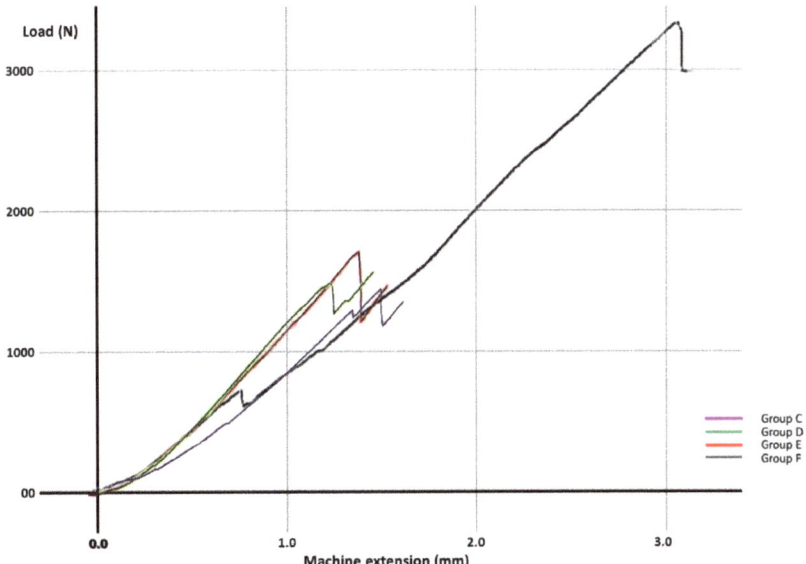

**Figure 8.** Result comparison for Groups C–F.

Table 3. The maximum force values at which the teeth in each of the six groups fractured.

| Group | Mean (N) | Standard Deviation | Median | Fracture Force (N) for Each Specimen | | | | | |
|---|---|---|---|---|---|---|---|---|---|
| | | | | 1 | 2 | 3 | 4 | 5 | 6 |
| A | 2902 | 114 | 2889 | 2780 | 2795 | 2835 | 2943 | 3010 | 3050 |
| B | 972 | 65 | 988 | 865 | 930 | 972 | 1004 | 1025 | 1040 |
| C | 1339 | 84 | 1348 | 1210 | 1286 | 1315 | 1382 | 1413 | 1430 |
| D | 1415 | 67 | 1408 | 1340 | 1358 | 1372 | 1445 | 1478 | 1500 |
| E | 1712 | 62 | 1716 | 1630 | 1655 | 1698 | 1734 | 1765 | 1790 |
| F | 2334 | 662 | 2112 | 1742 | 1795 | 1855 | 2370 | 2925 | 3320 |

Statistical analysis using the ANOVA method in order to understand the relevance of the study revealed a $p$ value of 0.000195, showing a statistically significant difference between Groups C–F restored with four different types of base materials (Table 4).

Table 4. ANOVA Method and $p$ value.

| ANOVA: Single Factor | | | | | | |
|---|---|---|---|---|---|---|
| SUMMARY | | | | | | |
| Groups | Count | Sum | Average | Variance | | |
| C-ZPC | 6 | 8036 | 1339.333 | 7126.267 | | |
| D-GIC | 6 | 8493 | 1415.5 | 4563.1 | | |
| E-RMGIC | 6 | 10,272 | 1712 | 3909.2 | | |
| F-FC | 6 | 14,007 | 2334.5 | 438,639.5 | | |
| ANOVA | | | | | | |
| Source of Variation | SS | df | MS | F | $p$-Value | F Crit |
| Between Groups | 3,682,527 | 3 | 1,227,509 | 10.80939 | | |
| Within Groups | 2,271,190 | 20 | 113,559.5 | | | |
| Total | 5,953,717 | 23 | | | | |

## 4. Discussion

Choosing the base material for medium-sized MOD cavities is difficult, because it can influence the long-term prognostic of the restored tooth. These cavities are involving both enamel and dentin; reducing the quantity of the dental tissues is a predisposing factor for fracture [1]. Studies reported that teeth with MOD cavities are losing their resistance in a proportion of 60%, compared to the non-prepared ones [22]. It has been reported that most recommended base materials for ensuring fracture resistance of the tooth are the ones presenting an elasticity modulus similar with the one of the dentin, such as composite resins [23,24], while the elasticity modulus of the zinc polycarboxylate cements and glass ionomer cements is smaller than that of the composite resins [25–27]. Some studies reported that using a base material with a low elasticity modulus presents the advantage of a higher deformation under occlusal forces, which reduces the fracture risk, while another study analyzing fracture resistance of non-vital teeth restored with different base materials showed that their different elasticity modulus did not influence fracture resistance of the teeth at all [28].

Other authors reported that conventional glass ionomer cement used as a base material had a positive influence on fracture resistance, teeth restored in such manner having a similar fracture resistance to the non-prepared ones [29,30]. Another study showed that glass ionomer cements used as base absorbed tensions generated during setting of the composite fillings [31]. Other authors showed that for non-vital teeth using glass ionomer cements as a base did not increase the fracture resistance [32,33], while another study concluded that using conventional glass ionomer cements as a base in MOD cavities can increase the resistance [34]. Eakle analyzed fracture resistance of adherent filling materials and showed that, although conventional glass ionomers have inferior mechanical properties compared to composite resins, using them as restoration materials did not decrease fracture resistance of the restored teeth [35]. Compared to conventional ones, new glass ionomers that are enriched with resins offer a better working time, due to the possibility to control the polymerization. The results of the study made by Oz et al. showed that the best fracture resistance was that of the teeth restored with MOD fillings that had bases of glass ionomer modified with resins, compared to conventional glass ionomers and flow composites [36]. Still, the results obtained by Taha et al. in a study on non-vital teeth having flow composite as a base showed that, using these materials, the fracture resistance of those teeth improved [37]; similarly, other studies observed the smallest fracture resistance for glass ionomer cements used as base, and the highest for flow composites [38–41]. In our study, the best fracture resistance was also obtained for the group having flow composite as a base, glass ionomer cements modified with resins being in the middle.

Using a base material under an adhesive composite filling increases the fracture resistance of the restored non-vital teeth [3,32,42]; still, the excessive thickness of the base has a negative influence on it [43]. Other studies showed that in case of teeth with massive loss of hard dental tissues the higher tensions appear in the remaining dental tissues and not to the interface between tooth and restoration, so the tooth can suffer a fracture [44,45]. In our in vitro experiment, the teeth were prepared in such manner that the resulting MOD cavities were medium-sized; within these limits, the highest fracture resistance was obtained using the flow composite as a base material. Additionally, our results showed that any restoration of teeth increased their fracture resistance, compared to the absence of the fillings. Further tests are necessary in order to assess how the results may change in case of larger, more profound cavities.

## 5. Conclusions

Regardless of the materials chosen for this study, the results showed that untouched molars (Group A) had the best fracture resistance, with much higher values obtained compared to the filled ones; also, the prepared but not filled at all molars (Group B) had the lowest values of all groups, showing that lost and not replaced fillings expose molars to significantly higher fracture risks. These results underline once more the importance of monitoring and prevention, especially in countries with poor or limited insurance systems. Within the limits of this study, for medium size mesial-occlusal-distal (MOD) cavities, filled with composite resins, the best base material that can be used in terms of fracture resistance proved to be the flow composite, followed by the glass ionomer modified with resin, and by the conventional glass ionomer cement. The smallest fracture resistance was obtained using zinc polycarboxylate cement as a base. It can be concluded that light-cured base materials are a better option for the analyzed use case, one of the possible reasons being their compatibility with the final restoration material, also light-cured.

**Author Contributions:** Conceptualization, G.C., R.M. and O.C.A.; methodology, C.F.; software, D.B., M.N.D. and D.C.; validation, D.I.T. and L.T.; formal analysis M.N.D.; investigation L.T.; supervision, O.C.A.; data curation D.B., D.C. and R.M.; writing—original draft preparation G.C. and C.F.; writing—review and editing, D.I.T. and O.C.A. All authors have read and agreed to the published version of the manuscript.

**Funding:** This research received no external funding.

**Institutional Review Board Statement:** Not applicable.

**Informed Consent Statement:** Not applicable.

**Data Availability Statement:** Data is contained within the article.

**Conflicts of Interest:** The authors declare no conflict of interest.

**Sample Availability:** Samples are not available from the authors.

## References

1. Nam, S.H.; Chang, H.S.; Min, K.S.; Lee, Y.; Cho, H.W.; Bae, J.M. Effect of the number of residual walls on fracture resistances, failure patterns, and photoelasticity of simulated premolars restored with or without fiber-reinforced composite posts. *J. Endod.* **2010**, *36*, 297–301. [CrossRef] [PubMed]
2. Meng, Q.F.; Chen, Y.M.; Guang, H.B.; Yip, K.H.; Smales, R.J. Effect of a ferrule and increased clinical crown length on the in vitro fracture resistance of premolars restored using two dowel-and-core systems. *Oper. Dent.* **2007**, *32*, 595–601. [CrossRef] [PubMed]
3. Soares, P.V.; Santos-Filho, P.C.; Martins, L.R.; Soares, C.J. Influence of restorative technique on the biomechanical behavior of endodontically treated maxillary premolars. Part I: Fracture resistance and fracture mode. *J. Prosthet. Dent.* **2008**, *99*, 30–37. [CrossRef]
4. Sorrentino, R.; Aversa, R.; Ferro, V.; Auriemma, T.; Zarone, F.; Ferrari, M.; Apicella, A. Three-dimensional finite element analysis of strain and stress distributions in endodontically treated maxillary central incisors restored with different post, core and crown materials. *Dent. Mater.* **2007**, *23*, 983–993. [CrossRef]
5. Mărgărit, R.; Suciu, I.; Bodnar, D.C.; Grigore, M.; Scărlătescu, S.A.; Andrei, O.C.; Măgureanu, C.M.; Chirilă, M.; Bencze, A.; Ionescu, E. Fracture resistance of molars with MOD cavities restored with different materials. *Rom. Biotechnol. Lett.* **2021**, *26*, 2323–2330. [CrossRef]
6. Mărgărit, R.; Tănăsescu, L.A.; Bodnar, D.; Ion, C.G.; Burlibaşa, M.; Bisoc, A.; Farcaşiu, C.; Dina, M.N.; Andrei, O.C. Comparison of fracture resistance of teeth presenting non-carious cervical lesions, restored with different composite materials. *Mater. Plast.* **2020**, *57*, 299–305. [CrossRef]
7. Soares, P.V.; Santos-Filho, P.C.; Gomide, H.A.; Araujo, C.A.; Martins, L.R.; Soares, C.J. Influence of restorative technique on the biomechanical behavior of endodontically treated maxillary premolars. Part II: Strain measurement and stress distribution. *J. Prosthet. Dent.* **2008**, *99*, 114–122. [CrossRef]
8. Krämer, N.; Reinelt, C.; Frankenberger, R. Ten-year clinical performance of posterior resin composite restorations. *J. Adhes. Dent.* **2015**, *17*, 433–441.
9. Pallesen, U.; Van Dijken, J.W. A randomized controlled 30 years follow up of three conventional resin composites in class II restorations. *Dent. Mater.* **2015**, *31*, 1232–1244. [CrossRef]
10. Eskitaşcioğlu, G.; Belli, S.; Kalkan, M. Evaluation of two post core systems using two different methods (fracture strength test and a finite elemental stress analysis). *J. Endod.* **2002**, *28*, 629–633. [CrossRef]
11. Mondelli, R.F.; Ishikiriama, S.K.; De Oliveira Filho, O.; Mondelli, J. Fracture resistance of weakened teeth restored with condensable resin with and without cusp coverage. *J. Appl. Oral Sci.* **2009**, *17*, 161–165. [CrossRef]
12. Plotino, G.; Buono, L.; Grande, N.M.; Lamorgese, V.; Somma, F. Fracture resistance of endodontically treated molars restored with extensive composite resin restorations. *J. Prosthet. Dent.* **2008**, *99*, 225–232. [CrossRef]
13. Alomari, Q.D.; Reinhardt, J.W.; Boyer, D.B. Effect of liners on cusp deflection and gap formation in composite restorations. *Oper. Dent.* **2001**, *26*, 406–411.
14. Cho, E.; Chikawa, H.; Kishikawa, R.; Inai, N.; Otsuki, M.; Foxton, R.M.; Tagami, J. Influence of elasticity on gap formation in a lining technique with flowable composite. *Dent. Mater. J.* **2006**, *25*, 538–544. [CrossRef]
15. Yoshida, Y.; Van Meerbeek, B.; Nakayama, Y.; Snauwaert, J.; Hellemans, L.; Lambrechts, P.; Vanherle, G.; Wakasa, K. Evidence of chemical bonding at biomaterial-hard tissue interfaces. *J. Dent. Res.* **2000**, *79*, 709–714. [CrossRef]
16. Feilzer, A.J.; De Gee, A.J.; Davidson, C.L. Curing contraction of composites and glass-ionomer cements. *J. Prosthet. Dent.* **1988**, *59*, 297–300. [CrossRef]
17. Kovarik, R.E.; Breeding, L.C.; Caughman, W.F. Fatigue life of three core materials under simulated chewing conditions. *J. Prosthet. Dent.* **1992**, *68*, 584–590. [CrossRef]
18. Jemt, T.; Stalblad, P.A.; Øilo, G. Adhesion of polycarboxylate- based dental cements to enamel: An in vivo study. *J. Dent. Res.* **1986**, *65*, 885–887. [CrossRef]
19. Cara, R.R.; Fleming, G.J.; Palin, W.M.; Walmsley, A.D.; Burke, F.J. Cuspal deflection and microleakage in premolar teeth restored with resin-based composites with and without an intermediary flowable layer. *J. Dent.* **2007**, *35*, 482–489. [CrossRef]
20. Roggendorf, M.J.; Kramer, N.; Appelt, A.; Naumann, M.; Frankenberger, R. Marginal quality of flowable 4-mm base vs. conventionally layered resin composite. *J. Dent.* **2011**, *39*, 643–647. [CrossRef] [PubMed]
21. Ilie, N.; Bucuta, S.; Draenert, M. Bulk-fill resin-based composites: An in vitro assessment of their mechanical performance. *Oper. Dent.* **2013**, *38*, 618–625. [CrossRef]
22. Taha, N.A.; Palamara, J.E.; Messer, H.H. Fracture strength and fracture patterns of root filled teeth restored with direct resin restorations. *J. Dent.* **2011**, *39*, 527–535. [CrossRef] [PubMed]
23. Jiang, W.; Bo, H.; Yongchun, G.; Longxing, N. Stress distribution in molars restored with inlays or onlays with or without endodontic treatment: A three-dimensional finite element analysis. *J. Prosthet. Dent.* **2010**, *103*, 6–12. [CrossRef]
24. Kinney, J.H.; Marshall, S.J.; Marshall, G.W. The mechanical properties of human dentin: A critical review and re-evaluation of the dental literature. *Crit. Rev. Oral Biol. Med.* **2003**, *14*, 13–29. [CrossRef] [PubMed]
25. Tam, L.E.; Pulver, E.; Mccomb, D.; Smith, D.C. Physical properties of calcium hydroxide and glass-ionomer base and lining materials. *Dent. Mater.* **1989**, *5*, 145–149. [CrossRef]
26. Akinmade, A.O.; Hill, R.G. Influence of cement layer thickness on the adhesive bond strength of polyalkenoate cements. *Biomater* **1992**, *13*, 931–936. [CrossRef]

27. Natale, L.; Rodrigues, M.; Xavier, T.; Simoes, A.; De Souza, D.; Braga, R. Ion release and mechanical properties of calcium silicate and calcium hydroxide materials used for pulp capping. *Int. Endod. J.* **2015**, *48*, 89–94. [CrossRef]
28. Chan, T.; Kucukkaya Eren, S.; Wong, R.; Parashos, P. In vitro fracture strength and patterns in root-filled teeth restored with different base materials. *Aust. Dent. J.* **2018**, *63*, 99–108. [CrossRef]
29. Hernandez, R.; Bader, S.; Boston, D.; Trope, M. Resistance to fracture of endodontically treated premolars restored with new generation dentine bonding systems. *Int. Endod. J.* **1994**, *27*, 281–284. [CrossRef] [PubMed]
30. Wendt, S.L., Jr.; Harris, B.M.; Hunt, T.E. Resistance to cusp fracture in endodontically treated teeth. *Dent. Mater.* **1987**, *3*, 232–235. [CrossRef]
31. Davidson, C.L. Glass-ionomer bases under posterior composites. *J. Esthet. Dent.* **1994**, *6*, 223–224. [CrossRef]
32. Taha, N.A.; Palamara, J.E.; Messer, H.H. Assessment of laminate technique using glass ionomer and resin composite for restoration of root filled teeth. *J. Dent.* **2012**, *40*, 617–623. [CrossRef]
33. Trope, M.; Tronstad, L. Resistance to fracture of endodontically treated premolars restored with glass ionomer cement or acid etch composite resin. *J. Endod.* **1991**, *17*, 257–259. [CrossRef]
34. Banomyong, D.; Harnirattisai, C.; Burrow, M.F. Posterior resin composite restorations with or without resin-modified, glass-ionomer cement lining: A 1-year randomized, clinical trial. *J. Investig. Clin. Dent.* **2011**, *2*, 63–69. [CrossRef]
35. Eakle, W.S. Increased fracture resistance of teeth: Comparison of five bonded composite resin systems. *Quintessence Int.* **1986**, *17*, 17–20.
36. Oz, F.D.; Ergin, E.; Gurgan, S. Comparison of different base materials on fracture strength of mesio-occlusal-distal composite restorations. *Eur. J. Gen. Dent.* **2018**, *7*, 25–30. [CrossRef]
37. Taha, N.A.; Maghaireh, G.A.; Ghannam, A.S.; Palamara, J.E. Effect of bulk-fill base material on fracture strength of root-filled teeth restored with laminate resin composite restorations. *J. Dent.* **2017**, *63*, 60–64. [CrossRef]
38. Ilie, N.; Hickel, R.; Valceanu, A.S.; Huth, K.C. Fracture toughness of dental restorative materials. *Clin. Oral Investig.* **2012**, *16*, 489–498. [CrossRef] [PubMed]
39. Rosatto, C.M.; Bicalho, A.A.; Verissimo, C.; Braganca, G.F.; Rodrigues, M.P.; Tantbirojn, D.; Versluis, A.; Soares, C.J. Mechanical properties, shrinkage stress, cuspal strain and fracture resistance of molars restored with bulk-fill composites and incremental filling technique. *J. Dent.* **2015**, *43*, 1519–1528. [CrossRef]
40. Ilie, N.; Hickel, R. Investigations on a methacrylate-based flowable composite based on the SDR™ technology. *Dent. Mater.* **2011**, *27*, 348–355. [CrossRef]
41. Kim, R.J.; Kim, Y.J.; Choi, N.S.; Lee, I.B. Polymerization shrinkage, modulus, and shrinkage stress related to tooth-restoration interfacial debonding in bulk-fill composites. *J. Dent.* **2015**, *43*, 430–439. [CrossRef]
42. Belli, S.; Erdemir, A.; Ozcopur, M.; Eskitascioglu, G. The effect of fibre insertion on fracture resistance of root filled molar teeth with MOD preparations restored with composite. *Int. Endod. J.* **2005**, *38*, 73–80. [CrossRef]
43. Hormati, A.A.; Fuller, J.L. The fracture strength of amalgam overlying base materials. *J. Prosthet. Dent.* **1980**, *43*, 52–57. [CrossRef]
44. Versluis, A.; Tantbirojn, D.; Pintado, M.R.; Delong, R.; Douglas, W.H. Residual shrinkage stress distributions in molars after composite restoration. *Dent. Mater.* **2004**, *20*, 554–564. [CrossRef]
45. Kahler, B.; Swain, M.V.; Kotousov, A. Comparison of an analytical expression of resin composite curing stresses with in vitro observations of marginal cracking. *Am. J. Dent.* **2010**, *23*, 357–364.

MDPI
St. Alban-Anlage 66
4052 Basel
Switzerland
Tel. +41 61 683 77 34
Fax +41 61 302 89 18
www.mdpi.com

*Materials* Editorial Office
E-mail: materials@mdpi.com
www.mdpi.com/journal/materials

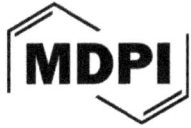

www.ingramcontent.com/pod-product-compliance
Lightning Source LLC
LaVergne TN
LVHW070405100526
838202LV00014B/1396